Contents

Preface to the third edition

Following the success of the second edition of *Essentials of Neonatal Medicine* we have been encouraged to extensively update the textbook. Neonatal medicine continues to develop, with improvements in survival and therapies better directed towards the prevention and management of complications in newborn babies. This third edition updates these new developments, and we have added an important new chapter on the ethical issues that arise as the result of our emerging technologies. We hope that this book will continue to be of value to the practitioners of the art and science of neonatal medicine: the doctors and nurses whose professional life is dedicated to the care of the newborn infant.

Malcolm I. Levene
David I. Tudehope
M. John Thearle

Note added in proof
Whilst this book was in production an important international agreement on the nomenclature of drugs was announced by the Medicines Control Agency. This announcement was made too late to be implemented in this book.

We would welcome and value any reader feedback. Let us know how you think this approach could be improved by emailing us at the following email address: authors@blacksci.co.uk which can then be forwarded to the authors.

Preface to the first edition

There has been an explosion of knowledge over the last decade in fetal physiology, antenatal management and neonatal intensive care. This has brought with it confusion concerning novel methods of treatment and procedures as well as the application of new techniques for investigating and monitoring high-risk neonates. The original idea for this book was conceived in Brisbane and a *Primer of Neonatal Medicine* was produced with Australian conditions in mind. We have now entirely rewritten the book and it is the result of cooperation between Australian and British neonatologists with, we hope, an international perspective.

We are aware of the need for a short book on neonatal medicine which gives more background discussion and is less dogmatic than other works currently available. We have written this book to give more basic information concerning physiology, development and a perspective to treatment which will be of value equally to neonatal nurses, paediatricians in training, medical students and midwives. Whilst collaborating on a project such as this we are constantly aware of the variety of ways for managing the same condition. This is inevitable in any rapidly growing acute special-

ity and we make no apologies for describing alternative methods of treatment where appropriate. Too rigid an approach will be to the detriment of our patients!

A detailed account of all neonatal disorders is not possible but common problems and their management are outlined giving an overall perspective of neonatology. Attention has been given to rare medical and surgical conditions where early diagnosis and treatment may be lifesaving. It is easy to be carried away with the excitement of neonatal intensive care and forget the parents sitting at the cotside. Our approach is to care for the parents as well as their baby and we have included two chapters on parent–infant attachment as well as death and dying. The final chapter deals with practical procedures and gives an outline of the commonly performed techniques used in the care of the high-risk newborn. We have also provided an up to date neonatal Pharmacopoeia as well as useful tables and charts for normal age-related ranges.

Malcolm I. Levene
David I. Tudehope
M. John Thearle

Acknowledgements

During the preparation of this book help and advice have been freely given by many of our colleagues, both medical and nursing. We are particularly grateful to Dr Henry Halliday and colleagues for permitting us to publish diagrams in Chapter 30 on Procedures. We also thank Mr Tim Milward and Dr John Parsons for allowing us to publish their illustrations.

We are indebted to Karen Brierly (a neonatal unit sister) for drawing a number of most helpful and clear diagrams of practical procedures, and to the Medical Graphics department at the Mater Misericordiae Public Hospitals for so generously giving their time to prepare high-quality photographs and diagrams.

We are most grateful to our secretaries, Christine Hildyard, Lyn Bavister and Trudy van Duivenvoorde, without whose support this edition would not have been completed.

1 Definitions and terminology

Conception, embryonic and fetal development, parturition and subsequent neonatal growth and development form a continuum. Obstetricians and neonatologists, however, have arbitrarily divided this into rigid categories, which are used to audit standards of care during the perinatal and subsequent periods. Unfortunately, international agreement regarding some of the terminology is lacking, and definitions within this developmental continuum given here are those used in the UK and Australia.

A *live birth* is one in which there are signs of life (breathing, heartbeat or spontaneous movement) after complete expulsion from the mother, irrespective of the gestational age or birthweight.

A *stillbirth*, or fetal death, is defined as an infant expelled from the birth canal at or after 24 weeks of pregnancy who shows no signs of life and has no heartbeat.

In Australia, stillbirth is defined as an infant born at or after 20 weeks' gestation and/or weighing ≥ 400 g with no signs of life. As the definition varies from country to country, comparison of figures may be misleading. The stillbirth rate is expressed as the number of infants born dead at or after 24 weeks (or ≥ 20 weeks in some countries) per 1000 live births and stillbirths.

Gestational age. This is calculated from the first day of the last normal menstrual period to the date of birth, and is expressed in completed weeks.

Term delivery occurs when the infant is born at or after 37 and before 42 weeks' gestation.

Preterm delivery occurs if the infant is born after less than 37 weeks' gestation. In the UK and Australia, 6–7% of infants are born preterm.

Post-term delivery occurs if the infant is born at or after 42 completed weeks of gestation. Approximately 3% of infants are born post-term.

Low birthweight (LBW) refers to any infant who weighs less than 2500 g at birth. In the UK and Australia, approximately 6% of live births are LBW. These infants are either born too early (preterm), or have grown inadequately in the uterus and are classed as 'small for gestational age'. Some low birthweight infants may be both preterm and small for gestational age.

Very low birthweight (VLBW) infants are those who weigh less than 1500 g at birth. Approximately 1–1.5% of liveborn infants are VLBW.

Extremely low birthweight (ELBW) infants are those who weigh less than 1000 g at birth. This category accounts for approximately 0.7% of all births.

Small for gestational age (SGA). The assessment of a baby depends on accurate assessment of gestational age (see pp. 77–78) and plotting of weight on an appropriate growth chart. There is no consensus on the definition of SGA, which varies from less than the 10th, 5th or 3rd percentiles or more than 2 standard deviations below the mean birthweight. Accordingly, incidence figures will vary.

Perinatal mortality rate (PMR)

$$PMR = \frac{\text{Number of stillbirths and neonatal deaths}}{\text{Number of stillbirths and live births}} \times 1000$$

For international comparisons, the rate refers to all births of at least 1000 g birthweight or, when birthweight is unavailable, of at least 28 weeks' gestation, and neonatal deaths occurring within 7 days of birth (as recommended by the World Health Organization (WHO)).

For Australian national statistics, the PMR refers to all births ≥ 500 g birthweight or ≥ 22 weeks' gestation, and the neonatal period is to day 28.

For the UK, the PMR refers to stillbirths ≥ 24 weeks and neonatal deaths in the first 7 days of life.

For Australian states, PMR refers to all births ≥ 400 g birthweight or ≥ 20 weeks' gestation, and the neonatal period is to day 28.

Neonatal death rate in the UK and Australia refers to the number of deaths within 28 days of birth of any child who had evidence of life after birth. Birthweight and/or gestational age criteria apply as for PMR.

Neonatal death is death occurring within 28 days of birth in an infant whose birthweight was at least 500 g or, if the weight was not known, an infant born after at least 22 weeks' gestation.

Postneonatal death rate (or late infant deaths) refers to the number of deaths of liveborn infants dying after 28 days but before 1 year of age per 1000 live births.

Infant death is death occurring within 1 year of birth in a liveborn infant whose birthweight was at least 500 g, or at least 22 weeks' gestation if the birthweight was not known. This category includes neonatal deaths as defined above.

Infant mortality rate (IMR) *(per 1000 live births)*

$$IMR = \frac{\text{Number of neonatal deaths + postneonatal deaths}}{\text{Total live births}} \times 1000$$

FACTORS AFFECTING PERINATAL DEATH RATES

Perinatal deaths relate to a wide variety of causes, either maternal or problems arising in the fetus or newborn. In both the UK and Australia in 1996 the PMR was 8.5 per 1000 live births, comprising 65% fetal deaths and 35% neonatal deaths (Fig. 1.1). The highest risk group was mothers aged < 20 and ≥ 40 years with PMRs of 12.0 per 1000 births. Social class is also an important factor. In the UK, there is almost a 100% difference in PMR between women in socioeconomic class I (professional groups) and those in class V (unskilled occupations).

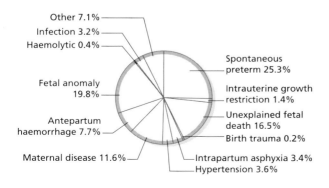

Fig. 1.1 Causes of perinatal death, Queensland 1996. These proportions are similar to those in many parts of the UK.

Other 7.1%
Infection 3.2%
Haemolytic 0.4%
Fetal anomaly 19.8%
Antepartum haemorrhage 7.7%
Maternal disease 11.6%
Spontaneous preterm 25.3%
Intrauterine growth restriction 1.4%
Unexplained fetal death 16.5%
Birth trauma 0.2%
Intrapartum asphyxia 3.4%
Hypertension 3.6%

Table 1.1 Cause of perinatal death, Whitfield classification

Classification
1 *Spontaneous preterm*
Multiple pregnancy
Previous bleeding
Previous spontaneous rupture of membranes
Incompetent cervix
Other
Idiopathic
2 *IUGR*
3 *Unexplained IUFD*
4 *Birth trauma*
5 *Intrapartum asphyxia*
6 *Hypertension*
Pre-eclampsia
Renal
Essential hypertension
7 *Maternal disease*
8 *Antepartum haemorrhage*
Placental abruption
Placenta praevia
Undetermined origin
9 *Fetal abnormality*
Chromosomal
CNS
CVS
Renal
Multiple malformations
Metabolic errors
Other
10 *Haemolytic disease*
Rhesus incompatibility
Other fetomaternal blood group incompatibility
Haemoglobinopathy of α-thalassaemia
11 *Infection*
12 *Other*

The sex of the fetus or infant is also important. In Australia, the male perinatal death rate was 8.6 per 1000 in 1993–95, compared to 7.4 per 1000 for females. Maturity is of course an important factor in the PMR: about half of all deaths occurred in babies who weighed less than 2000 g at birth, and of this group more than half weighed less than 1000 g. For twins the PMR is 4.3 times higher than for singletons. For higher order multiples it is nine times greater.

CLASSIFICATION OF PERINATAL DEATHS

It is difficult for doctors to agree on the cause of death in a diverse group of patients. Epidemiologists, obstetricians, neonatologists and pathologists may analyse deaths differently and report inconsistent rates. A traditional method for classifying perinatal deaths is based on the main maternal conditions or major obstetric antecedents.

The most reliable cause of death is obtained by an experienced perinatal pathologist conducting an autopsy examination, but even following such examination the precise cause of death may be undetermined, particularly when the infant dies before birth (see Fig. 1.1). For this reason, classification systems have been devised which identify the pathological processes occurring in the mother. A useful system is shown in Table 1.1.

REFERENCES

Perinatal Statistics, Queensland 1996 (1998) Queensland Health, Brisbane.

Whitfield, C.R., Smith, N.C., Cockburn, F. & Gibson, A.A.M. (1986) Perinatally related wastage—a proposed classification of primary obstetric factors. *British Journal of Obstetrics and Gynaecology* **93**, 694–703.

FURTHER READING

Avery, G.B., Fletcher, M.A. & MacDonald, M.G. (eds) (1994) *Neonatology: Pathophysiology and Management of the Newborn*, 4th edn. Lippincott-Raven, Philadelphia.

Day, P., Lancaster, P. & Huang, J. (1997) *Australia's Mothers and Babies 1995*. AIHW National Perinatal Statistics Unit, Sydney.

Office for National Statistics (1996) *Series DH3 (29) Mortality Statistics. Childhood, Infant and Perinatal*, The Stationery Office, London.

World Health Organization (1992) *International Statistical Classification of Diseases and Related Health Problems*, 1, 10th revision. WHO, Geneva.

2 Fetal physiology, assessment of fetal wellbeing and adaptation to extrauterine life

Perinatology is a term used to describe the study of diseases involving the fetus and newborn infant. This involves the clinical disciplines of fetal medicine and neonatology. The obstetrician must have a thorough knowledge of pregnancy and its effects on the mother and fetus, as well as fetal development and physiology. He or she must also have an understanding of fetal adaptation to the extrauterine environment. The neonatologist specializes in the medical care of the newborn infant but must have a thorough understanding of fetal development and physiology. This chapter briefly reviews some aspects of fetal assessment and physiology to provide the paediatrician and neonatal nurse with a better understanding of current obstetric practice.

PLACENTAL FUNCTION

The placenta is a fetal organ, which has two major functions: transport and metabolism. The trophoblast of the placenta acts as a barrier to prevent the maternal immune system from reacting against 'foreign' fetal antigens. Rejection does not occur because the trophoblastic cells appear to be non-antigenic.

The uterus is supplied by maternal blood from the uterine arteries which dilate throughout pregnancy, increasing fetoplacental blood supply 10-fold by term. Maternal blood bathes the intervillous space and is separated from fetal blood by the chorionic plate. Transport of nutrients and toxins occurs at this level. Oxygenated fetal blood in the capillaries of the chorionic plate leaves the placenta via the umbilical cord to the fetus (Fig. 2.1).

Transport

The placenta transports nutrients from the mother to the fetus as well as waste products in the other direction. This occurs in a number

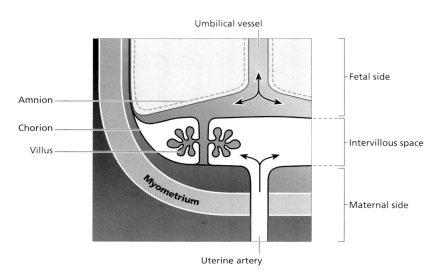

Fig. 2.1 Diagram of placental structures showing blood perfusion.

of different ways, including simple diffusion for small molecules and, for larger molecules, active transport, which is an energy-requiring carrier-mediated process.

The placenta also acts as a 'lung' and is responsible for gaseous exchange of O_2 and CO_2 as well as maintenance of acid–base status.

Metabolism

The placenta is metabolically active and produces hormones, including human chorionic gonadotrophin (HCG), human placental lactogen (HPL) and human chorionic thyrotrophin (HCT). It also detoxifies drugs and metabolites.

Oestriol cannot be produced by the placenta alone as it cannot hydroxylate pregnenolone. This is done by the fetal liver and adrenal glands. The metabolites are then sulphated by the placenta to form oestrogens, one of which is oestriol.

Because of its metabolic activity, the placenta has very high energy demands and consumes over 50% of the total oxygen and glucose transported across it.

FETAL FUNCTION

The placenta is an essential organ for maintaining fetal homeostasis but the fetus is capable of performing a variety of physiological functions.

1 The fetal liver is responsible for the production of albumin, coagulation factors and red blood cells.
2 The fetal kidney excretes urine, which contributes to amniotic fluid.
3 Fetal endocrine organs produce thyroid hormones, corticosteroids, mineralocorticoids, parathormone and insulin from 12 weeks' gestation.
4 Some immunoglobulins are produced by the fetus from the end of the first trimester.
5 The fetus breathes from about 11 weeks' gestation, but this is irregular until 20 weeks. It is not until 36 weeks that the fetus breathes regularly for 55–90% of the time. One purpose

of fetal breathing is to promote an intermittent tracheal flux of fetal lung fluid into the amniotic fluid. This explains why fetal lung maturity can be assessed by measuring the lecithin/sphingomyelin (L/S) ratio on amniotic fluid (see p. 93). With ultrasound techniques, fetal breathing *in utero* can be observed (see p. 9).

FETAL CIRCULATION

The fetal circulation consists of two umbilical arteries bringing deoxygenated blood to the placenta and a single umbilical vein carrying oxygenated blood back to the heart. The aorta of the fetus divides into the common iliac arteries and then the internal and external iliac arteries. The umbilical arteries are branches of the internal iliacs. The umbilical vein drains into the portal sinus and thence bypasses the liver via the ductus venosus to reach the inferior vena cava (Fig. 2.2).

The fetal circulation is quite different from the neonatal circulation. Deoxygenated blood is carried via the two umbilical arteries to the placenta, where it is oxygenated as it comes

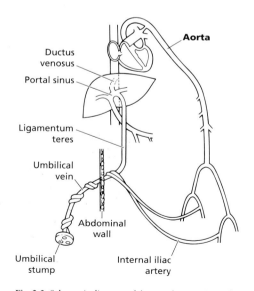

Fig. 2.2 Schematic diagram of the vessels comprising the fetal circulation.

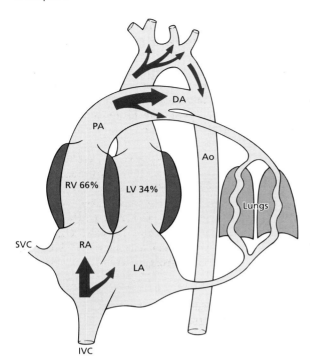

Fig. 2.3 Diagram of the fetal circulation through the heart and lungs, showing the direction of flow through the foramen ovale and ductus arteriosus (DA). The percentages refer to the proportion of the cardiac output from each ventricle. The size of the arrow represents the proportion of flow. IVC, inferior vena cava; SVC, superior vena cava; RA, right atrium, LA, left atrium; RV, right ventricle; LV, left ventricle; PA, pulmonary artery; Ao, aorta. (After Rudolph & Heymann 1970.)

into close apposition with maternal blood in the intervillous spaces. Oxygenated fetal blood is carried in the umbilical vein, where it bypasses the liver via the ductus venosus. The blood then passes into the inferior vena cava and right atrium of the heart (Fig. 2.3). At atrial level much of the blood is shunted across the foramen ovale from the right atrium to the left. Oxygenated blood is pumped by the right ventricle into the pulmonary artery, but the majority bypasses the lungs via the ductus arteriosus to flow into the aorta. Only 7% of the combined ventricular output of blood passes into the lungs. The right ventricle is the dominant ventricle, ejecting 66% of the combined ventricular output.

In summary there are three shunts.

1 The ductus venosus bypasses blood away from the liver.

2 The foramen ovale shunts blood from the right atrium to the left atrium, bypassing the lungs.

3 The ductus arteriosus shunts blood from the pulmonary artery to the aorta.

The last two shunts can only function because of the very high fetal pulmonary vascular resistance and high pulmonary artery pressure.

Umbilical vessels

Usually there are two umbilical arteries and one umbilical vein. Approximately 1% of babies have only one umbilical artery and this may be associated with growth retardation and congenital malformations, especially of the renal tract: 7% of babies with a single umbilical artery have significant renal anomalies. Chromosomal anomalies are also more common in infants with a single umbilical artery. An ultrasound assessment of renal anatomy is warranted for infants born with a single umbilical artery, and karyotype analysis where multiple anomalies are found.

Cardiovascular adaptations required for extrauterine life

While the fetus is breathing *in utero* the lungs are filled with fluid, but at the time of birth the baby generates enormous negative pressures of approximately 60–90 cmH$_2$O and fills the lungs with air. With the first two or three breaths much of the fetal lung fluid is expelled. The remainder is absorbed into pulmonary lymphatics and capillaries over the first 6–12 h. Sometimes these clearance mechanisms fail, or else there is too much fluid to start with and the baby develops symptoms. This condition is known as transient tachypnoea of the newborn (see p. 95) or retained fetal lung fluid. The stimulus for the first breath is not known with certainty, but is probably due to the bombardment of the baby with physical stimuli, such as cutaneous and thermal changes. It is also due in part to emptying of the lungs of fluid.

With the first few breaths the arterial oxygen tension (Pao_2) increases from the fetal level of 2–3.5 kPa (15–25 mmHg) to the newborn level of 9–13 kPa (60–90 mmHg). This relative hyperoxia results in closure of the ductus arteriosus: this is functionally closed by 10–15 h, but not anatomically closed until 4–7 days. There is a marked fall in pulmonary vascular resistance shortly after birth, so that pulmonary blood flow increases. Because of the decrease in pulmonary blood pressure, there is a drop in pressure on the right side of the heart, so that there is no longer shunting of blood from right to left atrium across the foramen ovale. This takes some time to close and in 10% it remains patent through life. After birth there is a marked decrease in blood flow in the inferior vena cava and the ductus venosus closes in response to this. It remains as a vestigial remnant—the ligamentum teres—throughout life. The umbilical vessels take longer to become obliterated and may still be cannulated for up to 10 days after birth.

Many factors may interfere with these changes at birth. If the baby has suffered from severe birth asphyxia or has respiratory distress syndrome, blood may continue to be shunted through fetal channels. A clinical syndrome of persistence of the fetal circulation, where pulmonary pressures remain elevated, is well recognized.

ASSESSMENT OF FETAL WELLBEING

There are many ways to assess the integrity of the fetoplacental unit. These include assessment of maturity, diagnosis of fetal abnormality, monitoring of fetal growth and evaluating wellbeing in the third trimester, as well as monitoring in labour (Fig. 2.4).

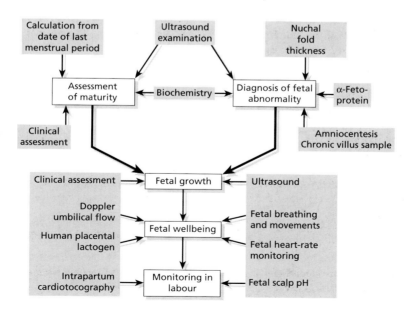

Fig. 2.4 A plan for the assessment of fetal wellbeing. See text for description.

Assessment of maturity

CLINICAL ASSESSMENT

Clinical assessment of maturity depends on the measurement of fundal height. This is most accurate in the first 10 weeks of pregnancy, and can be very unreliable later or in obese women. Fetal quickening can help in dating the duration of pregnancy: in primiparous women movements are first felt at about 20–21 weeks and in multiparous women at approximately 18 weeks.

ULTRASOUND

Early ultrasound measurement of fetal size is the most reliable way to estimate the duration of pregnancy and is considered to be even more reliable than calculation from the date of the last menstrual period. There are a number of ultrasonic measurements which correlate well with gestational age in the first trimester. These include crown–rump length (may be technically a difficult measurement to make), biparietal diameter (BPD) and femur length. The BPD measurement between 12 and 18 weeks' gestation appears to be amongst the best of all methods for assessing the duration of pregnancy.

FETAL RADIOGRAPHY

Radiography of the fetus is now rarely used as a method of establishing maturity. The talus ossifies at approximately 26 weeks and the lower femoral epiphysis appears at 37 weeks, but there is considerable variation and unnecessary exposure to radiation is undesirable.

Diagnosis of congenital abnormality

MATERNAL BLOOD SCREENING

Abnormally elevated α-fetoprotein (AFP) levels are associated with open neural tube disorders and may be used as a screening test in early pregnancy. Low levels of AFP correlate with increased risk of trisomy 21, and this in conjunction with other biochemical markers in the mother's blood (the triple test) is used to screen for this condition. The test does not give a definitive diagnosis but can be used to give a high or low risk for Down syndrome.

ULTRASOUND

Ultrasound examination of the fetus for congenital abnormalities is now highly developed and is offered as a routine procedure in many centres. Major malformations of the central nervous system, bowel, heart, genitourinary system and limbs should be detected and can be diagnosed in specialized centres early enough to consider termination of pregnancy. Down syndrome can often be detected by measurement of nuchal fold thickness.

AMNIOCENTESIS

Amniotic cell culture or fluid analysis is valuable for the diagnosis of a variety of fetal abnormalities. Cells can be cultured for chromosome analysis or to study enzyme activity. Measurement of the optical density in amniotic fluid at 450 nm will detect haemolysis occurring as a result of rhesus haemolytic disease (see p. 205). Decisions regarding early delivery or intrauterine transfusion can be made on the basis of serial amniocentesis measurements.

CHORIONIC VILLUS SAMPLING

Chorionic villus sampling (CVS) involves the transcervical or transabdominal passage of a needle or cannula into the chorionic surface of the placenta at 9–11 weeks' gestation to withdraw a small sample of tissue into a syringe. Because of the 1% risk of abortion related to the procedure, the test is reserved for detection of genetic or chromosomal abnormalities in at-risk pregnancies, rather than as a mere screening test. There is concern that CVS may cause damage to the developing embryo and it is less commonly performed than previously.

FETAL BLOOD SAMPLING (CORDOCENTESIS)

Fetal blood sampling is an ultrasound-guided technique for sampling blood from the umbilical cord to assist in the diagnosis of chromosome abnormality, intrauterine infection, coagulation disturbance, haemolytic disease or fetal compromise.

Fetal growth

CLINICAL ASSESSMENT

Monitoring uterine size is a time-honoured clinical method of assessing fetal growth. Unfortunately, up to 50% of growth-restricted infants are not detected clinically.

ULTRASOUND

Serial estimates of BPD, abdominal circumference and head-to-abdomen ratios are widely used to monitor fetal growth. In fetuses suffering intrauterine growth retardation, head growth is usually the last to slow down. In some centres, estimates of fetal weight by ultrasound are becoming reliable.

Fetal wellbeing

BIOCHEMICAL ASSESSMENT

Assessment of fetal wellbeing by biochemical surveillance has now ceased in most centres as its sensitivity and specificity are very poor. Consistent unrecordably low levels of oestriols suggest either placental sulphatase deficiency or adrenal hypoplasia (see p. 179).

DOPPLER FLOW VELOCITY ANALYSIS

Doppler flow velocity waveforms of the umbilical artery are now used as a major determinant of fetal wellbeing. In fetuses who show growth restriction, abnormal Doppler waveforms are a reliable prognostic feature. Reversed flow velocity during diastole is an ominous sign and is associated with the risk of imminent fetal demise. The significance of absent diastolic flow velocity is uncertain but may not be bad.

FETAL BREATHING MOVEMENTS

These can be assessed by ultrasound and show marked variability. Abnormalities include gasping-type respiration, extreme irregularity of breathing in a term fetus and complete cessation of breathing. This technique has not yet been fully evaluated and its practical value is limited.

ANTEPARTUM MONITORING OR NON-STRESS TEST (NST)

The response of the fetal heart trace to naturally occurring Braxton Hicks contractions or fetal movements provides information on fetal health during the third trimester. The fetal heart trace is classified as reactive or non-reactive, depending on whether there is a minimum of two accelerations of 15 beats per minute or more, lasting at least 15 s, in response to fetal movements over a 20-min observation period.

Monitoring in labour

INTRAPARTUM MONITORING

Continuous monitoring of the fetal heart rate can be performed non-invasively with a cardiotocograph strapped to the abdominal wall, or invasively with a fetal scalp electrode inserted after the membranes have ruptured. The three common abnormalities detected on heart monitoring are illustrated in Fig. 2.5.

1 *Early decelerations (type 1).* Slowing of the fetal heart occurs coincident with the uterine contraction and is probably due to compression of the fetal head, causing vagal stimulation. Early decelerations are not associated with fetal hypoxia and are not serious.

2 *Late decelerations (type 2).* There is a transient slowing of the fetal heart after the contraction, and the heart rate does not resume its baseline until after the contraction has ceased. It is due to impaired blood flow through the

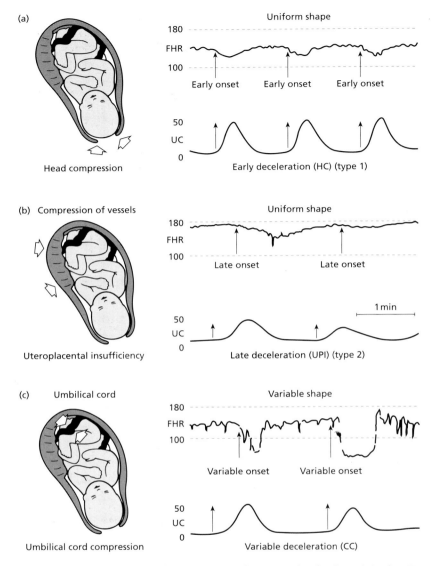

Fig. 2.5 Commonly recognized variations in fetal heart rate recordings. (Reproduced with permission from Hon *et al.* 1975.)

intervillous spaces of the placenta and reflects fetal hypoxia.

3 *Variable decelerations.* There is a short-lived irregular dip in the fetal heart rate, starting at the onset of a contraction and of variable duration. This is probably due to cord compression.

In addition to these three patterns, the variability of baseline heartbeat must be considered. The baseline rate is considered normal between 120 and 160 beats per minute. A flat baseline with little or no beat-to-beat variability is an ominous pattern. A baseline variability of more than 10–15 beats is a healthy sign. The most serious abnormal pattern is decelerations superimposed on a fetal tachycardia.

Despite the widespread use of fetal heart rate monitoring for over 20 years it has not been shown to reduce morbidity in term infants.

It has, however, increased the rate of delivery by caesarean section. There is no evidence that routine fetal heart rate monitoring in the low-risk fetus improves outcome. Careful monitoring with intermittent auscultation in these cases seems to be as reliable.

FETAL SCALP pH

This technique should be used in conjunction with intrapartum cardiotocograph monitoring. In the presence of abnormal fetal heart rate patterns, fetal scalp pH measurement may be helpful. It is believed that a pH of less than 7.20 is associated with the development of fetal compromise and that a pH greater than 7.25 is satisfactory. A pH value between 7.20 and 7.25 is suspicious and should be remeasured after a short time. Maternal acidosis may influence the fetal pH, which should be more than 0.2 units less than the maternal pH for the diagnosis of fetal distress.

FETAL DISTRESS

This is a commonly used clinical term, although there are difficulties with its definition. Fetal distress usually means a stressed fetus showing signs of compromise due to lack of oxygen or undernutrition. It may also be used to describe an investigatory finding, such as failure of head growth on serial biparietal ultrasound examinations.

Used here, the term describes the 'at-risk' fetus. Fetal distress may be related to the following basic underlying causes:

1 maternal: hypotension, hypertension, diabetes mellitus, cardiovascular disease, anaemia, malnutrition and dehydration;
2 uterine: hypertonia, usually due to excessive use of Syntocinon;
3 placental: premature separation, vascular degeneration; and
4 umbilical: prolapse, knot or cord around fetal neck.

The features of fetal distress are:
1 reduction in fetal movements (this has a weak correlation with adverse outcome);
2 passage of thick meconium into the amniotic fluid;
3 fetal scalp pH less than 7.20;
4 fetal heart rate abnormality as defined above.

REFERENCES

Hon, E.H., Zanini, B. & Cabal, L.A. (1975) *An Introduction to Neonatal Heart Rate Monitoring.* University of California, Los Angeles Press.
Rudolph, A.M. & Heymann, M.A. (1970) The circulation of the fetus *in utero*: methods for studying distribution of blood flow, cardiac output and organ blood flow. *Circulation Research* **26**, 298.

FURTHER READING

Behrman, R.E. (ed.) (1983) *Neonatal–Perinatal Medicine. Diseases of the Fetus and Infant*, 3rd edn. C.V. Mosby, St Louis.
Nijhuis, J.G. (ed.) (1992) *Fetal Behaviour. Developmental and Perinatal Aspects.* Oxford University Press, Oxford.

3 Neonatal depression at birth and resuscitation of the newborn

Perinatal asphyxia is the most frequent and serious preventable problem of the fetus and newborn infant. Severe, inadequately treated perinatal asphyxia may lead to major problems after birth, with major long-term sequelae such as mental retardation, spasticity and epilepsy. Good perinatal care can prevent or minimize fetal and neonatal hypoxia.

Neonatal depression at birth (Apgar score ≤ 6 at 1 min) occurs in about 14% of all births, and so a person expert in neonatal resuscitation must be available within 2 min for all births. Perinatal asphyxia remains as a major source of neonatal morbidity in developed countries, and ranks together with perinatal infection as the cause of at least two-thirds of neonatal mortality in developing countries. Owing to problems with definition, reported incidences in full-term neonates vary from 2 to 4/1000 live births, and even more so for very low birthweight (VLBW) infants, with rates of up to 60%.

The terms 'birth' and 'perinatal asphyxia' were previously loosely used to describe depression at birth, but because of the potential medicolegal implications certain criteria need to be satisfied before a specific diagnosis is made.

FETAL RESPONSES DURING LABOUR

Every contraction during labour may cause relative hypoxia and hypoperfusion, a condition which can be considered as mild asphyxia. During these episodes the fetus has a repertoire of responses which protects him from injury (Table 3.1). It is only if these responses become overwhelmed that the fetus suffers injury. These reflexes are designed to maintain function in vital organs such as the brain and

Table 3.1 Responses of the normal fetus to transient episodes of 'asphyxia' in labour

Redirection of blood flow towards:
  brain
  myocardium
  adrenals

and away from:
  skin
  bowel
  muscles

'Diving seal reflex' comprising:
  bradycardia
  increased blood pressure

Episodes of anaerobic metabolism resulting in metabolic acidosis

myocardium. In addition, episodes of fetal bradycardia may occur during contractions. These are part of the 'diving seal reflex' and are normal, but episodes of fetal bradycardia may be mistaken for fetal distress. Anaerobic metabolism may also occur during transient periods of asphyxia, and is again a normal physiological adaptation.

IMMEDIATE EFFECTS OF PERINATAL ASPHYXIA

Asphyxia is usually an intrapartum event: birth liberates the fetus from a hostile environment and adequate resuscitation may restore the infant to a normal physiological state. The asphyxiated baby follows a predictable sequence of reactions, and both the respiratory and cardiovascular systems are directly involved.

Respiratory activity

Initially, there is a stage of increased respiratory

activity which is followed by a period of apnoea (primary apnoea). This is then followed by a series of rhythmic gasps, which increase in frequency for a short time and then become less frequent until secondary (or terminal) apnoea occurs. Spontaneous recovery will occur if the baby is rescued before the secondary apnoea phase. Once terminal apnoea has occurred, active resuscitation is required to save the baby's life. The precise time at which terminal apnoea occurs in the human fetus or newborn is not known, for obvious reasons.

Cardiovascular activity

Heart rate and blood pressure changes occur simultaneously with the respiratory changes described above. Initially, there is a rise in blood pressure and heart rate, followed by a decline until the onset of primary apnoea. This fall is probably mediated by vagal stimulation. A transient rise in heart rate and blood pressure occurs when gasping develops, but this then rapidly falls again as secondary apnoea develops. This is due to myocardial anoxia, and without resuscitation the fetus/newborn dies. The pulmonary vascular resistance increases dramatically with the stage of secondary apnoea and the newborn circulation generally tends to revert to a fetal state. Figure 3.1 summarizes these changes in graphical form.

A baby with primary apnoea will appear blue with some tone and reflex activity and the heart rate will be accelerating. The baby will usually recover spontaneously, but this can be accelerated by physical and chemical stimulation. Traditionally, this condition was called asphyxia livida.

In contrast, the baby with secondary (or terminal) apnoea has passed his last gasp and will not recover without vigorous resuscitation. In this case the baby is white or intensely cyanosed, unresponsive and flaccid, the heart rate is less than 100 and perfusion is poor. This condition was referred to as asphyxia pallida.

Unfortunately, in the delivery room one often cannot distinguish between primary and

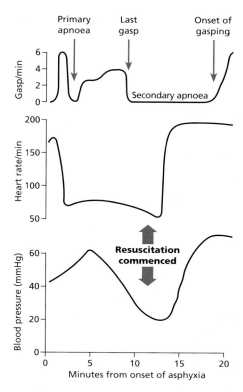

Fig. 3.1 The physiological effect of acute asphyxia and the response to resuscitation. (Redrawn from Dawes 1968, with permission.)

secondary apnoea, so that energetic resuscitation of all apnoeic infants should be undertaken on the assumption that all these infants have secondary apnoea.

After resuscitation it can usually be determined whether the apnoea was primary or secondary. Babies with primary apnoea have an accelerating heart rate, develop spontaneous respiration before 'pinking up', and are often observed to gasp or cry before becoming apnoeic. In contrast, babies with secondary apnoea 'pink up' while being manually ventilated before establishing spontaneous respiration.

It should be noted that the longer the time to initiate adequate resuscitation, the longer the time to the first gasp. For every 1-min delay there will be a 2-min delay before the first gasp.

Table 3.2 The Apgar score

Sign	0	1	2
Heart rate	Absent	< 100/min	> 100/min
Respiratory effort	Absent	Weak cry	Strong cry
Muscle tone	Limp	Some flexion	Good flexion
Reflex irritability (suctioning pharynx)	No response	Some motion	Cry
Colour	Pale. Overall cyanosis	Centrally pink, periphery blue	Pink

ASSESSMENT OF INFANT AT BIRTH

The quantitative Apgar score (Table 3.2) performed at 1 min, 5 min and, if necessary, 10 min, and first described by Virginia Apgar in 1953, remains the most reliable and reproducible way of assessing the infant's condition. The Apgar score must be done accurately and objectively for each of the five items at exactly 1 and 5 min if it is to be of use in assessing the severity of neonatal depression.

A useful way of scoring the Apgar is by deleting points from 10 for a baby who is in good condition at birth and giving points from zero for a baby who is depressed at birth.

Generally the first sign to be lost, and the last one to be regained after resuscitation, is muscle tone. Probably the single most useful sign in judging the need for resuscitation is the heart rate, and if there is bradycardia less than 100/min the baby will usually require positive-pressure ventilation.

Other factors to be considered when assessing birth asphyxia are:
1 time to establish spontaneous, regular respirations;
2 time when infant 'pinked up'; and
3 time before heart rate was 100/min.

The Apgar score and the above three factors have some limited prognostic significance (see p. 19).

Generally an Apgar score of 7–10 at 1 min is normal, 4–6 is moderately depressed and 0–3 is severely depressed. Many infants can be resuscitated despite an Apgar score of 0 at birth, and may sustain no long-term neurological damage.

WHAT IS ASPHYXIA?

Virginia Apgar introduced the scoring system which now bears her name in an attempt to describe the condition of the infant shortly after birth. Although she did not intend it to refer to asphyxia, it has nevertheless become widely used for that purpose and in many centres asphyxia is defined by a low Apgar score. Using this criterion (an Apgar score of 3 or less at 5 min), the incidence of asphyxia is 3–9/1000 full-term infants (Nelson & Ellenberg 1981; Ergander *et al.* 1983). If asphyxia is defined as the requirement for intermittent positive-pressure ventilation for more than 1 min, then 5/1000 full-term infants had this condition (MacDonald *et al.* 1980).

The terms 'birth asphyxia' and 'perinatal asphyxia' were previously loosely used to describe depression at birth, but because of the potential medicolegal implications stringent criteria must be satisfied for their use.

The essential characteristics of the newborn response to asphyxia of such a degree as to be likely to cause harm are:
1 Apgar score 0–3 at > 5 min;
2 neonatal neurological sequelae (e.g. hypotonia, seizures, coma);
3 evidence of multiorgan system dysfunction in the immediate neonatal period;
4 umbilical cord arterial pH < 7.0; and

5 umbilical cord arterial base deficit ≥ 16 mmol/L.

To objectively state that there was a likelihood of a prolonged acute hypoxic–ischaemic event in labour causing permanent brain injury to a previously healthy fetus in labour, one also needs:

1 evidence of a major 'sentinel' hypoxic event, e.g. a ruptured uterus, antepartum haemorrhage, cord prolapse or amniotic fluid embolism, i.e. something that significantly changes normal fetal oxygenation in labour;

2 evidence of possible fetal compromise ('distress') from the time of the sentinel event, e.g. major changes in the fetal heart rate and/or fetal acidosis on fetal blood sampling; and

3 neonatal ultrasound evidence of recent cerebral oedema and/or intracerebral haemorrhage.

Assuming this evidence is present, to show that such objectively proven acute asphyxial brain damage was preventable, one needs to show that:

1 it could reasonably be detected;

2 an unnecessary delay of some hours then occurred; and

3 there was another mechanism of delivery that could reasonably have been achieved in a very much shorter time without major risk to the mother.

The communication between clinicians caring for the woman and those caring for the neonate is best served by replacing the term 'fetal distress' with 'non-reassuring fetal status', followed by a further discription of findings, e.g. repetitive variable decelerations, fetal bradycardia or biophysical profile score of > 2.

FETAL RESPONSES TO HYPOXIA

Most perinatal hypoxic–ischaemic cerebral injury (90% of cases) originates antepartum, with only a small but highly controversial component being solely attributed to intrapartum events. The fetus has highly efficient protective reflexes to combat hypoxia and hypoperfusion which are active antepartum but particularly so during labour.

PERINATAL ASPHYXIA

Causes of perinatal asphyxia

The most common clinical settings associated with hypoxic–ischaemic injury are listed in Table 3.3.

Prevention of perinatal asphyxia

The prevention of perinatal asphyxia involves the following:

1 recognition of high-risk pregnancies;

2 accurate assessment of gestation;

3 assessment of fetoplacental function, e.g. oestriols, ultrasound, fetal movements;

4 assessment of pulmonary maturity (see p. 97);

5 intrapartum fetal heart rate monitoring;

6 treatment of fetal distress *in utero*;

7 ensuring a paediatrician, anaesthetist or other trained person is available to resuscitate the infant if necessary. This should be done before the infant is born to give the doctor time to read the notes, check the equipment and, if possible, introduce him- or herself to the parents.

Communication with the paediatrician during labour or prior to delivery by caesarean section is the key to a successful resuscitation.

A person experienced in neonatal resuscitation should be present at the following types of delivery:

- *High-risk pregnancy*—rhesus isoimmunization, moderate to severe pre-eclampsia, growth-retarded fetus, insulin-dependent diabetic, antepartum haemorrhage, prolonged rupture of the membranes.
- *Abnormal labour*—fetal distress, deep transverse arrest, cephalopelvic disproportion.
- *Abnormal delivery*—caesarean section, moderate or heavy meconium staining of liquor, prolapsed cord, vacuum, mid or high forceps, rotation forceps.
- *Abnormal presentation*—breech, face, brow, compound, shoulder.
- *Abnormal gestation*—preterm delivery.
- *Abnormal fetus*—hydramnios, known abnormality, past history of serious abnormality, multiple births.

Table 3.3 Major causes of neonatal depression in delivery room

Cause	Major effect	Examples
Drugs	Respiratory depression	Anaesthetics, narcotics, $MgSO_4$, tranquillizers
Uteroplacental failure	Hypoxia, acidosis	PET, IUGR, placenta praevia, tetanic contractions
Haemorrhage	Hypovolaemia/shock	Abruptio placentae, fetomaternal transfusion
Developmental anomalies	Cardiac, pulmonary insufficiency	Congenital heart disease, diaphragmatic hernia
Oligohydramnios	Pulmonary insufficiency	Potter's syndrome, PROM
Physical/mechanical	Interruption of blood supply	Prolapsed cord, breech with head entrapment
Severe immaturity	Pulmonary insufficiency	RDS, inadequate respiratory effort
Post-maturity	Meconium passage, placental deterioration	Meconium aspiration syndrome, persistent pulmonary hypertension of newborn
Environmental	Hypothermia	Unplanned home birth
Iatrogenic	Hypoxia, vagal stimulation, excessive ventilation	Pulmonary air leak, intubation of oesophagus/bronchus, apnoea/bradycardia
Extrinsic pulmonary compression	Pulmonary insufficiency	Pleural effusion, pulmonary hypoplasia
Precipitate delivery, abnormal presentation	Birth trauma	Intracranial haemorrhage
Premature, prolonged rupture of membranes	Perinatal infection, chorioamnionitis, pneumonia	

Preparation of equipment is of the utmost importance prior to a successful resuscitation. The nursery personnel should be notified and the necessary equipment prepared. If the mother has had an antepartum haemorrhage, and especially if the Kleihauer test reveals fetal blood, or if a severely rhesus-immunized infant is expected, fresh O-negative blood should be to hand. The history of analgesics and sedatives administered to the mother should be obtained. When preparing for an asphyxiated infant, it is appropriate always to expect the worst possible situation so that all equipment will be ready.

Resuscitation equipment should include: oxygen line and attachment for bag-and-mask ventilation, pharyngeal airway, laryngoscope, suction apparatus for pharynx, stomach and endotracheal tube, meconium aspirator, overhead radiant warmer, sterile warm towels, endotracheal tubes of the appropriate size, a stopwatch and drugs (sodium bicarbonate, 1/10 000 adrenaline, naloxone (Narcan), calcium gluconate).

Routine resuscitation of a non-asphyxiated infant (Apgar 7–10) should consist of:
1 pharyngeal suction as the head delivers, prior to clamping of the umbilical cord;
2 placing the baby with the head lower than the rest of the body;
3 keeping the baby warm by radiant heater or wrapping in warmed blankets. Liquor, blood, vernix and meconium are wiped off baby's skin to prevent excessive evaporative heat loss;
4 pharynx and nares are gently suctioned;
5 heart is auscultated and 1- and 5-min Apgar scores accurately assessed;
6 oxygen may be administered by face mask at a flow rate of 1–2 L/min if baby is still blue;
7 vitamin K (1 mg) is given intramuscularly or orally (see p. 213) to prevent haemorrhagic disease of the newborn, cord blood is sampled and stored for subsequent investigations; and

8 baby is labelled and handed to mother for cuddling or breastfeeding if desired.

Suctioning of the airway

A frequent reason for failure to establish adequate respirations in the newborn is obstruction of the airway with mucus, blood, meconium or amniotic fluid. The baby is held and then placed in a head-down position, and the pharynx is gently suctioned with a size 8 FG catheter with controlled wall suction not exceeding −150 mmHg pressure, or via a suction catheter. Mouth suction should no longer be used because of the risk of viral infections such as human immunodeficiency virus (HIV) (see p. 67). Both nostrils should then be gently suctioned. If there has been moderate or heavy meconium staining of the liquor, the pharynx should be suctioned under laryngoscopic vision by a doctor. If meconium is seen at or below the vocal cords, the trachea should be intubated and suctioned with a size 5 FG catheter or a meconium aspirator. If large amounts of thick meconium are present in the trachea, then the endotracheal tube should be withdrawn, together with its core of meconium, and a fresh tube introduced. Depending on the amount of meconium present, a number of tubes may need to be inserted during the course of resuscitation.

After establishment of regular respirations and when the infant's condition is stable, a large nasogastric tube should be passed to exclude oesophageal atresia. The tube should also be passed through both nostrils to exclude choanal atresia. If gastric aspirate is greater than 25 mL, it may suggest small bowel obstruction, hydramnios or an infant of a diabetic mother. If the liquor is meconium stained, the stomach should be aspirated and lavaged with saline to prevent gastritis and vomiting. If there has been prolonged rupture of the membranes, a sample of gastric aspirate should be sent for Gram staining and bacteriological culture.

Resuscitation of the infant with moderate depression

If the 1-min Apgar score is 4–6, or the infant has not established respirations by 1 min or is persistently cyanosed, then ventilation with O_2 will be necessary in addition to previous resuscitation.

Bag-and-mask ventilation

All medical and nursing staff who work in a delivery suite should be proficient at bag-and-mask ventilation. A tight-fitting face mask (Bennett, Laerdal type) should be selected of the appropriate size for the baby's face. This should fit snugly around the bridge of the nose and chin, and not obstruct the nares. The jaw should be held forward as the operator squeezes the bag at a rate of about 35 breaths/min. The chest should be watched for adequate inflation and should also be auscultated for air entry. Heart rate and colour should be continuously reassessed. The Laerdal and Penlon bags are designed not to deliver high pressures when used in the recommended way. If air entry is unsatisfactory, a pharyngeal airway may need to be inserted. It should be possible to ventilate all infants adequately with a bag and mask until more experienced help arrives (see Chapter 30 for a more detailed description).

Intubation and positive-pressure ventilation (see Chapter 30)

Intubation and positive-pressure ventilation will be required for:
1 babies with Apgar scores of 0–3 at 1 min;
2 if baby is still blue following bag-and-mask ventilation;
3 if Apgar score is less than 6 at 5 min.

Intubation may be orotracheal with a tapered tube such as Warne's size 8, 10, 12 or 14 (sizes 8 and 10 require an introducer), oro- or nasotracheal with Portex size 2.5, 3.0 or 3.5 (Magill forceps necessary for nasotracheal). An infant laryngoscope is necessary.

External cardiac massage (see Chapter 30)

If the baby has a heart rate less than 30/min in spite of adequate ventilation, or if the heart rate is less than 40/min at any time, the baby requires external cardiac massage. Both hands are placed around the infant's chest with the fingertips on the back and the thumbs touching over the sternum, and the thumbs are pressed down at a rate of 80–100/min. The heart massage should be interspersed with ventilation so that there are three beats for each breath.

In summary, the priorities in neonatal resuscitation are described in the order 'ABC':

A **Airway**—first establish an adequate airway;
B **Breathing**—then institute appropriate ventilation;
C **Circulation**—then ensure adequate circulation.

Drugs required in resuscitation

Naloxone (Narcan) is a specific opiate antagonist and is used in the treatment of infants depressed at birth as a result of narcotics given to the mother within 4–6 h of delivery. The dose recommended by the manufacturers is 0.01 mg/kg of the 0.02 mg/mL strength (Neonatal Narcan). In cases of neonatal depression thought likely to be due to maternal narcotics, a larger dose (0.1 mg/kg) is now recommended, either intravenously or intramuscularly. This drug appears to be safe and has no depressant effects itself.

Other drugs are rarely used but include the following:

1 sodium bicarbonate (8.4% or M) is given as a slow dilute intravenous infusion in a dose of 2–5 mmol/kg for severe metabolic acidosis when the baby has not responded to oxygenation and ventilation (see also Chapter 11). This may be given directly into the umbilical vein or preferably via an umbilical catheter (1 mL is equivalent to 1 mmol of 8.4% sodium bicarbonate). Bicarbonate should only be administered for metabolic acidosis and only when the baby is being adequately ventilated and oxygenated; and

2 adrenaline (1 in 10 000) in a dose of 0.3–1 mL into the umbilical vein. It is also effective if given down an endotracheal tube. Calcium gluconate (100 mg/kg) and isoprenaline (0.1–0.5 mg/kg/min) may be used for severe bradycardia or cardiopulmonary arrest.

Sequelae of birth asphyxia

The sequelae of birth asphyxia may be divided into early and late.

EARLY

These may involve any organ system:
1 *Metabolic*
  (a) metabolic acidosis (infants respond with tachypnoea which may mimic respiratory distress syndrome (RDS));
  (b) inappropriate antidiuretic hormone secretion (see p. 250).
2 *Respiratory*
  (a) RDS—acidosis/hypoxia in the perinatal period increases the severity of RDS, or if surfactant production was marginal it may even cause RDS;
  (b) transient tachypnoea of the newborn—retained fetal lung fluid worsened by birth asphyxia;
  (c) aspiration of meconium.
3 *Cardiac*
  (a) myocardial ischaemia, often with tricuspid insufficiency and congestive heart failure due to a severe hypoxic–ischaemic insult to the myocardium. Characteristically changes are seen on the electrocardiogram (ECG) which include flat or inverted T waves, ST segment depression, abnormal Q waves, and sometimes complete bundle branch block. Real-time echocardiography may show a poorly contracting myocardium;
  (b) persistent pulmonary hypertension (persistence of fetal circulation);
  (c) patency of ductus arteriosus.
4 *Central nervous system*
Hypoxic–ischaemic encephalopathy (see below).
5 *Renal impairment* (see p. 253)
The kidney is very vulnerable to hypoxic–ischaemic insults, and either glomerular or tubular function (or both) may be affected. In its most extreme form acute anuria occurs, but more commonly the baby is oliguric

(passes < 1 mL of urine/kg/h). Up to 20% of asphyxiated full-term infants develop significant renal compromise and almost all will demonstrate oliguria, proteinuria, haematuria and elevated creatinine levels.

6 *Haematological*
Disseminated intravascular coagulation (see p. 214).

7 *Gastrointestinal*
8 *Necrotizing enterocolitis* (see p. 267).
9 *Other*
Adrenal haemorrhage; pulmonary haemorrhage.

LATE

The long-term outlook depends on the severity of the asphyxia. There have been few good studies giving clear indications for prognosis. The clinical severity of hypoxic–ischaemic encephalopathy is a better predictor of long-term outcome than Apgar scores or cord blood arterial pH. Many studies have analysed cranial ultrasound, computed tomography (CT) scan, cerebral blood flow velocity and intracranial pressure as predictors of outcome. Other research tools have included magnetic resonance imaging (MRI) and spectroscopy and near infrared spectroscopy. One study revealed that only two of 31 infants with Apgar scores of 0 at 1 min or 3 and less at 5 min who survived were severely handicapped (Scott 1976). The duration of the asphyxial episode is likely to correlate best with outcome. In another study of infants who had an Apgar score of 0–3 at 10 min, one-third died and 17% had cerebral palsy, but if the Apgar was still 0–3 at 20 min then almost 60% died and almost 60% of the survivors developed cerebral palsy

(Nelson & Ellenberg 1981). If the infants had not established spontaneous respiration by 20 min, then 44% died and 31% were severely handicapped. As well as cerebral palsy, mental retardation, epilepsy, deafness, blindness, microcephaly or hydrocephaly may all occur. Minor handicaps such as specific learning difficulties, behavioural problems and clumsiness may not manifest until many years after birth.

HYPOXIC–ISCHAEMIC ENCEPHALOPATHY

Clinical features

Asphyxia is the simultaneous combination of hypoxia and ischaemia, and the clinical neurological syndrome associated with this is referred to as hypoxic–ischaemic encephalopathy (HIE).

After the initial resuscitation, the infant may be flaccid, hypotonic and unresponsive. The clinical signs characteristically progress over the first 12–24 h, and then gradually improve in all but the most severe cases.

The severity of the HIE syndrome is ascribed retrospectively to one of three grades: mild, moderate or severe (Table 3.4).

Grade I includes increasing irritability with some degree of hypotonia, together with poor sucking, which recovers completely by 3 days of age. These infants often appear to be 'hyper-alert', a state in which they seem hungry but feed poorly and respond vigorously to minimal stimuli. Other causes of irritability, such as hypoglycaemia and infection, must be excluded.

Table 3.4 A scheme for the clinical severity of hypoxic–ischaemic encephalopathy (Levene *et al.* 1985)

Grade I (mild)	Grade II (moderate)	Grade III (severe)
Irritability	Lethargy	Coma
Hyperalert	Seizures	Prolonged seizures
Mild hypotonia	Marked abnormalities of tone	Severe hypotonia
Poor sucking	Requirement for tube feeding	Failure to maintain spontaneous respiration

Grade II includes more marked abnormalities of tone, with marked lethargy and usually a lack of interest in feeding. Seizures often develop between 12 and 24 h but are not severe. These infants classically show a differential increase in tone, in the neck extensors more than in the neck flexors, and leg tone greater than that in the arms. Improvement in these symptoms over the first week of life is essential before allocation to this group.

Grade III describes the most severely affected infants. They may initially breathe normally but rapidly become comatose, requiring ventilatory support. At this time they are profoundly hypotonic and often have multiple seizures, which are frequent and difficult to control. They are often areflexic. Fatalities should occur only in this group, and there may be no improvement prior to death.

In Leicester, 6 of 1000 liveborn full-term infants showed clinical features of HIE; 1.1 in 1000 were grade II, and 1 in 1000 grade III. One-quarter of infants with HIE had normal Apgar scores (Levene *et al.* 1985).

The severity of HIE is the best guide to prognosis (Levene *et al.* 1986). Babies with mild encephalopathy have an excellent prognosis; those with moderate encephalopathy have a 25% risk of serious sequelae, including cerebral palsy and mental retardation. Severe encephalopathy has a poor prognosis, with 80% of infants dying or surviving to be severely handicapped, but about 20% of such infants may survive without significant disability.

Cerebral neuroprotection

It is now recognized that the immature brain is remarkably resistant to the effects of acute brain injury such as hypoxic–ischaemic insult (asphyxia). The acute asphyxial insult may cause some initial neuronal injury, but sets in train a process of abnormal biochemical events that leads to delayed neuronal death, which may occur over days rather than hours. There is no one single route to neuronal death, but rather a whole series of pathways which may be interconnected. These involve damage to the cerebral vasculature (in part mediated by macrophages), free radical generation, excessive calcium entry due to glutamate neurotransmitter overstimulation and apoptosis. Apoptosis is 'programmed cell death', a normal function of any cell that does not receive survival signs from adjacent cells. This process is energy requiring and is different from neuronal necrosis. Apoptosis is a normal process in the developing brain, but insults such as asphyxia may exacerbate the process, leading to delayed neuronal loss. Table 3.5 summarizes mechanisms of neural loss which assist the reader in understanding the background to the potential therapies.

A number of potential therapies are being explored to reduce postasphyxial brain injury. These include allopurinol to block free radical generation, glutamate blockers to limit excessive calcium entry and hypothermia to reduce apoptotic losses. To date these are all experimental therapies and cannot be recommended in clinical practice. Hypothermia is a promising

Table 3.5 Mechanism of neural loss

	1° intracellular insult	Reactive reperfusion	2° delayed response
Na/H$_2$O flux/neural instability	+++	–	–
Calcium influx	+++	+	+
Glutamate receptor	+++	–	+
Free radical	++	–	++
Macrophage	++	++	+
Apoptosis	–	–	+++

research technique but should not be introduced before there is evidence of efficacy and safety from well-conducted randomized controlled studies.

WHEN TO STOP RESUSCITATION

As mentioned above, babies born apparently dead with an Apgar score of 0 can be resuscitated and survive without significant neurodevelopmental sequelae. Vigorous resuscitation should be attempted on all infants who were believed to be alive immediately prior to delivery. Yeo and Tudehope (1994) reported that all infants who have Apgar scores of 0 at 1 and 5 min, who survive with the aid of vigorous resuscitation, either subsequently die (80%) or are moderately to severely disabled.

If there is no cardiac output after 10 min, resuscitation should be abandoned.

Ergander *et al.* (1983) have shown that, in surviving infants who did not breathe for more than 20 min, about two-thirds were without major handicap. There are other possible reasons apart from asphyxia for a delay in establishing spontaneous respiration, and we advise that if there is doubt as to whether to continue resuscitation, and if a senior experienced doctor is not available, the baby should be taken to the neonatal unit for further care until more detailed assessment by a consultant can be undertaken.

'Brain death' cannot be diagnosed in the neonatal period. A condition referred to as 'irreversible brain injury' is a better concept in that in many cases those babies with massive brain insult likely to cause permanent and major brain damage can be detected within the first 24 h of life. The two methods which are available in most neonatal units are electroencephalogram (EEG) or cerebral function monitoring (CFM) and Doppler assessment of cerebral haemodynamics. A very abnormal EEG/CFM at 6 h after birth and sustained at 24 h is a good predictor of severe adverse outcome. Abnormalities in mature babies include an isoelectric or very low voltage trace and burst suppression. Doppler assessment of the

anterior or middle cerebral arteries has also been found to be a good predictor of bad outcome, but is only reliable at 24 h after birth. A Pourcelot Resistance Index (PRI) of < 0.5 on Doppler assessment accurately predicts adverse outcome (Gray *et al.* 1993). In practice a severely abnormal EEG/CFM at 6 h, together with a repeat EEG/CFM and abnormal Doppler at 24 h, will predict adverse outcome which can be described to parents as representing 'irreversible brain damage'.

TREATMENT OF ENCEPHALOPATHY

Treatment is largely directed towards complications. General measures include:
1 adequate tissue oxygenation;
2 maintenance of environmental temperature;
3 treatment of possible infection;
4 correction of coagulation disturbances;
5 correction of electrolyte imbalance; and
6 avoidance of hypoglycaemia.
Specific complications include:
1 intracranial haemorrhage;
2 hypotension;
3 seizures;
4 cerebral oedema.

Intracranial haemorrhage is not common in full-term asphyxiated babies, and subdural collection is the most important. This may be suspected on ultrasound examination if there is midline shift, but CT and MRI are the most sensitive investigations for this.

Hypotension will lead to further cerebral hypoperfusion, and low systemic blood pressure must be rapidly recognized and effectively treated with plasma or dopamine. Continuous intravascular blood pressure monitoring is most reliable, but frequent assessment with non-invasive techniques such as oscillometry or a Doppler probe is also satisfactory in most cases.

Seizures are common and may be subtle, at least in their early stages. Their recognition and treatment are fully discussed in Chapter 19.

Treatment aimed at minimizing cerebral oedema is traditional in birth asphyxia, but there are few good data on its beneficial effects. Fluid restriction (20% less than usual requirements) is probably reasonable, but we can find no reasons for recommending dexamethasone treatment. Mannitol 20% (1 g/kg) has been shown to be effective in lowering intracranial pressure (ICP) in infants known to have intracranial hypertension (Levene & Evans 1985), and can be used if there is clinical evidence of raised ICP (bulging fontanelle or acute deterioration in neurological condition).

CT scans correlate well with the presence of cerebral oedema, but ultrasound is much less reliable. An abnormal CT or MRI scan in the first or second week of life is a predictor of adverse outcome.

REFERENCES

Apgar, V. (1953) A proposal for a new method of evaluation of the newborn infant. *Current Research in Anesthesia and Analgesia* **32**, 253–267.

Dawes, G. (1968) *Fetal and Neonatal Physiology.* Year Book Publishers, Chicago.

Ergander, U., Eriksson, M. & Zetterstrom, R. (1983) Severe neonatal asphyxia. Incidence and prediction of outcome in the Stockholm area. *Acta Paediatrica Scandinavica* **72**, 321–325.

Gray, P.H., Tudehope, D.I., Masel, J.P., Burns, Y.R., Mohay, H.A., O'Callaghan, M.J. & Williams, G.M. (1993) Perinatal hypoxic–ischaemic brain injury. Prediction of outcome. *Developmental Medicine and Child Neurology* **35**, 965–973.

Levene, M.I. & Evans, D.H. (1985) Medical management of raised intracranial pressure after severe birth asphyxia. *Archives of Disease in Childhood* **60**, 12–16.

Levene, M.I., Bennett, M.J. & Punt, J. (eds) (1986) *Fetal and Neonatal Neurology and Neurosurgery.* Churchill Livingstone, Edinburgh.

Levene, M.I., Kornberg, J. & Williams, T. (1985) The incidence and severity of post-asphyxial encephalopathy in full-term infants. *Early Human Development* **11**, 21–26.

MacDonald, H.M., Mulligan, J.C., Allen, A.C. & Taylor, P.M. (1980) Neonatal asphyxia. I. Relationship of obstetric and neonatal complications to neonatal mortality in 38,405 consecutive deliveries. *Journal of Pediatrics* **96**, 898–902.

Nelson, K.B. & Ellenberg, J.K. (1981) Apgar scores as predictors of chronic neurological disability. *Pediatrics* **68**, 35–44.

Scott, H. (1976) Outcome of very severe birth asphyxia. *Archives of Disease in Childhood* **51**, 712–716.

Yeo, C.L. & Tudehope, D.I. (1994) Outcome of resuscitated apparently stillborn infants: a ten year review. *Journal of Paediatrics and Child Health* **30**, 129–133.

FURTHER READING

Avery, G.B., Fletcher, M.A. & MacDonald, M.G. (eds) (1994) *Neonatology: Pathophysiology and Management of the Newborn*, 4th edn. Lippincott-Raven, Philadelphia.

Levene, M.I. (1986) *Current Reviews in Neonatal Neurology.* Churchill Livingstone, Edinburgh.

Levene, M.I., Lilford, R.J., Bennet M.J. & Punt, J. (eds) (1994) *Fetal and Neonatal Neurology and Neurosurgery*, 2nd edn. Churchill Livingstone, Edinburgh.

Spitzer, A.R. (1994) *Intensive Care of the Fetus and Neonate.* Mosby, St Louis.

Volpe, J.J. (1995) *Neurology of the Newborn*, 3rd edn. W.B. Saunders, Philadelphia.

4 Examination of the newborn

CLINICAL EXAMINATION

The newborn infant is usually examined by a variety of people. The birth attendant will notice major congenital abnormalities, and the mother will closely scrutinize the baby for congenital defects, birthmarks, etc. Consequently, most obvious defects will be detected shortly after birth. It has been said that the newborn physical examination is the most valuable screening test performed at any time during life, as the early detection of various occult abnormalities (congenital heart disease, hip dislocation, cataracts, etc.) may allow early and effective treatment before morbidity occurs.

Measurement

It is important to ensure that the infant is kept warm during the examination and that appropriate hand-washing is done to avoid cross-infection.

The baby should be measured and the results recorded.

1 Birthweight (naked) is measured to the nearest 10 g.

2 Head circumference is recorded as the maximum occipitofrontal circumference. A number of measurements should be made and only the maximum or mean of the largest two measurements is recorded. A non-stretchable tape measure should be used for this purpose, and the measurement recorded to the nearest millimetre.

3 Length. The crown–heel measurement is recorded and is only reliable if performed on a neonatal measuring board (e.g. Harpenden neonatometer). This requires two people: one to secure the infant's head at the top of the board and a second to extend the legs so that the foot board firmly touches the infant's soles. An average of three measurements should be made and the figure recorded to the nearest millimetre.

All these measurements should be plotted on standard charts appropriate to the infant's gestational age and sex.

Physical examination

The newborn clinical examination must be carried out in a regular sequence so that items are not forgotten. A useful approach is the 'head to toe' technique. Whenever possible the infant should be examined in the presence of at least one parent. For a meaningful examination to be made it is essential to review the maternal history, method of delivery and difficulties at birth.

The physical examination can be considered under the headings below, and normal variations are discussed in the appropriate sections. The following descriptions include various common congenital abnormalities.

GENERAL APPEARANCE

Facies

There is a wide range of recognizable patterns of abnormalities based on facial features. These are well described by Jones (1997). Many are rare, but chromosomal disorders such as trisomies 21, 18 and 13 should be recognized (see p. 156). In addition, the following are often obvious: fetal alcohol syndrome (see Fig. 14.2, p. 150), Crouzon syndrome (Fig. 4.1), Treacher–Collins' syndrome (Fig. 4.2) and Potter's syndrome (see Fig. 22.1, p. 251).

Colour

The infant should be uniformly pink, but acrocyanosis (blueness of the hands and feet) is not

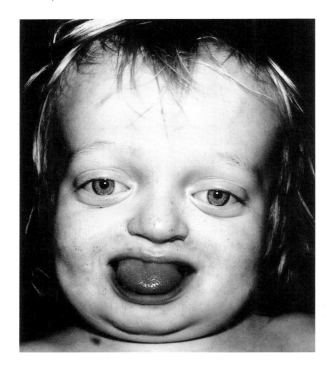

Fig. 4.1 Crouzon syndrome.

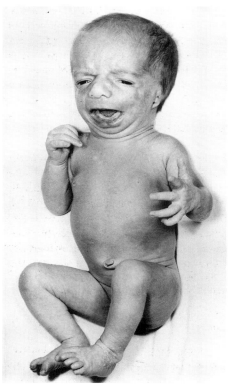

Fig. 4.2 Treacher–Collins' syndrome.

abnormal. Generalized cyanosis, pallor, jaundice, plethora, bruises and petechial haemorrhages are abnormal and should be recorded and investigated further.

Posture

The infant's posture and range of spontaneous movements observed during the examination should be noted. In the term infant the normal position is one with the hips abducted and partially flexed, the knees flexed, and the arms adducted and flexed at the elbow. Limited movement, exaggerated or asymmetrical movements, hypotonia or stiffness must be recorded.

Cry

This should be vigorous and sustained after stimulation, but it should be possible to console the infant by cuddling. A cry which is weak, high-pitched or hoarse is abnormal.

Skin appearance

This varies with gestation, and mild peeling in mature babies is not abnormal. Abnormal appearances, pigmentation and naevi are described in Chapter 24. African and Asian babies may show little generalized pigmentation at birth, except for the genitalia.

Head shape

Moulding and caput succedaneum (oedematous thickening of the scalp due to passage through the vagina) is normal in newly born infants and disappears within 2–3 days.

Plagiocephaly (parallelogram head) is usually seen as a flattening of the occipital region on one side. It is thought to be due to the position the infant has been lying in *in utero* and has no pathological significance. It usually improves with age. Plagiocephaly seen in older infants suggests limitation of neck rotation on the same side as the occipital flattening.

Scaphocephaly (long head with flattened temporoparietal regions) occurs commonly in premature infants and becomes less obvious with age.

Cephalhaematoma occurs when bleeding over the outer surface of a skull bone elevates the periosteum, causing a soft fluctuant swelling confined to the limits of the bone (Fig. 4.3). It may be bilateral, but only crosses the midline in the uncommon occipital variety.

Head size should be measured and hydrocephaly (see p. 223) and microcephaly (see p. 222) diagnosed.

Fontanelles. The anterior and posterior fontanelles are very variable in size and are normally soft and flat. Visible pulsation of the anterior fontanelle is normal. Bulging of the fontanelle may be due to raised intracranial pressure and is always abnormal.

Craniosynostosis. This term refers to premature fusion of one or more of the skull bones. Any bones may be affected, but the sagittal suture is most commonly involved. Facial bones may be affected and cause dysmorphism, such as is seen in Crouzon syndrome (Fig. 4.1). On examination of the head, the anterior fontanelle is usually small and the suture is ridged on palpation. Craniosynostosis causes abnormal head growth; if the sagittal suture is involved, the head becomes scaphocephalic. If this condition is suspected, X-ray will confirm the synostosis.

Craniotabes (ping-pong ball skull) refers to the softening of the skull bones, and with pressure the skull may be momentarily indented before springing out again. It is more common in preterm infants but also occurs in full-term babies. It usually has no significance, but congenital rickets and, more rarely, osteogenesis imperfecta or congenital hypophosphatasia may cause it.

EYES (see also Chapter 20)

Site

The position of the eyes in relation to the nasal bridge should be noted. If they are too far apart,

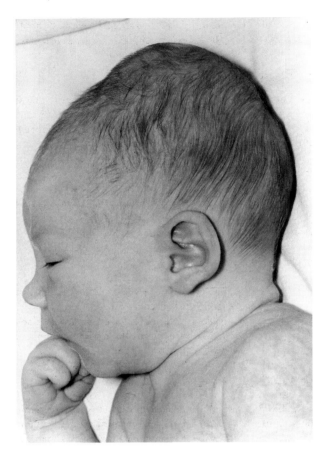

Fig. 4.3 Cephalhaematoma of the left parietal bone.

this is referred to as hypertelorism; if too close together, hypotelorism. These conditions are usually part of a more generalized syndrome.

Conjunctiva

This is usually clear, but subconjunctival haemorrhages are not uncommon in otherwise normal infants.

Conjunctivitis is a serious symptom and infection (e.g. gonococcus, chlamydia; see p. 73) must be excluded. Excessive lacrimation may be associated with a blocked nasolacrimal duct.

Cornea and iris

The cornea should be clear and a red reflex elicited (see p. 242). The pupils should constrict to light both directly and consensually.

Eyelids

Mild lid oedema may be present following a long labour, particularly in a face or brow presentation.

EARS

Shape

There is a wide familial variation.

Preauricular skin tags or sinuses are common. The tags should not be tied off if large or multiple, and the opinion of a plastic surgeon should be sought. Ear malformation may be part of Treacher–Collins' syndrome (see Fig. 4.2, p. 24).

Position

The top of the pinna should be above a horizontal line from the inner and outer canthi. Low-set ears are seen in a variety of conditions, including Potter's syndrome (see p. 251).

NOSE

Patency

Choanal atresia is excluded by gently passing a feeding catheter through both nostrils. Atresias may be bilateral or, more commonly, unilateral, and may be membranous or bony.

MOUTH

Lips

There is wide familial variation. Unilateral or bilateral cleft lip is a common congenital abnormality (1/1000 births). An absent philtrum (groove in the upper lip) and thin vermillion border (red part of the upper lip) are seen in *fetal alcohol syndrome* (see Fig. 14.2, p. 150).

Palate

Epstein's pearls (small inclusion cysts in the midline of the hard palate) are normal and eventually disappear.

Cleft palate. Use a torch to examine the mouth for cleft palate, bifid uvula or high arched palate. A submucous cleft palate can only be diagnosed by inserting the little finger into the mouth to feel for a mucous membrane-covered bony cleft.

Tongue

If large and protruding consider hypothyroidism (see p. 176), Down syndrome (usually accompanied by a small mouth (see p. 157) and Beckwith–Wiedemann syndrome (see p. 170).

Tongue tie is due to a short frenulum. It should not be cut, and rarely causes speech problems.

Jaw

Micrognathia (small underdeveloped jaw) is seen in Pierre Robin syndrome (see p. 259) and associated with cleft palate and cyanotic spells due to tongue prolapse.

Teeth

Natal teeth, mostly lower incisors, are not uncommon and if loose are best removed to prevent aspiration.

Mucous membranes

White patches suggest candida, which need to be distinguished from milk curd.

Ranulas are bluish-white mucous gland retention cysts on the floor of the mouth and usually require no treatment.

Saliva

Drooling or excessive saliva suggests an inability to swallow. Oesophageal atresia, or more rarely a neuromuscular disorder, should be excluded.

NECK

Sternomastoid tumour. Check for a full range of neck movements. Limitation of lateral rotation (turning) suggests shortening of the sternomastoid muscle due to haemorrhage. Sternomastoid tumour occurs in the middle third of that muscle and is best treated with physiotherapy.

Turner syndrome (see p. 156) and *Down syndrome* (see p. 156) are associated with redundant skin at the back of the neck. A low hairline is seen in Turner syndrome.

Klippel–Feil syndrome is associated with a short neck with limited movement. It is a rare condition.

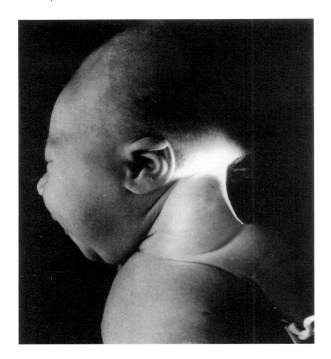

Fig. 4.4 Cystic hygroma of the neck
(transilluminated).

Cystic hygroma. Swelling of the side of the
neck which usually transilluminates brilliantly
(Fig. 4.4). Branchial clefts may give rise to a
branchial cyst, a branchial sinus or branchial
fistula.

Goitre may be present at birth and is always in
the midline.

CHEST

Shape

The chest should be symmetrical in shape and
move equally on respiration.

Respiratory distress of any cause will cause
sternal and intercostal recession.

Size

A small chest occurs in infants with hypoplastic
lungs and in a variety of rare syndromes.

Breast

Engorgement occurs commonly in both sexes
and is due to an oestrogen effect. 'Milk' may be
secreted from the nipple and this is not abnormal. Palpation and expression of the engorged
breast should be discouraged in order to prevent infection.

Supernumerary nipples are a common finding.

Lungs

Respiratory distress. The features of respiratory distress are tachypnoea (normal respiratory rate in the newborn is 30–60 breaths/
min), retraction, cyanosis, grunting and flaring
of the alae nasi. Chest retractions (sternal, substernal, intercostal or subcostal) suggest pulmonary disease.

Stridor (see p. 131) indicates upper airway
obstruction. An inspiratory stridor implies

extrathoracic obstruction, whereas expiratory stridor implies intrathoracic obstruction. Other signs of upper airway obstruction include suprasternal retraction, croupy cough and a hoarse cry.

Breath sounds should be symmetrical (if unilateral, suspect pneumothorax or diaphragmatic hernia). Auscultate with the diaphragm of the stethoscope for symmetry, air entry and adventitial breath sounds. Crepitations may be normal in the first hours of life.

CARDIOVASCULAR SYSTEM

Pulses

The normal heart rate varies between 100 and 175/min, but can drop to 90/min during quiet sleep. The cause of tachycardia and bradycardia is discussed in Chapter 12. The radial and femoral pulses should be palpable. Generally reduced peripheral pulses suggest hypoplastic left heart or cardiogenic shock (see p. 196), and absent femorals suggest coarctation of the aorta (see p. 196). Collapsing or bounding pulses are a feature of delayed closure of the ductus arteriosus (see p. 198).

Apex beat

This should be localized to the fourth intercostal space in the midclavicular line. The left ventricular impulse, palpated at the apex, and the right ventricular impulse, palpable at the lower left sternal edge, are recorded as normal or, if increased, as +, ++ or +++.

A right-sided heart suspected on auscultation may be primary or due to left-sided pneumothorax, left diaphragmatic hernia or true dextrocardia.

Auscultation

A triple or gallop rhythm is always abnormal. Systolic murmurs may be normal in the first 24 h of life. Congenital heart disease is discussed in Chapter 17. Auscultation of a heart murmur in systole is ascribed as $^1/_6 \rightarrow {^5/_6}$ according to intensity, site of maximal intensity and radiation.

ABDOMEN

Distension suggests an *intestinal obstruction* or intra-abdominal mass. A scaphoid abdomen suggests diaphragmatic hernia. A lax abdominal wall with much redundant skin is seen in the 'prune-belly' syndrome. *Divarication* of the rectus muscles may produce a bulge in the abdominal wall between the medial edges of the rectus muscles. No treatment is required and the condition disappears with age.

Liver

This is normally palpable up to 1 cm below the right costal margin. Hepatomegaly may be due to lung hyperinflation, cardiac failure, sepsis, hepatitis, intrauterine infection or haemolysis.

Spleen

The tip can be palpated in about a quarter of normal infants. Splenomegaly suggests infection (prenatal or postnatal) or haemolysis.

Kidney

May be palpable normally, particularly if the baby is relaxed. Moderate kidney enlargement may be due to hydronephrosis, dysplastic or cystic kidneys or rarely a Wilms' tumour. An adrenal mass (e.g. haemorrhage or neuroblastoma) may be very difficult clinically to distinguish from a renal mass. Massive kidney enlargement occurs in bladder neck obstruction or cystic disease.

Anus

This should be patent (tested with a rectal thermometer) and normally situated. Imperforate anus is usually associated with a fistula into the vagina or bladder (in males).

UMBILICUS

Vessels

Normally two thick-walled arteries and a thin-walled vein are seen. One to two per cent of infants have a single umbilical artery, and other congenital malformations may rarely be present in conjunction with this. If there is a single umbilical artery a renal ultrasound should be undertaken to exclude an anomaly of the renal tract.

Colour

Normally translucent due to Wharton's jelly. Green colouration occurs due to meconium staining, or yellow staining due to hyperbilirubinaemia.

Stump

The cord usually separates by 10 days, leaving a yellow or greenish eschar. Reddening of the skin around the umbilicus is abnormal and suggests significant infection. Discharge and cellulitis are also signs of infection. Discharge of urine or meconium from the stump suggests a patent urachus or patent omphalomesenteric duct, respectively. Exomphalos and gastroschisis are discussed in Chapter 23.

Umbilical granulomata are caused by excessive granulation tissue at the umbilical stump. They look like small red swellings resembling a strawberry, and are best treated by the application of a silver nitrate stick on one or two occasions.

Umbilical hernia of the healed umbilicus is particularly common in black babies or those born prematurely, and usually develops in the first month or so of life. A small hernia requires no treatment and spontaneous regression by 6–18 months is the most usual outcome.

GENITALIA

Ambiguous genitalia are discussed in Chapter 16.

Testes

The testes are present in the scrotum in 98% of full-term male infants. Failure to descend by 6 weeks is abnormal.

Ectopic testicles or arrest in the line of normal descent should also be referred for surgical opinion.

Penis and urethra

The foreskin in infants is not retractable and must not be forced. The urethral meatus normally opens at the tip of the glans penis.

Hypospadias occurs if the meatus opens abnormally on the ventral surface of the penis, and is most commonly glandular.

Epispadias occurs when the urethra opens on the dorsal surface of the penis.

Scrotum

A *hydrocoele* may be present at birth, and transilluminates brilliantly. It may extend upwards along the spermatic cord. Most disappear spontaneously during the first year of life and require no treatment other than reassurance.

Inguinal hernia rarely presents at birth but is common in infants who have been born prematurely due to a patent processus vaginalis. The scrotal swelling can usually be reduced. Surgery is required in all cases to prevent incarceration or strangulation of the hernia.

Testicular torsion. A swollen, tender or red scrotum suggests either strangulated inguinal hernia or testicular torsion. Both require an urgent surgical opinion.

Pink nappies

Occasionally, urates may react with the urine in the newborn period, leaving a pinkish-red stain on the napkin which may be confused with haematuria. The condition is usually self-limiting and only occurs in the first few weeks of life.

Hymen

Hymenal skin tags are common in the newborn female infant and are associated with a protrusion of redundant vaginal mucosa. No specific treatment is required and the condition usually regresses spontaneously in the first few weeks of life.

Hydrometrocolpos describes a bulging imperforate hymen, caused by the accumulation of vaginal secretions.

Vagina and vulva

The size of the labia majora depends on gestational age, but by term they should completely cover the labia minora.

Labial fusion occurs in the adrenogenital syndrome and labial adhesions are also not uncommonly seen in otherwise normal infants.

Mucoid vaginal discharge occurs in most mature female infants shortly after birth. It is white and thick and may continue for 2–3 weeks.

Vaginal bleeding may occur in normal infants.

Clitoris

This is variable in size. If large, consider adrenogenital syndrome (see p. 178), a maternal progesterone effect or an intersex state (see p. 183).

EXTREMITIES

Feet

Mild postural deformities may be present, but if the ankle joint can be passively moved through the entire range of normal movements no treatment is necessary. Abnormalities include talipes equinovarus, talipes calcaneovalgus and metatarsus varus (see Chapter 21).

Hips

The hips should be carefully examined to detect a dislocated or dislocatable hip (see p. 246).

Arms

The range of normal movements should be passively tested. The fingers and palms should be examined for abnormalities. A single palmar crease may be present in Down syndrome.

Clinodactyly is a lateral curvature of the fifth finger and may be part of more generalized abnormalities.

Brachial plexus injury. Spontaneous arm movement should be observed: if abnormal, brachial plexus injury (see p. 39) or bony fractures may be present.

NEUROLOGICAL SCREENING EXAMINATION

A simple screening examination should be done in all newborn infants. It consists essentially of assessment of muscle tone and primitive reflexes. Absence or abnormality indicates pathology and a more detailed neurological examination will be indicated (Table 4.1).

Table 4.1 Neurological screening examination

	Normal	Abnormal
Primitive reflexes	Moro, sucking, rooting, grasping, walking, pupillary	Absence of appropriate reflexes
Movement/tone	Spontaneous symmetrical movement	Flaccidity, rigidity, convulsions, tremors, asymmetrical movement

NEUROLOGICAL EXAMINATION OF THE NEWBORN

The neurological evaluation is an essential part of the examination of the newborn, but is often poorly performed and recorded. *The behavioural state* of the infant will severely affect the neurological signs elicited. Ideally, the baby should have been fed 1 h previously and needs to be fully exposed, at least in the initial phase of the examination, and warmed with a radiant heat warmer. The state needs to be recorded using Brazelton's classification (Brazelton 1973).

State I: Quiet sleep.
State II: Active sleep.
State III: Semi-wakefulness.
State IV: Awake, alert and cooperative.
State V: Awake, fussing and uncooperative.
State VI: Crying.

The assessment consists of the observation, examination and recording of the following.

1 *Abnormal movements* such as tremors, jitteriness or convulsions. Tremulousness or jitteriness must be distinguished from convulsions (see Chapter 20).

2 *Spontaneous movements*. The quality and quantity of spontaneous movements are observed and described. Absence of movements may occur in one limb only (monoplegia), two limbs on the same side of the body (hemiplegia), or two legs (paraplegia). The absence of spontaneous movements is often suggestive of a 'sick baby' and very rarely a sign of a paralysed baby.

3 *Posture*. The posture of a baby will depend on the gestational age (see Assessment of maturity, p. 33). A *hypotonic* baby will tend to be in the 'frog position' with reduced spontaneous movement. A *hypertonic* baby may be in a state of predominant flexion or extension. Excessive crowding *in utero* may result in joint contractures. A baby with cerebral irritation may have extensor posturing with arching of the back, opisthotonus, scissoring of the legs and thumbs tightly adducted in the cortical position.

4 *Assessment of tone*. Limb tone is assessed by posture and the amount of resistance to passive movement. In the evaluation of tone a comparison is made between the two sides of the body and between the upper and the lower limbs. The head must be held in the midline to prevent eliciting a tonic neck response. *Hip adductor* tone is assessed by the hip adductor angle with the legs passively abducted. *Head or neck tone* is assessed with the arms held in traction. *Truncal tone* is assessed with the baby held in ventral suspension.

5 *Deep tendon reflexes*. The knee, biceps, ankle and hip adductor jerks are elicited by tapping the appropriate tendons with the fingers. These jerks are usually easily demonstrable, but asymmetrical responses, overactive or absent jerks may be significant.

6 *Ankle clonus*. Ankle clonus may be demonstrated by pressing the thumbs with a rapid, abrupt movement against the distal part of the soles of the feet. Up to six beats of clonus may be normal, but sustained ankle clonus suggests neurological impairment.

7 *Primitive reflexes*. There are some 33 primitive reflexes described in the newborn infant. Primitive reflexes generally first appear at about 32 weeks' gestation but are not well developed until 36 weeks and not readily repeatable until term. In a sick or neurologically depressed term infant the primitive reflexes may be absent. These reflexes usually start to disappear or integrate by 6 weeks and should have disappeared completely by 12 weeks in the term infant. The persistence of primitive reflexes beyond 12 weeks after birth in the term infant, especially when associated with hypertonia, hyperreflexia and sustained ankle clonus, might suggest developing cerebral palsy. These reflexes may reappear in elderly patients who have sustained a cerebral insult. Primitive reflexes may be used to demonstrate:

(a) asymmetry of function;
(b) gestational age of baby;
(c) abnormal neurological function.

Only a few reflexes need to be used by the examiner, but they must be used consistently and their interpretation fully understood. The reflexes recommended are:

(a) *Moro reflex*—elicited by placing one

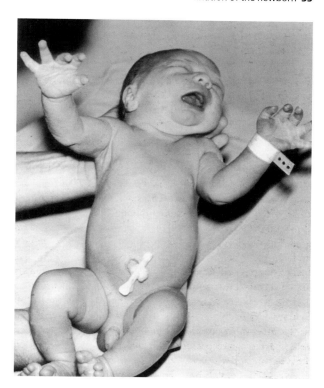

Fig. 4.5 Eliciting the Moro reflex.

hand under the infant's shoulders and the other under his head and then suddenly dropping the head by several centimetres. A full response consists of abduction and extension of the arms, followed by adduction and flexion (Fig. 4.5). An asymmetry would suggest a brachial plexus palsy or a bone injury;

(b) *palmar grasp*—elicited by applying pressure to the palm of the hand, resulting in flexion of the fingers and a firm grasp of the object. If traction is then applied the infant should lift his head off the bed and head lag can be assessed;

(c) *tonic neck reflex*—elicited by turning the head to one side and consisting of extensor and increased tone in the arm and leg on that side. The opposite side often shows a flexion response. This is not always demonstrable at birth, but is pathological or obligatory if the infant cannot 'break' the posture after a few seconds;

(d) *stepping reflex*—the infant is held upright and, as his weight is applied to the foot in contact with the bed, that leg extends while the other leg flexes;

(e) *rooting reflex*—as the cheek is touched the head turns to the stimulus and mouthing movements commence.

8 *Cranial nerves.* The examination of the cranial nerves may be difficult in the newborn (Table 4.2).

ASSESSMENT OF MATURITY

An accurate estimate of gestational age is necessary in the management of the ill or premature infant. An obstetric estimate of the duration of pregnancy may be inaccurate for a number of reasons, and assessment of gestational age should be part of the routine examination of any infant in whom this is in doubt. Gestational age is assessed on both

Table 4.2 Cranial nerves

I Impossible to test.

II The term infant, when in the right behavioural state, can fixate and follow through about 60°. No conclusions can be drawn if this is not demonstrable.

III, IV and VI A fixed squint may suggest a nerve lesion. Asymmetric or non-reacting pupils are abnormal.

V Absent corneal reflex and rooting reflexes are abnormal.

VII Facial nerve palsies are common following birth, and facial asymmetry on crying or sucking should be looked for.

VII The demonstration of a startle response to a loud noise is a crude test of auditory function. An absent response is not diagnostic of a hearing deficit. Brain stem-evoked responses to auditory stimuli provide a definitive test of auditory function. Conventional audiometric testing can be misleading in the newborn infant.

IX, X and XII These are usually examined together. Infants with lesions of these nerves generally exhibit features of gross bulbar palsy with absent gag, suck and swallow reflexes and palatal insufficiency. They cannot swallow their secretions and have obstructive apnoea.

XI The sternomastoid muscle is visualized with the head extended and the infant lying in the supine position. The strength of the muscle is determined by the infant's attempts to right the head.

physical and neurological criteria. The New Ballard Score (NBS) (1991) has been shown to be a valid, accurate assessment tool (see Chapter 8).

REFERENCES

Ballard, J.L., Khoury, J.C., Wedig, K., Wang, L., Eilers-Walsman, B.L. & Lipp, R. (1991) New Ballard Score, expanded to include extremely premature infants. *Journal of Pediatrics* **119**, 417–423.

Brazelton, T.B. (1973) Neonatal behavioural assessment scale. *Clinics in Developmental Medicine*, no. 50. SIMP, London.

Jones, K.L. (ed.) (1997) *Smith's Recognizable Patterns of Human Malformation*, 5th edn. W.B. Saunders, Philadelphia.

FURTHER READING

Korones, S.B. (ed.) (1981) *High-Risk Newborn Infants. The Basis for Intensive Nursing Care*, 3rd edn. C.V. Mosby, St Louis.

5 Birth trauma

Injuries may be sustained either during labour or at delivery, and may occur despite skilled obstetric care.

The decreased incidence in birth trauma over recent years has been attributed to changing trends in obstetric management, such as caesarean section instead of difficult vaginal delivery. Despite the falling incidence, birth injury is still a cause for concern to the obstetrician and neonatal paediatrician. Parents sometimes attribute birth injury to obstetric mismanagement, and this may result in litigation. Unfortunately, such events encourage the practice of defensive obstetrics and a high caesarean section rate may be a consequence of this.

Illingworth (1985) maintained that it may be inappropriate to ascribe a child's so-called 'brain damage' solely to labour or delivery without considering other causative factors. 'Brain damage' can occur without difficult labour or perinatal hypoxia, and despite caesarean section. It is simplistic to relate brain damage to single factors such as breech delivery or hypoxia at birth without considering the many interacting prenatal, perinatal and postnatal factors.

An increasing number of traumatic lesions are due to iatrogenic insult, sustained in the neonatal unit.

INCIDENCE

It is estimated that significant birth injury (excluding asphyxia) occurs in 0.2/1000 live births (Curran 1981) and is more likely in breech deliveries and premature infants. Birth trauma as a cause of neonatal death has declined dramatically in both term and preterm infants in recent years.

RISK FACTORS FOR BIRTH INJURY

The effect of changing patterns of obstetric practice on birth-associated mechanical injuries is difficult to evaluate. However, a number of risk factors for birth injury have been identified (Table 5.1).

Specific birth injuries are detailed below.

Soft tissue injuries

ERYTHEMA, ABRASIONS AND LACERATIONS

These are seen following forceps and vacuum delivery, episiotomy, uterine incision at caesarean section, cephalopelvic disproportion and scalp electrode monitoring (Fig. 5.1).

TRAUMATIC CYANOSIS (TRAUMATIC PETECHIAE)

These occur over the head, neck and upper chest following a difficult delivery. They often occur with breech presentation and in infants born with the umbilical cord tightly around the neck. They may be related to a sudden increase in intrathoracic pressure during passage of the chest through the birth canal. These petechiae usually fade within 2–3 days and require no treatment other than parental reassurance. Traumatic petechiae must be clearly distinguished from generalized petechiae associated with coagulation disturbances.

ECCHYMOSES (BRUISING)

Bruising may be seen with traumatic deliveries, precipitate labour, preterm infants, poorly

Table 5.1 Risk factors for birth injury

Fetal condition

Prematurity

Small for gestational age

Multiple pregnancy

Fetal distress

Malpresentation

Breech presentation (see Table 5.2)

Brow, face, compound presentation

Malposition

Occipitoposterior arrest

Deep transverse arrest

Cephalopelvic disproportion

Macrosomia, e.g. infant of diabetic mother, hydrops fetalis

Macrocephaly

Contracted pelvis
   Shoulder dystocia
   Severe moulding
   Unengaged head

Prolonged labour

Delay—cervix fully dilated

Delay—cervix not fully dilated

Precipitate labour

Maternal factors

Nulliparity

Short stature

Obesity

Inexperienced accoucheur

controlled deliveries or abnormal presentations, e.g. face, brow, breech.

SUBCUTANEOUS FAT NECROSIS

This term is applied to well-demarcated indurated areas in the skin occurring where pressure has been applied, e.g. forceps blades on the face. No treatment is required.

STERNOMASTOID TUMOUR

See p. 27.

Injuries to the head

CAPUT SUCCEDANEUM

See p. 25.

CEPHALHAEMATOMA (see Fig. 4.3)

This occurs in about 1% of newborn infants and is due to bleeding between the periosteum and the cranial bones (usually parietal, less commonly occipital) as a result of shearing or tearing of communicating veins during delivery. The extent of the swelling is limited by the underlying skull bone and does not cross suture lines. It is due to buffeting of the fetal skull against the maternal pelvis, which is seen especially in prolonged labour. It may also occur following a forceps or vacuum delivery. Subperiosteal bleeding is slow and may not appear until the second day of life. Enlargement may occur during the first week and the swelling may persist for several weeks. This edge may be confused with a depressed fracture of the skull.

Complications associated with a cephalhaematoma may include:
1 an underlying linear skull fracture;
2 jaundice due to resorption of the blood;
3 calcification at its edge, which may occur some weeks later during the resorption process. This should not be confused with a depressed skull fracture;
4 intracranial haemorrhage may rarely be associated with cephalhaematoma.

SUBAPONEUROTIC HAEMORRHAGE (SUBGALEAL HAEMORRHAGE)

On rare occasions haemorrhage may occur beneath the aponeurotic sheet joining the two portions of the occipitofrontalis muscle of the scalp. It is seen particularly in black infants. It may be the consequence of trauma during

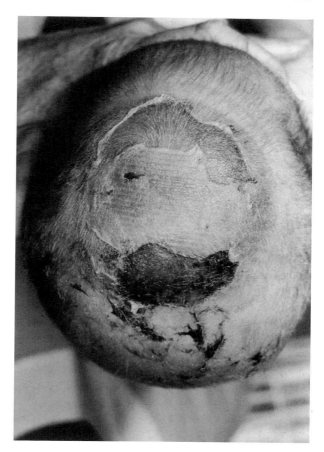

Fig. 5.1 Scalp lacerations and
bruising following vacuum delivery.

Table 5.2 Injuries more likely to occur in infants delivered by breech

Haemorrhage

Subdural tears due to tentorial rupture (see p. 231)

Rupture of intra-abdominal viscus (usually liver or kidney)

Occipital osteodiastasis with cerebellar haemorrhage

Orthopaedic
   Dislocation: shoulder, cervical vertebrae, hip, knee

Fracture: clavicle, humerus, femur; damage to sternomastoid muscle

Neurological
   Asphyxia secondary to cord prolapse

Cervical plexus injury: Erb's or Klumpke's paralysis

Facial nerve palsy

Soft tissue injury

Extensive bruising, particularly genitals

delivery, especially with vacuum extraction, or may indicate the presence of a coagulation defect. These haemorrhages can spread over the scalp and may be fluctuant. Shock may result from the blood loss of a large sub-aponeurotic haemorrhage and transfusion may be required.

SKULL FRACTURES

Generally linear fractures require no specific treatment. Depressed fractures are usually associated with forceps application or head compression produced by the maternal sacral promontory. Large fractures may be associated with cerebral contusion and neurosurgical consultation may be necessary. Depression of the skull may remain for many months after birth.

INTRACRANIAL HAEMORRHAGES

See Chapter 20.

Peripheral nerve injuries

Nerve injuries in the newborn infant may be due to stretching, compression, twisting, hyperextension or separation of the nervous tissue. They may be classified pathologically as:
1 *neuropraxia* (swelling of the nerve);
2 *axonotmesis* (complete peripheral degeneration with total recovery);
3 *neurotmesis* (complete division of all structures).

Electromyography and nerve conduction studies can distinguish a neuropraxia from a neurotmesis. The following nerve injuries occur in the newborn.

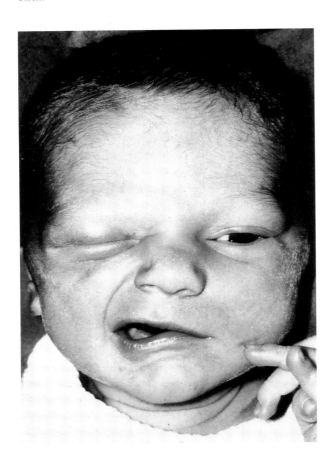

Fig. 5.2 Left-sided facial palsy.

FACIAL NERVE PALSY (Fig. 5.2)

This may be due to an upper or lower motor neuron lesion, but clinical distinction is difficult. Lower motor neuron facial palsy due to oblique application of the forceps blade is a common injury. The nerve may also be damaged by prolonged pressure on the maternal sacral promontory. Upper motor neuron lesions are much less common and are due to brain injury or nuclear agenesis (Moebius syndrome).

The lesion is recognized clinically by an inability to close the eye and a lack of lower lip depression on crying. These are seen on the affected side. This must be distinguished from 'asymmetrical crying facies' caused by an absence of the depressor anguli oris muscle. In this condition eye closure is normal but there is failure of the mouth to move downward and outward on the affected side when the infant cries. Asymmetry usually remains into adult life but becomes less obvious with time. It is commonly seen in other members of the family as well.

In most cases complete recovery occurs; only rarely is permanent facial palsy seen. If the eye cannot be closed, patching and 1% methylcellulose (artificial tears) eyedrops should be used to prevent corneal damage.

BRACHIAL PLEXUS PALSY

Injury to the brachial plexus may be due to excessive lateral flexion, rotation or traction upon the neck. Such trauma may be seen with normal delivery, with impacted shoulders or during delivery of the aftercoming head of a breech.

Three types of brachial plexus injury can be described:

Erb's palsy (upper brachial plexus palsy) (Fig. 5.3). In this lesion the fifth and sixth cervical nerve roots are injured and the arm will be held in adduction, with the elbow extended and the forearm pronated with the wrist flexed. This is traditionally known as the 'waiter's tip' position.

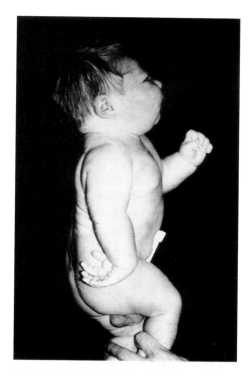

Fig. 5.3 Right-sided Erb's palsy showing the typical 'waiter's tip' position of the hand.

Klumpke's paralysis (lower brachial plexus palsy). In this uncommon lesion the seventh and eighth cervical and first thoracic segment nerve roots are injured: this involves the small muscles of the hand, with localized wrist drop and flaccid paralysis of the hand. The grasp reflex will be absent.

Total paralysis of the arm. Where all trunks of the brachial plexus have been damaged there will be complete paralysis of the arm, with flaccidity and sensory, trophic and circulatory changes. Spinal injury should be suspected when paralysis is bilateral.

For the three types described, active treatment is unnecessary as it does not hasten recovery. Passive movement of the joints will prevent contractures. Mild injuries recover within a few days, and more severe lesions can be expected to recover spontaneously in 2–4 months. In some cases early surgery to the nerve may be beneficial. In a large study of brachial plexus paralysis, 85% of cases were normal by 4 months of age, 92% by 12 months and 93% by 4 years (Gordon *et al.* 1973).

RADIAL NERVE INJURY

Rarely radial nerve paralysis may result from fracture of the humerus, as may occur when there is difficulty in delivering the arm during breech extraction. The use of the 'deltoid region' as a site for intramuscular injection (now usually avoided) has resulted in radial nerve injury, because the deltoid muscle of the newborn infant is so small that correct localization of the needle point is difficult. It may also be seen following repeated brachial artery sampling of arterial blood.

SCIATIC NERVE INJURY

Misplacement of the needle tip during intramuscular injection into the buttock region carries with it a risk of injuring the sciatic nerve.

PHRENIC NERVE PALSY

This is caused by injury to cervical nerve roots C3, 4 and 5, and is generally associated with brachial plexus palsy. As the newborn infant predominantly breathes with the diaphragm rather than the intercostal muscles there is often severe respiratory distress, especially when the lesion is bilateral. The clinical diagnosis is confirmed by chest X-ray, which shows an elevated hemidiaphragm, and X-ray or ultrasound screening shows an immobile diaphragm.

RECURRENT LARYNGEAL NERVE PALSY

This is a rare cause of congenital laryngeal stridor and is due to birth trauma associated with excessive lateral traction of the neck. The diagnosis is made by laryngoscopy and treatment is expectant.

SPINAL CORD INJURY

This is rare and usually associated with difficult breech deliveries involving internal version and breech extraction; rarely it may occur with shoulder dystocia. The injury is due to stretching of the cervical spinal cord. There are three modes of clinical presentation:
1 poor condition from birth, respiratory depression, shock and hypothermia, death;
2 normal at birth but later develops respiratory depression, paralysed legs and urinary retention;
3 paralysis from birth, and the extent of the paresis depends on the spinal level involved.

The investigation of choice is spinal magnetic resonance imaging (MRI). Neurosurgical decompression is necessary for a large haematoma in the spinal canal. Somatosensory potentials may help to localize the level of the spinal injury.

Bone and joint injuries

Traumatic fractures of bones are frequently associated with the classic signs of fracture, e.g. swelling, avoidance of movement, deformity and crepitus. Fractures of the upper limb bones may be suspected by an asymmetrical Moro reflex or failure to spontaneously move one arm.

CLAVICLE

This is the bone most frequently fractured during the birth process. It may be associated with impacted shoulders, especially in the infant of a diabetic mother or a difficult breech delivery. Specific treatment is not required.

HUMERUS

This is generally a fracture of the upper third of the shaft and there is usually considerable deformity. Radial nerve injury sometimes also occurs. Treatment consists of an immobilizing plastic backslab or immobilization with a binder to the chest.

FEMUR

This occurs rarely during breech extraction, either vaginally or at caesarean section. It occurs predominantly in the breech with extended legs as flexion occurs. Treatment consists of immobilization in a plaster case, gallows traction or cutaneous traction, and a Thomas splint.

MULTIPLE OR UNUSUAL FRACTURES

When these occur, osteogenesis imperfecta or non-accidental injury should be suspected.

DISLOCATION OF JOINTS AND SEPARATION OF EPIPHYSES

These are difficult to diagnose and require specialized treatment.

Organ injuries

LIVER AND SPLEEN

Subcapsular haematoma of the liver can occur after a breech extraction or following external cardiac massage. It may also result from 'atraumatic' vertex deliveries. Rupture of the liver or spleen is more likely to occur where there is hepatosplenomegaly (rhesus haemolytic disease, diabetic mother).

ADRENAL

Adrenal haemorrhages may occur with breech extraction, although they are usually a post-mortem finding and are unsuspected in live infants. They are more commonly associated with overwhelming bacterial infection and disseminated intravascular coagulopathy.

Table 5.3 Iatrogenic disease occurring in newborn infants

Skin lesions

Fetal scalp electrode lacerations

Transcutaneous Po_2 monitor burns

Calcified heel nodules from heel-stick venepuncture

Chemical burns from skin antiseptics

Extravasation lesions due to leakage of intravenous solutions

Oxygen toxicity, retinopathy of prematurity (see p. 240)

Bronchopulmonary dysplasia (see p. 110)

Hearing deficits

Antibiotics

Incubator noise

Cardiac failure from patent ductus arteriosus

Necrotizing enterocolitis (see p. 267)

Rickets (see p. 172)

Digit damage, nerve palsies, nasal deformities, oral deformities and bowel disturbance from catheters, tubes and needles

Premature thelarche

Postural deformities

Scaphocephaly

Narrow arched grooved palate

External rotation of hips and feet

KIDNEYS

Ruptured kidneys may occur very rarely during delivery in breech preterm infants.

TESTICLES

Testicular bruising and haemorrhage are commonly seen in breech presentations. No treatment is necessary.

INJURIES SUSTAINED IN THE NEONATAL UNIT

An increasing number and range of traumatic lesions are due to iatrogenic insults sustained in the modern neonatal intensive care unit. These lesions predominantly occur in preterm infants and relate to the invasive procedures and technology necessary to salvage increasingly small infants (see Table 5.3).

REFERENCES

Curran, J.S. (1981) Birth associated injury. *Clinics in Perinatology* 8, 111–130.

Gordon, M., Rich, M., Deutschberger, J. & Even, M. (1973) The immediate and long term outcome of obstetric birth trauma, brachial plexus paralysis. *American Journal of Obstetrics and Gynecology* 117, 51.

Illingworth, R.S. (1985) A paediatrician asks why it is called birth injury? *British Journal of Obstetrics and Gynaecology* 92, 122–130.

FURTHER READING

Fanaroff, A.A. & Martin, R.H. (eds) (1997) *Neonatal-Perinatal Medicine: Diseases of the Fetus and Infant*, 6th edn. Mosby, St Louis.

Schaffer, A.J. & Avery, M.E. (eds) (1983) *Diseases of the Newborn*, 5th edn. W.B. Saunders, Philadelphia.

Spitzer, A.R. (1994) *Intensive Care of the Fetus and Neonate*. Mosby, St Louis.

Volpe, J.J. (1994) *Neurology of the Newborn*, 3rd edn. W.B. Saunders, Philadelphia.

6 Infant feeding and nutrition

The ideal food for healthy full-term infants is breast milk (p. 47). If the baby is born growth restricted, the volume of milk required is higher than a normally grown baby of the same weight (see below). Premature infants have different nutritional requirements from full-term infants and require to be fed either directly into the bowel or intravenously (p. 58). Infant feeding and nutrition can conveniently be discussed under the following headings:
1 specific nutritional requirements;
2 breastfeeding;
3 formula feeding;
4 feeding the very low birthweight (VLBW) infant;
5 common feeding disorders;
6 total parenteral nutrition;
7 specialized feeding regimens.

SPECIFIC NUTRITIONAL REQUIREMENTS

Fluids

Water is the major constituent of infants but its proportion varies with maturity (Fig. 6.1). For this reason, the daily requirement of the newborn is relatively higher than that of older children, and that of the premature infant higher still. Mechanisms for conserving water are often poorly developed in immature infants, and their requirements depend on conceptual age, postnatal age and environment.

A healthy breastfed infant will consume as much fluid as is required, given ready access to the breast. Healthy bottle-fed infants will also 'know' how much fluid they need and should be allowed to consume milk when they want it, to the volume that satisfies them. Unfortunately, many mothers feel that their baby should take all his or her milk at every feed, and overfeeding may become a problem. In addition, ill or premature babies need to be given their requirements as they cannot be relied upon to take what they need. For these reasons, recommended feeding schedules have been devised (Table 6.1). These fluid requirements will be maintained up to 3 months of age, and then slowly reduced to 100 mL/kg by the age of 1 year.

Infants who have suffered intrauterine growth restriction should be fed to an expected weight as if they had grown normally *in utero*. This is usually a figure halfway between the 50th centile weight for gestational age and their actual weight. Ill premature infants, particularly those with lung disease, may tolerate less than their recommended volume. Excessive fluid volume in these infants may predispose to delayed closure of the

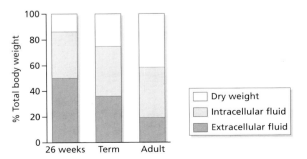

Fig. 6.1 Total body water and extracellular fluid expressed as percentages of body weight. (Redrawn from Dear 1984, with permission.)

Table 6.1 Recommended feeding schedules (fluid volume mL/kg according to day of life)

	Day of life						
	1	2	3	4	5	6	7
Term infant	30	60	90	120	130	140	150
Preterm infant	60	80	100	120	140	160	180
'Sick' preterm infant	60	70	80	90	100	110	120

Add 20 mL/kg for open radiant heat source incubator and for phototherapy.

ductus arteriosus and congestive cardiac failure (see p. 195). Some very immature infants may lose large amounts of water through their kidneys or skin. In such cases a significantly higher fluid intake may be required.

For these reasons, recommended feeding schedules are of little value in sick infants: the fluid intake must be tailored to the infant's requirements and his or her state of hydration. Clinical assessment of hydration is made by skin turgor, fontanelle tension, moistness of the mucous membranes and urine output. In practice clinical methods for assessing fluid requirements are unreliable: laboratory investigations are more helpful. Serum sodium, potassium, creatinine, osmolality and haemoglobin (haematocrit) should be measured daily. In addition, urinary osmolality or specific gravity (SG) is an important measurement. Daily weighing is a most valuable assessment of hydration and growth.

Serum osmolality may be affected by hyponatraemia, hyperglycaemia or uraemia, and may be unreliable under these circumstances. Similarly, glycosuria or proteinuria may affect urinary SG. We have found measurement of SG with Multistix SG (Ames Ltd) reliable as an approximation to urinary SG and it is not affected by glycosuria. In practice we aim to keep the urinary SG between 1005 and 1010, increasing the fluid volume if the urine becomes more concentrated, and considering reduction in the presence of very dilute urine.

Inappropriate antidiuretic hormone (IADH) secretion is a relatively common condition in both premature and full-term infants with severe lung or cerebral disorders. It may also be seen following neonatal surgery. The hallmark is dilute serum (low serum sodium and osmolality) with concentrated urine. Peripheral oedema is often present. The treatment is fluid restriction until the serum osmolality returns to the normal range (270–285 mmol/L).

Energy

Energy requirements for optimal growth depend on the baby's birthweight, gestational age and state of health. Ill babies are likely to be more catabolic and will have greater energy requirements. In addition, the smaller the infant the greater the requirements, and this is particularly so in infants who have suffered intrauterine growth restriction. Table 6.2 gives the energy requirements of various groups of infants for optimal growth.

CARBOHYDRATE

Lactose is the sole carbohydrate source in human milk and must be metabolized to glucose for energy utilization in the brain and other organs. Approximately 40% of the infant's total energy requirement comes from the carbohydrate in milk.

FAT

Fat in milk provides approximately half of the infant's energy requirements. Human milk fat is better absorbed than cows' milk fat. The

Table 6.2 Energy requirements for optimal growth (at end of first week of life)

	Energy (kcal) kcal/kg/day	Energy (kJ) kJ/kg/day
Premature infant	120	516
Small for gestational age	140+	602
Term infant	100	403

Table 6.3 Recommended enteral intake of minerals for term and VLBW infants (Koo & Tsang 1993)

	Enteral mineral intake (mmol/kg/day)	
	Term infant	VLBW infant
Sodium	2.5–3.5	3.0–4.0
Potassium	2.5–3.5	2.0–3.0
Chloride	5.0	1.5–4.5
Phosphorus	1.0–1.5	1.9–4.5
Calcium	1.2–1.5	3–5.5
Magnesium	0.6	0.3–0.6

mature infant absorbs about 90% of the fat in human milk, but infants weighing less than 1300 g absorb only 75–80% of fat from human milk, and less from artificial milk. Unsaturated fatty acids are better absorbed than saturated fatty acids, and medium-chain triglycerides better than long-chain triglycerides. Infants require 4–6 g fat/kg/day.

Recently, considerable interest has developed in the role of long-chain polyunsaturated fatty acids (LC-PUFAs) in milk and their role in brain development. LC-PUFAs are present in human but not bovine milk, and fish oils are a particularly rich source. As accumulation of fetal LC-PUFAs is increased up to five times in the last trimester, prematurely born infants are thought to be particularly at risk of deficiency. Supplementation of milk with fish oils has shown enhanced maturation of the visual system in prematurely born infants, but this does not seem to confer long-term benefit. Routine supplementation of human milk with LC-PUFAs is the subject of ongoing research and is not currently routinely recommended.

PROTEIN

Approximately 10% of the infant's energy requirements is provided by protein. The recommended daily intake is 2.5–3.5 g/kg/day for full-term infants and 3.0–3.8 g/kg/day for very premature infants. Milk protein is divided into curd (mainly casein) and whey (predominantly lactalbumin). Human milk contains more whey and cows' milk considerably more curd. There are also important differences in the amino acid profile of human and cows' milk. Some low birthweight infants fed a formula high in protein and especially high in the casein component develop a feeding acidosis or late metabolic acidosis. This is due to the inability of the preterm kidney adequately to excrete the acid produced from protein metabolism.

Minerals

The recommended minimal mineral requirements for optimal nutrition are shown in Table 6.3. In sick infants, particularly those receiving intravenous nutrition, it is important

Table 6.4 Recommended daily enteral intake of some trace minerals (Ehrenkranz 1993)

	Daily requirement (mmol/kg)	Daily requirement (µg/kg)
Zinc	7.7–12.3	500–800
Copper	1.9	120
Manganese	0.01	0.75
Chromium	0.001	0.05

to monitor serum levels of these minerals, and adjust intakes accordingly. Extra sodium may be required by the VLBW infant, as there may be a high urinary loss for the first weeks of life. Potassium should not be given until adequate renal function has been established.

Trace elements

Recommended enteral requirements are shown in Table 6.4. Copper and zinc have been shown to be essential trace elements for newborn infants. Other trace elements thought to be essential are chromium, manganese, iodine, cobalt and selenium. Breast milk and modern formula feeds contain some of these elements.

Fluoride is important in tooth development. Supplementation for infants and children is recommended in areas where drinking water is not fluoridated. The dose should be 0.1 mg/kg/day. Excessive fluoride intake during infancy may result in dental enamel fluorosis.

Iron

Both preterm and term infants born to healthy mothers have sufficient iron stores at birth to double their haemoglobin mass. Depletion of these stores occurs at 3 months in premature and 5 months in term infants. If the baby is not receiving adequate iron in the diet by this age, iron deficiency anaemia will develop. Breast milk provides sufficient iron for a term infant up to 6–9 months of age. Preterm infants (irrespective of which milk they receive) should be supplemented with oral iron from 6 weeks until the age of 12 months. They require approximately 2–4 mg of elemental iron daily, or about 45 mg of ferrous gluconate.

Table 6.5 Recommended daily dosage for vitamin supplementation

	Recommended daily dosage
Vitamin A	500–1500 iu
Vitamin D	400 iu
Vitamin E	5 iu
Vitamin C (ascorbic acid)	35 mg
Folate	50 µg
Niacin	5 mg
Riboflavin	0.4 mg
Thiamine	0.2 mg
Vitamin B_6	0.2 mg
Vitamin B_{12}	1 µg
Vitamin K	15 µg

Vitamins

The daily vitamin requirements for the newborn and young infant are shown in Table 6.5. The preterm infant probably requires more vitamin D (1000 iu). This is discussed in the section on rickets of prematurity (see p. 172). Much has been written about the supplementation of premature infants with vitamin E. However, there is no good evidence that this prevents late anaemia, or bronchopulmonary dysplasia. Its role in the prevention of retinopathy of prematurity is discussed on p. 240. Vitamin K is the only vitamin in which the normal breastfed infant may become seriously deficient. Vitamin K deficiency may cause haemorrhagic disease of the newborn (see p. 213).

BREASTFEEDING

Breast milk is the ideal food for normal full-term babies, but unfortunately in many western societies its advantages are not fully utilized. The advantages of breastfeeding can be considered as those for the baby and those for the mother, although these are of course interrelated.

Advantages to the baby

1 Nutritional. It provides the baby with a source of nutrition that changes with the baby's changing metabolic needs.
2 It confers an advantage in intellectual attainment (see below).
3 Anti-infective (see below).
4 Antiallergic. The avoidance of foreign proteins in formula feeds reduces the risk of asthma and eczema in infants predisposed to these conditions.
5 Protection against various illnesses (e.g. gastroenteritis), but apparent protection against SIDS (sudden infant death syndrome) probably relates to maternal education, socio-economic status and birthweight, rather than to breastfeeding *per se*.

Advantages to the mother

1 Successful breastfeeding brings a sense of pride and achievement which she alone can provide.
2 Promotion of a close mother–baby relationship which provides security, warmth and comfort to her baby.
3 Lactation helps the mother lose weight acquired in pregnancy.
4 Convenience, as there is no preparation of formula. It can also be simply expressed, stored and given to the baby by others.
5 Lactational amenorrhoea remains the world's most important contraceptive by delaying the return of ovulation.
6 Oxytocin release during breastfeeding contracts the uterus and helps its involution.
7 Financial benefit, as breastfeeding is free.
8 It is possible to continue breastfeeding if a mother needs to return to paid work.
9 Breastfeeding confers some health advantages on the mother, as there appears to be some protection against ovarian and premenopausal breast cancer and osteoporosis.

In the UK, in 1990, nearly 40% of women never breastfed their babies and over 60% who started breastfeeding had stopped by the time their baby was 6 weeks old. In 1991 UNICEF and the World Health Organization introduced the global baby-friendly hospital initiative to improve these figures. The '10 steps' (Table 6.6) to successful breastfeeding are intended as a standard of good practice.

Table 6.6 The '10 steps' to successful breastfeeding (Vallenas & Savage-King 1997)

Step 1	Have a written breastfeeding policy that is routinely communicated to all healthcare staff
Step 2	Train all healthcare staff in the skills necessary to implement this policy
Step 3	Inform all women (face to face and with leaflets) about the benefits and management of breastfeeding
Step 4	Help mothers initiate breastfeeding shortly after delivery
Step 5	Show mothers how to breastfeed and how to maintain lactation (by expressing milk) even if they should be separated from their infants
Step 6	Give newborn infants no food or drink unless 'medically' indicated. No promotion of formula milks
Step 7	Practise 'rooming-in'. All mothers should have their infant's cots next to them 24 h a day
Step 8	Encourage breastfeeding on demand
Step 9	Give no artificial teats or pacifiers to breastfeeding infants
Step 10	Foster the establishment of breastfeeding support groups and refer mothers to them

The physiology of lactation

During pregnancy there is a marked increase in the number of ducts and alveoli within the breast in response to oestrogens, progesterone and placental lactogen. In the third trimester prolactin secreted by the anterior pituitary sensitizes the glandular tissue with the secretion of small amounts of colostrum. The flow of milk after birth is under the control of the let-down reflex. The baby rooting at the nipple causes afferent impulses to pass to the posterior pituitary, which secretes oxytocin. This stimulates the smooth muscle fibres surrounding the alveoli to force the milk into the large ducts. After birth there is an increase in prolactin levels which maintains milk production. The hormonal maintenance of lactation is summarized in Fig. 6.2.

Stress inhibits oxytocin release and may reduce milk production. This may cause the baby to cry more, thereby heightening maternal stress and further inhibiting milk production. This may be an important factor in the failure of long-term lactation (see below).

Milk production is controlled by endogenous (maternal) and exogenous (baby) factors.
1 *Endogenous.* In the first weeks of lactation, prolactin secretion occurs in response to feeding and controls milk production.
2 *Exogenous.* After a few weeks of successful breastfeeding the baby exerts the major control on breast milk production. The amount of milk produced is related to effective and frequent removal of milk from the breast by the baby.

Nutritional aspects

Human milk is uniquely adapted to the requirement of babies, with low levels of protein and minerals compared to the milks of other species. The energy content of human milk (67 kcal/100 mL) is provided by fat (54%), carbohydrate (40%) and protein (6%). Human milk has a very low protein content of only 0.9 g/100 mL, with a casein : whey ratio of 0.3. A larger proportion of the nitrogen in human milk is derived from non-protein

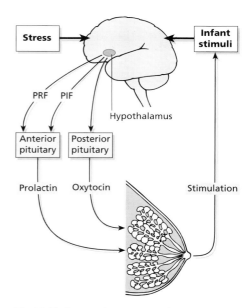

Fig. 6.2 The hormonal maintenance of lactation. PIF, prolactin inhibiting factor; PRF, prolactin releasing factor.

sources compared to cows' milk. Human milk contains twice the amount of lactalbumin as cows' milk (and is immunologically different), but no lactoglobulin, which is a significant component of the protein constitution of cows' milk. The levels of amino acids such as taurine, aspartic acid, glutamic acid and asparagine are especially high. Human milk fat is better absorbed than cows' milk fat because of the smaller size of the emulsified fat globules and the presence of lipase in human milk.

The main differences between human and cows' milk are shown in Table 6.7. There is a higher proportion of unsaturated fatty acids and a lower proportion of saturated fatty acids in human milk than in cows' milk. Human milk contains more vitamins A, C and E and nicotinic acid than does cows' milk, but less vitamin B_1, B_2, B_6, B_{12} and K. The low mineral level in human milk results in a low renal solute load for the immature kidney. Although calcium and phosphate levels in cows' milk are higher than in human milk, their absorption in cows' milk is much lower.

Table 6.7 Proteins in human milk and cows' milk (g/100 mL). (Reproduced from Hambraeus *et al.* 1984)

	Human milk	Cows' milk
Total protein	0.89	3.30
Caseins	0.25	2.60
Total whey protein	0.64	0.70
α-Lactalbumin	0.26	0.12
α-Lactoglobulin	–	0.30
Lactoferrin	0.17	Trace
Serum albumin	0.05	0.03
Lysozyme	0.05	Trace
IgA	0.10	0.003
IgG	0.003	0.06
IgM	0.002	0.003
Others	0.07	0.15

Variations in breast milk

Early breast milk contains a higher sodium and protein concentration than milk from mothers who have fed their infants for several months. The high sodium content in early milk reflects the young infant's inability to fully conserve sodium by the kidneys, a mechanism which matures in the weeks following birth. The amount of lactose in breast milk increases with postnatal age as the intestinal disaccharidase enzyme mechanism matures. Interestingly, up to 90% of milk is taken from the breast in the first 4 min of feeding; the rest of the 'feed' is largely non-nutritive. Bottle-fed infants have quite a different pattern of intake, less than 40% of the feed being taken in the first 5 min.

It is now known that the milk constituents of mothers who deliver prematurely are different from those of women who deliver at full term. Preterm milk contains a higher protein and sodium content than term milk, supporting the suggestion that preterm milk is better suited to premature infants than milk from established breastfeeding mothers. In addition, preterm milk contains considerably more immuno-globulin A (IgA) than term milk. The amount of lactose and fat (and consequently energy) is less in milk from mothers delivering prematurely. This may reflect the immaturity of the digestive and absorptive mechanisms of premature infants.

Anti-infective properties of breast milk

Breastfeeding is an effective method of protection from infection while a baby's immunological system is developing. Breastfed infants are less likely to develop gastroenteritis, necrotizing enterocolitis (NEC) (see p. 267), otitis media and other serious infections, such as septicaemia and meningitis. This is due to numerous host resistance factors in human milk, which include:

Immunoglobulins. IgA is the most important immunoglobulin secreted in breast milk, and is in very high concentrations in colostrum.

Cells. Breast milk contains vast numbers of macrophages, polymorphs, and both T and B lymphocytes.

Lysozyme. This acts to lyse the *Escherichia coli* cell membrane.

Lactoferrin. This binds iron, which is necessary for some bacteria to multiply.

Antiviral properties possibly due to secretory IgA or interferon production by lymphocytes.

Bifidus factor. The stool of breastfed babies is more acid than that of artificially fed infants. This, together with the carbohydrate bifidus factor, encourages lactobacilli to flourish, which has the effect of inhibiting the growth of *E. coli.* Unfortunately, a single artificial feed is enough to upset this delicate balance and the gut flora changes as a result.

Contraindications to breastfeeding

These are uncommon and can be divided into maternal and infant contraindications.

IN THE MOTHER

1 Acute illness—a relative contraindication, as illness is usually over quickly.
2 Chronic illness—neoplasms, mental illness, tuberculosis.
3 Breast infection/abscess temporary expression of that breast is necessary.
4 Human immunodeficiency virus (HIV) infection in the mother can be transmitted to the baby through the cells in breast milk. In developing countries the risk of gastroenteritis from contaminated feeds outweighs the risk of acquiring HIV infection from breast milk, but in developed countries, where clean water is taken for granted, breastfeeding by HIV-positive women is discouraged (see also p. 67).

IN THE INFANT

1 Acute illness—this may be temporary and the expression of breast milk should be encouraged.
2 Mechanical problems—severe cleft lip, cleft palate.
3 Metabolic problems—galactosaemia, phenylketonuria, lactose intolerance.
4 Breast milk jaundice (see Chapter 13)—interruption of breastfeeding may rarely be considered for a few days in order to make a diagnosis or until the jaundice falls to a safer level.

EXCRETION OF DRUGS IN BREAST MILK

The question of excretion of drugs (medically administered or illicit) as well as environmental toxins in breast milk has caused great concern and anguish to many mothers. Unfortunately, there is little scientific information on this subject. The factors that enhance the transfer of drugs in breast milk include:
1 the lipid solubility of the drug;
2 the pH of milk is 6.6–7.4, so that basic drugs such as antihistamines, aminophylline, opiates and antidepressants are more likely to be excreted in higher concentrations;
3 unionized drugs;
4 those not protein bound; and
5 those of low molecular weight.

Table 6.8 gives a guide to the safety of drugs given to breastfeeding mothers.

In addition, infants with glucose-6-phosphate dehydrogenase deficiency (see p. 208) may haemolyse if exposed to nitrofurantoin, sulphonamides or sulphasalazine via breast milk.

Techniques of breastfeeding

ESTABLISHMENT OF LACTATION

Preparation for breastfeeding should begin in the antenatal period. It has been shown that antenatal expression of colostrum results in an increase in the duration of breastfeeding and a reduction in milk engorgement.

The infant should be put to the breast as soon as possible after delivery and the timing and duration of feeds should be responsive to the needs of the baby. Breastfeeding at night should be encouraged. The time the baby spends on the breast should be gradually increased so that the nipples get used to the baby's sucking. Supplementing breast milk with water or glucose reduces the duration of breastfeeding with no compensating benefit, and should be strongly discouraged.

The baby should never be pulled off the breast. The jaw should be released by depressing with the finger at the corner of the baby's mouth. Each feed should be started on alternate breasts. Nipple creams and sprays are unnecessary.

PROBLEMS WITH BREASTFEEDING

Ill or preterm baby

The mother should be encouraged to express by hand within a few hours of birth, as frequent breast expression up to six to eight times a day increases lactation. A pump should only be used if it is comfortable and convenient and the nipples are not already traumatized.

Jaundiced baby

The sleepy, jaundiced baby may need to take

Table 6.8 A guide to the use of common drugs in breastfeeding mothers. (Reproduced from Read *et al.* 1984)

Unsuitable for breastfeeding mothers	Only use if mother and infant can be monitored	Safe to use in breastfeeding mothers
Gold salts	Aminoglycosides	Codeine
Indomethacin	Cotrimoxazole	Non-steroidal anti-inflammatories
Phenylbutazone	Ethambutol	Paracetamol
Chloramphenicol	Isoniazid	Salicylates*
Tetracyclines	Clonidine	Cephalosporins
Phenindione	Diuretics	Erythromycin
Lithium	Antidepressants	Metronidazole*
Iodides	Carbamazepine	Penicillins
Oestrogens (high dose)	Phenytoin	Rifampicin
Antimetabolites	Primidone	Beta blockers
Atropine	Carbimazole	Digoxin
Ergotamine	Oral contraceptives	Heparin
Opiates (high dose)	Thiouracils	Hydralazine
Amiodarone	H_2 antagonists	Methyldopa
Dapsone	Antihistamines	Warfarin
Doxepin	Theophylline	Barbiturates*
Vitamin D (high dose)		Benzodiazepines*
		Sodium valproate
		Corticosteroids*
		Progestogens
		Bulk laxatives
		Kaolin
		Inhaled bronchodilators

* Only if low-dose regimens.

expressed breast milk from a bottle, so that an adequate intake of milk may be given and documented.

Test weighing

This is a technique performed to assess the volume of milk obtained while the baby is suckling at the breast. The weight of the infant (dressed or undressed) before a feed and after a feed is compared. If the baby is gaining weight satisfactorily and seems contented, test weighing is unnecessary. If there is genuine concern regarding the volume obtained at the breast,

test weighs may be indicated. However, it must be emphasized that an isolated test weigh may be very misleading and provoke anxiety: it is unlikely to produce a realistic indication of the amount or nature of milk a baby is receiving because of variations in intake from feed to feed and the changing composition of milk within the feed.

Insufficient breast milk

While in hospital the mother will require a great deal of support and reassurance and continued nipple stimulation to establish an adequate supply of milk. After discharge social and emotional problems may influence the milk supply.

Reasons for low supply include maternal anxiety, inadequate sucking stimulus due to inappropriate feeding routines and behaviours, and inadequate glandular response.

Milk engorgement

This can largely be prevented by demand feeding. Once breast engorgement has occurred, hot packs before feeding and cold packs after feeding are helpful. The mother should only express sufficient milk to soften the areola, to enable the baby to latch on to the breast.

Overfeeding

If there is an excessive amount of milk and the baby receives it too quickly, posture feeding, with the mother lying on her back, is recommended.

Cracked nipples

Cracks are caused by incorrect positioning of the baby on the breast. Nipple soreness may be due to positional soreness, nipple fissure, infection such as candida, and dermatitis. Rarely is it necessary to take the baby off the breast, and there is little evidence that this practice accelerates healing. Nipple care with the application of lanolin or Masse cream and exposure to sunlight and fresh air may help heal the cracks. Hindmilk left on the nipples to dry after a feed may aid the healing process.

Inverted or retracted nipples

There is no evidence that inverted or retracted nipples inhibit the woman's ability to breast-feed her baby successfully, or that treatment prior to birth with nipple exercises or shields improves breastfeeding rates.

Sleepy babies

This may be present in the first day or two after delivery and may relate to analgesia and anaesthesia or mild birth asphyxia.

'Fighting the breast'

This is often associated with maternal anxiety and is aggravated if there are difficulties in getting the baby to the breast. Careful support and reassurance are necessary to establish successful lactation under these circumstances.

Twin feeding

If the twins are full term and vigorous, twin feeding should be possible even from day 1. Often the twins are small and do not readily suckle at the breast, so that expression may be necessary initially. It is an individual choice as to whether the babies are fed together or separately.

Weaning (changing from breast milk to another milk)

The decision on when to wean is an individual one between mother and baby. If breastfeeding has been established for more than 3–4 months, weaning should be a gradual process over at least 2–3 weeks. The last feed to be stopped should be the evening feed. If weaning takes place before 6 months, it is advisable to put the infant on a formula milk. Mutual weaning has many advantages, but often there are overwhelming reasons for maternal-led weaning.

ADVICE TO BREASTFEEDING MOTHERS

If there are problems with breastfeeding after discharge from hospital, midwives and/or health visitors can provide help and support. Most countries have a wide range of community resources well equipped to deal with the mother under stress.

SUPPLEMENTS TO BREASTFEEDING

Full-term infant

Babies receive sufficient supplemental iron in

breast milk alone, at least until 6 months of age, and probably until 9 months. At about 6 months some iron-containing foods, such as cereal, egg yolk and meat broths, should be slowly introduced. Breast milk contains sufficient vitamins for the full-term infant until solids are introduced.

Preterm infant

The preterm infant needs supplemental iron whether breastfed or not. Ferrous gluconate is introduced on day 21 of life in a dose of 0.5 mL/day. Similarly, the premature infant requires extra vitamins, which can be commenced on day 14.

Breast milk bank

There are many advantages to feeding infants breast milk, namely its nutritional balance, its antimicrobial properties and the avoidance of foreign protein. For these reasons, milk banks have been established in order to provide breast milk for infants in whom artificial feeds may be disadvantageous. The practice of breast milk banking was placed in doubt with the worldwide epidemic of acquired immunodeficiency syndrome (AIDS), but by carefully screening donor mothers, milk banking is enjoying renewed enthusiasm. Donor mothers are invariably those who are well established breastfeeders. Many are encouraged to collect the drip milk (that issuing from the non-feeding breast). This milk has a considerably lower fat content, which can be boosted by expressing any excess of milk from the breasts after the infant has completed a feed. The milk is collected in sterile plastic bottles and stored in the mother's own domestic refrigerator at 4°C for not longer than 48 h. It is then delivered to the milk bank and frozen (−20°C) prior to heat treatment.

A major advantage of breast milk is its antimicrobial properties. Sterilization of the milk by boiling destroys all these properties. Pasteurization by the Holder method (62.5°C for 30 min) preserves IgA and lysozyme, but unfortunately cells are very sensitive and

easily destroyed. A bacteriological sample is taken prior to pasteurization, and if any toxin-producing organisms are cultured the milk is discarded. A second sample is taken after pasteurization and, if free of pathogens and with a cell count below 100 000 organisms/mL, it is refrozen until required. Milk is not accepted from women who are HIV or hepatitis B positive.

Breast milk and intelligence

There has been considerable debate as to whether babies who have been breastfed subsequently have a higher intelligence (IQ) than those given formula milk in the early months of life. This debate is beset with the difficulties of self-selection, as it is often women of higher socioeconomic class who elect to breastfeed, and intelligence has a major genetic influence.

Lucas *et al.* (1992, 1994) have conducted a number of intervention studies on premature babies. In one study mothers who elected not to breastfeed, with their agreement, had their babies randomized to receive either banked donor milk or preterm formula. A second group of babies was studied where the mother had elected to breastfeed, but if complements were required the baby would be randomly allocated to receive either banked donor milk or preterm formula. These studies show as clearly as is currently possible that at 7–8 years babies who had received human milk had a 10-point higher IQ than those who had never received breast milk.

Breast milk fortifiers

Recently manufacturers have produced sachets to add to breast milk which enhance it nutritional content. Table 6.9 lists the constituents of two commonly used fortifiers. Studies have not shown any long-term benefit in terms of growth at 18 months.

ARTIFICIAL FEEDING

If a mother fails in her attempts to breastfeed

Table 6.9 Composition of breast milk fortifiers. Amounts given are what would be added to each 100 mL breast milk

	Enfamil human (4 sachets)	Cow & Gate (Karical) (2 sachets)	Nestle (FM 85) (1 scoop)	S26 Human milk fortifier (2 sachets)
Protein (g)	0.7	0.7	0.9	1.0
Fat (g)	0.05	0	0	0.15
CHO (g)	2.73	2.0	3.6	2.3
Energy (kcal)	14	14	14	14.6
Calcium (mg)	90	60	51	90
Phosphorus (mg)	45	40	34	45
Sodium (mg)	7	3		

or does not wish to undertake breastfeeding, she must not be made to feel inadequate or guilty. Successful bottle feeding is much better than unsuccessful breastfeeding.

Commercially produced infant formulae which are reconstituted with water are sold as powders or 'ready-to-feed' liquids. The infant milk manufacturers produce milks which are similar to mature breast milk and are often marketed as 'breast milk substitutes'. The World Health Organization has set down very strict criteria in the International Code of Marketing of Breast-milk Substitutes. More recently, formula feeds have been developed which are better suited to the needs of premature infants.

Most infant formulae in the UK are prepared from cows' milk and all contain added iron and vitamins A, C and D; some also contain trace elements. They may be classified into two categories (DHSS 1980):

1 *modified milk formulae (cows' milk with added carbohydrate)*, either lactose or maltodextrins, e.g. Ostermilk Complete Formula, Ostermilk Two, Cow and Gate Plus, SMA White Cap, Milumil;

2 *demineralized whey-based formulae (skimmed cows' milk with added carbohydrate and mixed fats, animal and vegetable)*. In this type of milk the protein has been altered to more closely resemble the ratio of whey protein to casein in breast milk. The use of demineralized whey allows the mineral content of the milk to approach more closely that in breast milk, e.g. Cow and Gate Premium, Osterfeed, SMA Gold Cap, Aptamil.

Table 6.10 shows the constituents of various infant milk formulae available in the UK.

Table 6.10 Typical contents of various milks fed to mature and immature infants (contents per 100 mL of milk)

	Mature human milk	Modified milk formula	Demineralized whey formula	Preterm formula
Energy (kcal)	70	65	68	80
Protein (g)	1.34	1.7	1.45	2.0
Sodium (mg)	15	25	19	35
Calcium (mg)	35	61	35	90
Phosphorus (mg)	15	49	29	50
Carbohydrate (g)	7.0	2.8	7.0	6.6–8.6
Fat (g)	4.2	2.6	3.82	4.8

Unmodified cows' milk or evaporated milks should not be given to infants less than 6 months of age.

Techniques of artificial feeding

VOLUMES

The amounts suggested in the first section of this chapter should be given.

INTERVAL BETWEEN FEEDS

In general, term infants weighing less than 3 kg are fed 3-hourly initially. Infants over 3 kg can be 'demand' fed or fed 4-hourly. It is reasonable to delete the night feed if the infant does not wake, once he is over 3 kg in weight.

STERILIZATION

A suitable technique for teats and bottles should be followed. One commonly used is the 'Milton method'. Water used in the preparation of feeds must be bacteriologically safe. This may be conveniently achieved by boiling the water for 10 min before it is used for feed preparation.

PREPARATION OF FEEDS

Guidelines suggested by milk manufacturers for their products should be carefully followed. The preparation of too concentrated feeds is an important cause of hypernatraemic dehydration.

FEEDING THE VLBW INFANT

Few subjects in neonatal medicine generate as much controversy as the appropriate way to feed the very premature infant. Some ill VLBW infants will not tolerate milk feeds and require total parenteral nutrition (see p. 58). For those to whom milk may safely be given there is a choice between breast milk (expressed from the infant's own mother—EBM—or banked breast milk—BBM) or a formula feed. Specially adapted formula milks have been developed

for the needs of premature babies which meet their nutritional requirements better than do standard formula feeds.

The following are the general principles on which feeding the VLBW baby is based.

Breast milk

It is known that human milk, including that from the mother who delivers preterm, is not nutritionally adequate for very immature infants. However, breast milk has important properties that make it attractive to feed to preterm infants. These include:
1 reduced risk of infection owing to the anti-infective properties described earlier (p. 49);
2 breast milk is thought to reduce the risk of NEC in premature infants (p. 267);
3 the presence of growth factors in milk, which may be absorbed intact through the baby's gut;
4 probably confers an advantage for cognitive development (p. 53).

Low birthweight formula

Table 6.10 shows the typical contents of low birthweight formulae compared to formulae for mature infants. These often contain more sodium, potassium, protein and carbohydrate than breast milk and regular artificial feeds. We continue one of these formulae until the infant is 35 weeks' postconceptual age, and then change to a regular formula feed.

Enteral vs. parenteral feeds

Early exposure of the baby's gut to enteral feeds has been shown to mature gut function. Low-volume hypocaloric feeds (20 mL/kg) reduce the time to reach full feeding to significantly lower than in babies who do not have early feeding. This effect is probably mediated through the stimulation of gut hormones.

Practical management

In developing a policy for feeding the VLBW

infant, the following principles should be considered:

1 early introduction of breast milk is beneficial even if given in small volumes (hypocaloric);

2 avoid milk feeding in the first 5–7 days in babies at very high risk of NEC (critically ill, severe intrauterine growth restriction, particularly if absent diastolic flow on antenatal Doppler studies);

3 once feeding with breast milk is established, supplement the milk with either breast milk fortifiers or low birthweight formula;

4 the nasogastric route is preferred. Nasojejunal feeding is associated with a significantly higher risk of death and should not be used unless there is a particular indication;

5 there appears to be no advantage of continuous feeding over bolus feeding, which is more physiological. In babies with gastro-oesophageal reflux continuous feeding may be more appropriate to reduce reflux;

6 total parenteral nutrition (TPN) (p. 58) should be used only when milk feeding is contraindicated, or as a supplement to milk feeding where a low volume of milk is indicated. Use TPN for the shortest acceptable period of time.

Rickets of prematurity

This occurs in rapidly growing premature infants and is at least in part related to imbalance in the calcium and phosphate in the infant's feeds. The condition is fully discussed in Chapter 16.

COMMON FEEDING DISORDERS

The most frequent problems are possetting, vomiting, colic, constipation, diarrhoea and failure to thrive, and will be discussed below.

Vomiting

Possetting. Many babies have small spills of feed (posset) and this is considered normal.

Vomiting. This is a common symptom in the newborn and its causes may be non-organic or organic.

1 *Non-organic*: overfeeding; incorrect preparation of feeds; overstimulation or excessive handling of baby; crying; air swallowing.

2 *Organic*: infection (urinary tract infection, gastroenteritis, meningitis, otitis media); gastro-oesophageal reflux, gastritis (meconium, blood), hiatus hernia; organic bowel obstruction, pyloric stenosis, small bowel obstruction, large bowel obstruction; transient gastrointestinal intolerance (e.g. prematurity, metabolic disorders); food allergy (cows' milk). Bile-stained vomiting must always be urgently investigated to exclude malrotation of the bowel (p. 263).

INVESTIGATION

The cause of infant vomiting can usually be determined if a careful history of feeding technique, description of the vomiting, preparation of the infant formula and other symptoms are assessed. The physical examination must be complete. A test feed is often necessary. If there is a possibility of underlying pathology but the history and physical examination are inconclusive, then appropriate investigations are necessary, e.g.:

1 abdominal X-ray (erect, supine): bowel obstruction;

2 ultrasound examination is very useful in the investigation of malrotation;

3 barium swallow: hiatus hernia, gastro-oesophageal reflux;

4 urine microscopy: urinary tract infection;

5 septic screen: infection;

6 stool cultures and microscopy: infection.

MANAGEMENT OF THE VOMITING BABY

1 Identify and treat the cause wherever possible.

2 Maintain fluid balance: parenteral therapy may be indicated.

ORGANIC CAUSES OF VOMITING

It is appropriate to discuss some organic causes of vomiting.

Gastritis

This may be due to meconium or blood swallowed before or during birth. Characteristically it is associated with mucous vomiting.

Treatment. The routine aspiration of the stomach after birth, followed by lavage with normal saline where blood or mucus is present, may prevent the occurrence of vomiting. Where established mucus vomiting exists, gastric lavage with normal saline is usually all that is necessary.

Gastro-oesophageal reflux/hiatus hernia

Gastro-oesophageal reflux is a common cause of vomiting in the newborn infant. It is caused by an incompetent lower gastro-oesophageal sphincter and is particularly prevalent in preterm infants, as well as neurologically abnormal infants with severe hypo- or hypertonia. It frequently occurs following repair of diaphragmatic hernia and oesophageal atresia. The vomiting usually occurs at the end of a feed, and particularly when 'winding' the baby.

The character of the vomiting varies from small spills occurring just after feeds to large, sometimes projectile, occasionally bloodspecked vomits. The natural history is for gradual improvement with growth of the infant, and cessation usually by the end of the first year of life in normal children.

Complications

These include:
1 persistent vomiting leading to failure to thrive;
2 oesophagitis, hiatus hernia, oesophageal stricture;
3 obstructive apnoea, SIDS and 'near miss' SIDS;
4 recurrent aspiration of milk, with the development of a brassy cough, wheeze and stridor;
5 Sandifer's syndrome. This occurs in older, mentally retarded children who show head-cocking trait associated with iron-deficient anaemia and reflux oesophagitis.

Investigations

Infants with mild symptoms do not require investigation. Many tests have been used to evaluate reflux. One commonly used is a barium swallow with inversion of the infant during the procedure to show the degree of reflux present. Other investigations include a technetium milk scan, which is more sensitive to the detection of reflux than a barium study, and a pH probe inserted into the middle third of the oesophagus. Oesophagoscopy may be useful in a few infants.

Treatment

1 Studies have demonstrated the prone position with a 30–40° head-up tilt to be the position of choice. Mild cases usually improve when the infant is nursed in a more upright position. Special chairs have been used, but are often inappropriate.
2 Thickening the feeds with an agent such as Nestargel, Carobel or Thixo-D is usually effective, in combination with upright feeding. Sometimes the feed needs to be so thick that it must be spooned into the baby.
3 Antireflux milks utilize carob, rice or starch thickeners.
4 Drugs. Infant Gaviscon (1–2 g with each feed) has been used, but this treatment may cause constipation. The use of prokinetic drugs which increase the rate of gastric emptying (cisapride) may be particularly effective but should be used carefully because of potential cardiac arrhythmias. If gastritis occurs, antacid therapy or cimetidine may be effective.
5 Surgery. Rarely fundoplication will be necessary when medical treatment fails or when respiratory complications occur.

Pyloric stenosis

This condition usually presents after the first month of life: rarely it may occur in the first week. It is characterized by projectile vomiting, more commonly in boys, and is associated with visible peristalsis and a palpable 'tumour'. There is often a family history.

Treatment is surgical and consists of a muscle-splitting operation of the pylorus (Ramstedt's operation).

Infant colic

Some apparently healthy infants, who are feeding well and gaining weight, cry at certain times during the day, but especially in the evening around 6 pm. The condition tends to disappear spontaneously at about 3 months. There is often no obvious cause, although many explanations have been given including: overfeeding, underfeeding, milk allergy, spoiling and boredom.

Treatment includes attention to feeding techniques, posture feeding and warmth to the abdomen, e.g. baths. The removal of dairy products from the maternal diet when breastfeeding occasionally helps. Dicyclomine hydrochloride (Merbentyl) 2–5 mL given 15 min before feeds may be useful. The daily maximum dose should not exceed 20 mL. Recently the manufacturers of Merbentyl have recommended avoiding this agent in infants under 6 months of age because of several case reports of apnoea.

Constipation

This term means hard, dry stool without regard to the frequency. Often when mothers talk of constipation they mean an absence of stools for 2–3 days, which may be normal. Breastfed babies are unlikely to be constipated and yet may not have a stool for several days.

AETIOLOGICAL FACTORS

1 Inadequate or improper feeding, e.g. too concentrated milk formula.
2 Anatomical abnormalities, e.g. anal stenosis, Hirschsprung's disease, fissure *in ano*.

TREATMENT

The management will depend on the underlying cause. Local anaesthetic cream (e.g. xylo-caine) is used for fissure *in ano*. Alteration of the feeds may be indicated, e.g. giving prune juice, orange juice or extra water. The addition of a stool-wetting agent such as dioctyl sodium increases the fluid in the stools. Milk of magnesia may be used as a mild laxative. Glycerine suppositories and/or small enemas may occasionally be indicated.

Diarrhoea

This term is used to mean loose frequent stools. Stools initially change colour from a dark green–black (meconium), through a greenish-yellow transitional stage, and attain the typical yellow colour by 4–5 days. Stools may be very frequent initially, especially in breastfed babies, and should not be confused with diarrhoea. Infants under phototherapy commonly have greenish loose stools and these must be distinguished from diarrhoeal stools.

When an infant is having loose frequent stools, the following causes of diarrhoea should be considered:
1 maternal diet in a breastfed infant, e.g. excessive chocolate, Coca Cola, etc.;
2 incorrect formula preparation, overfeeding;
3 infective (viral, bacterial, protozoan);
4 sugar intolerance: transient or permanent;
5 steatorrhoea, e.g. cystic fibrosis.

Management will involve treatment of the specific cause whenever possible, and attention to fluid balance as necessary. Antidiarrhoeal drugs are not used in the newborn period.

Failure to thrive

This is a term used to describe infants whose weight gain is inadequate. Weight gain in the first year of life is not linear, but frequently occurs in spurts. Generally babies at least double their birthweight by 5 months, and treble it by 1 year. The infant who fails to thrive shows a characteristic fall-off in weight gain and linear growth. These measurements cross centile lines in a downward direction, and this is more significant than an infant whose measurements are on or below the third centile but who grows along a line parallel to the centile line. A fall in the incremental growth curve when gluten is introduced into the diet is very suspicious of coeliac disease. Normal head growth may continue despite poor weight gain, as brain growth is the last to fail.

TOTAL PARENTERAL NUTRITION

TPN is not the preferred method for feeding infants and should be used only when appropriate enteral feeding is not possible.

Indications

1 Gastrointestinal obstruction.
2 Following gastrointestinal surgery.
3 NEC.
4 Severe malabsorption.
5 Severe recurrent apnoea.
6 The tiny infant.

Methods

Some of the solutions used in TPN are highly irritant and may cause severe tissue damage if subcutaneous extravasation occurs. For this reason, administration of TPN through a long-line (see p. 319) is advisable.

The TPN regimen aims to provide carbohydrate, fat, protein, electrolytes, minerals and vitamins.

CARBOHYDRATE

This is usually in the form of 5%, 7.5% or 10% dextrose, and it is to this that the electrolyte and mineral mixture is added. Dextrose is mixed with the amino acid solution in the ratio of 3 : 1. This combined solution is both acidic and hypertonic.

PROTEIN

This is provided as a mixture of either crystalline L-amino acids or, less commonly, a solution of fibrin or casein hydrolysate. The provision of amino acids in these solutions does not closely match the amino acid requirements of ill infants, and regular serum and urinary amino acid profiles should be measured. The maximum rate of infusion for protein is 3.0 g/kg/day, and is mixed with the dextrose electrolyte solution prior to infusion.

FAT

Intralipid 10% or 20% fat emulsion is most commonly used. This is made from soya bean oil, egg yolk lecithin and glycerol, and contains a high proportion of essential long-chain fatty acids. Intralipid is protein bound in the plasma and may displace bilirubin from albumin. For this reason, it should not be used if the unconjugated serum bilirubin is more than 100 µmol/L. Some infants, particularly those who are very ill with respiratory disease, appear to fail to clear the fat emulsion from the circulation and it accumulates in the lungs. The serum should be regularly examined for opalescence and Intralipid stopped if the serum is cloudy. Intralipid is commenced at 1 g/kg/day and, if tolerated, increased to a maximum of 3 g/kg/day. It is recommended that the hourly infusion rate does not exceed 4 g/kg for any one hour. Intralipid should be infused simultaneously with carbohydrate through a 'Y' connector distal to a bacterial filter.

MINERALS

Sodium and potassium requirements are estimated daily and added to the dextrose as required. A mineral mix (e.g. Pedel) provides the necessary trace minerals.

VITAMINS

Water-soluble vitamins (e.g. Solvito 0.5 mL/kg/day) and fat-soluble vitamins (e.g. Vitlipid 1 mL/kg/day) are added to the solutions. Vitlipid is mixed with Intralipid, but is photosensitive and the syringe into which it is added should be protected from light.

Investigations

The following investigations should be performed at regular intervals throughout the duration of TPN:
1 *4–6-hourly*: glucose estimations by stick tests;
2 *daily*: weight, electrolytes, urea, serum and urinary osmolality, acid–base, and observations of serum for lipaemia;
3 *weekly*: length, head circumference, calcium, phosphate, liver transaminases, total protein, albumin, total bilirubin, alkaline phosphatase, amino acid profile and haemoglobin.

Complications

1 Infection. There is a constant risk of septicaemia when giving TPN. *Staphylococcal epidermidis* is the commonest cause of systemic infection, especially in infants fed through a long-line. Regular cultures should be taken.
2 Hyperglycaemia. Premature babies do not tolerate glucose well. Four-hourly stick tests for glucose should be carried out. Insulin (0. 1 U/kg) may be necessary.
3 Metabolic disturbances. Careful biochemical surveillance is essential in all infants receiving TPN (see above).
4 Cholestatic jaundice.
5 Hyperammonaemia.
6 Lipaemia and fat accumulation in the lungs.
7 Metabolic acidosis.
8 Venous thrombosis (long-line).
9 Tissue injury due to extravasation (peripheral line).

SPECIALIZED FEEDING REGIMENS

There are a number of gastrointestinal or metabolic problems that may require a special milk diet. These include:
1 cows' milk protein intolerance;
2 lactose intolerance;
3 fat malabsorption (cystic fibrosis, biliary atresia);
4 phenylketonuria;
5 galactosaemia;
6 inborn errors of amino acid metabolism.

A variety of specialized milk formulae are available for treating these conditions. These include:

Soya bean milks. These contain soya bean protein instead of cows' milk protein. Most commercially available soya protein-based milks exclude lactose as well as cows' milk protein and are suitable for use in babies with galactosaemia or lactose intolerance. Examples include Cow and Gate Formula S, Mead Johnson Prosobee and Wyeth Wysoy.

Lactose-free milks. These are used in lactose intolerance and some may be suitable for the treatment of galactosaemia. Examples of this type of milk include Galactomin 17, Pregestimil and Nutramigen.

Low protein. There are a variety of milks suitable for infants with inborn errors of amino acid metabolism, such as phenylketonuria and maple syrup urine disease. These rare conditions require the close support of an experienced dietitian.

Additional energy. There are several methods of providing energy in excess of 120 kcal/kg without exceeding 180–200 mL milk/kg. These may be used when it is difficult to obtain energy for growth with standard formulae.
1 MCT oil 9 kcal/g (39 kJ/g).
2 Caloreen 4 kcal/g (17 kJ/g). This is a polymer of glucose which exerts only 20% of the osmotic pressure of an isoenergetic solution of glucose and can be added to the infant's milk. Dose 2–6 g/kg/day.
3 Duocal (628 kJ/100 mL). This is an emulsion of carbohydrate (non-lactose) and fat.
4 Human milk fortifier (see p. 53).

REFERENCES

Dear, P.R.F. (1984) Nutritional problems in the newborn. *Hospital Update* **November**, 915–917.

DHSS (1980) *Present Day Practice in Infant Feeding*. HMSO, London.

Ehrenkranz, R.A. Iron, folic acid and vitamin B$_{12}$.

In: *Nutritional Needs of the Preterm Infant*. Eds: Tsang, R.C., Lucas, A., Uauy, R., Zlotkin, S. pp. 177–194. Waverly Europe Ltd, Williams & Wilkins, Baltimore 1993.

Hambraeus, L., Fransson, G.B. & Lönnerdal, B. (1984) Human milk composition. *Nutrition and Abstracts and Reviews* **54**, 4.

Koo, W. & Tsang, R.C. (1993) Calcium, magnesium, phosphorus, and vitamin D. In: *Nutritional Needs of the Preterm Infant* (senior eds, M.I. Levene, R.J. Lilford; associated eds, M.J. Bennett, J. Punt). Williams & Wilkins, London, Baltimore.

Lucas, A., Morley, R., Cole, T.J. & Gore, S.M. (1994) A randomised multicentre study of human milk versus formula and later development in preterm infants. *Archives of Disease in Childhood* **70**, F141–F146.

Lucas, A., Morley, R., Cole, T.J., Lister, G. & Leeson-Payne, C. (1992) Breast milk and subsequent intelligence quotient in children born preterm. *Lancet* **339**, 261–264.

Read, M.D., Golightly, P.W. & Grant, E. (1984) A Guide to Drugs in Breast Milk. Boehringer, Ingelheim.

FURTHER READING

Phillips, V. (ed.) (1976) *Successful Breast Feeding*. Nursing Mothers' Association of Australia, Hawthorn, Victoria.

Sauer P.J.J., Saenz de Pipaon Marcos, M. & Baartmans, M.G.A. (1997) Nutrition of the very-low-birth weight infant. In: *Advances in Perinatal Medicine* (ed. F. Cockburn). Parthenon Publishing, New York.

Tsang R.C., Lucas A., Uauy, R. & Zlotkin, S. (eds) (1993) *Nutritional Needs of the Preterm Infant. Scientific Basis and Practical Guidelines*. Williams & Wilkins, Baltimore.

Wood, C.B. & Walker-Smith, J. (eds) (1981) *MacKeith's Infant Feeding and Feeding Difficulties*. Churchill Livingstone, Edinburgh.

7 Infection

Infection is an ever-present problem in the newborn. Not only is it common, but it presents in many different ways and must therefore be considered in the differential diagnosis or as a possible complication of almost every condition affecting the newborn. The incidence of infection is approximately 5 per 1000 live births, and is more common in premature infants.

HISTORICAL ASPECTS

Sepsis has always been one of the prime causes of neonatal mortality, and the history of neonatology runs hand in hand with the history of neonatal sepsis. The major nursery pathogens have been:

1 1930s and 1940s—group A β-haemolytic streptococcus;
2 1940s and 1950s—coliform organisms;
3 late 1950s and early 1960s—*Staphylococcus aureus* emerged as the major nursery pathogen, but towards the end of this era was largely eradicated by the routine use of hexachlorophene (Phisohex);
4 1960s—coliform organisms. These will always present a problem because there is no passive maternal immunization;
5 1970s—group B β-haemolytic streptococcus became the major pathogenic organism in the neonatal nursery;
6 1980s—coagulase-negative staphylococci were recognized to be serious nosocomial pathogens, especially in extremely preterm, sick infants. Other 'new' pathogens included *Acinetobacter*, *Citrobacter*, *Serratia* and *Enterobacter* species.

THE IMMATURE IMMUNE SYSTEM

The immune system develops from early in fetal life, but is not functionally fully integrated until about 1 year of age. Immunity can be considered to be specific and non-specific.

Specific immunity

Specific immunity is mediated through lymphocytes, of which there are two types: B and T cells.

B CELLS

When stimulated, B lymphocytes transform to plasma cells and produce immunoglobulin (Ig). IgM is the first type to be produced at 15 weeks' gestation, and IgG is first produced at 20 weeks. Initially fetal levels of the three major Ig types are at minimal levels and remain very low at birth. Adult levels of IgM are found by 1 year and of IgG at 5 years. IgG is the only Ig that crosses the placenta, and consequently at birth the baby has high levels of maternally derived IgG. This gives the neonate effective passive immunity, but the levels fall in the months after birth.

T CELLS

T cells are produced in the fetal bone marrow and migrate to the thymus; hence the term thymus (or T)-related lymphocytes. When stimulated by an infective agent they transform to perform one of three functions:

1 helping the immune response of other cells;
2 suppressing the immune response of other cells;
3 killing target cells.

On stimulation, these cells also produce chemical messengers called lymphokines, such as interleukin and interferon, which have a role in amplifying the immune response. Neonatal lymphocytes do not function as efficiently as mature lymphocytes owing to a reduced production of lymphokines.

Non-specific immunity

White blood cells (other than lymphocytes) are the predominant non-specific immune cells. In particular, the granulocyte has a phagocytic function of engulfing bacteria. These white cells are also called phagocytes and are attracted to sites of inflammation by chemotactic chemicals such as complement and leukotriene.

Opsonins are chemical agents necessary for the phagocyte to engulf bacteria and the main opsonins are complement and fibronectin. Opsonic activity is impaired in the neonate.

SUSCEPTIBILITY OF THE NEONATE TO INFECTION

The neonatal immune system is much less efficient in a number of fundamental ways, predisposing the infant to infection. Exogenous factors may also predispose the infant to infection.

Endogenous factors

1 Low levels of Igs, particularly IgM and IgA.
2 Premature infants fail to receive normal passive IgG transfer during the last trimester of pregnancy.
3 Phagocytic action is less effective in the newborn.
4 Opsonic activity is impaired and, in particular, complement levels are low.
5 As well as the premature infant being more prone to infection, intrauterine growth-restricted infants also appear to be more susceptible.

Exogenous factors

1 The baby is born bacteriologically sterile, with little competition from existing bacterial flora when exposed to potential pathogens. Babies exposed to very early antibiotic use,

either as newborns or as fetuses, may be predisposed to colonization with potentially pathogenic organisms.
2 Drugs may further impair immune function, with corticosteroids being the main offenders.
3 Fat emulsions. Agents such as Intralipid appear to impair the phagocytic function of the white cells.
4 Hyperbilirubinaemia reduces immune function in several different ways.

Origins

Infections may be acquired *in utero* (congenital), intrapartum or postnatally.

CONGENITAL (INTRAUTERINE)

Transplacental

First trimester: TORCH infections. This is an acronym derived from the first letter of the following conditions:
Toxoplasmosis
Other, e.g. Coxsackie B virus, varicella, human immunodeficiency virus (HIV),
Rubella
Cytomegalovirus (CMV)
Herpes simplex type 2

Second trimester: Treponema pallidum (syphilis).

Third trimester and labour:
1 Viral—varicella zoster, hepatitis B, Coxsackie B, echovirus, HIV.
2 Bacterial—group B β-haemolytic streptococcus, *Listeria monocytogenes, Haemophilus influenzae,* pneumococcus.
3 Protozoan—malaria.

Ascending infections

These occur after rupture of the membranes and represent the most common form of ante- and intrapartum infection. The most frequent pathogens are: bowel organisms (e.g. *Escherichia coli, Klebsiella, Pseudomonas,*

Proteus, Enterococcus fecalis), group B β-haemolytic streptococcus, group A streptococcus and rarely *Staphylococcus aureus*.

INTRAPARTUM

These organisms colonize the infant during passage through the birth canal, but only cause infection in a relatively small proportion. Prolonged rupture of the membranes predisposes to intrapartum infection. Pathogens include: herpes simplex 2, *Neisseria gonorrhoeae*, hepatitis B, group B β-haemolytic streptococcus, *Chlamydia trachomatis*, *Candida albicans* and perhaps HIV.

ACQUIRED

In the nursery (nosocomial):
1 bacteria—coagulase-negative staphylococci, *Staphylococcus aureus*, group B β-haemolytic streptococcus, coliforms, *Salmonella* sp., *Shigella* sp., anaerobic bacteria, *Pseudomonas* sp.;
2 viruses—coxsackie, rotavirus, respiratory syncytial virus, adenovirus, echovirus;
3 fungal—*Candida albicans*.

CONGENITAL (TORCH) INFECTIONS

Devastating effects on the fetus may result from intrauterine infections. Fortunately, such occurrences are rare, but constant vigilance is necessary to keep the incidence low. There are many similarities in the clinical picture between some congenital infections and it is convenient to think about, and investigate, the TORCH group as a whole.

Clinical features

Infection at the embryonic stage (first 12 weeks) may lead to multiple abnormalities (Fig. 7.1). With infection occurring later, the baby may be born with a viraemia and may have neonatal illness associated with jaundice, enlarged liver and spleen, anaemia and thrombocytopenia. The predominant features of the three most common prenatal infections are shown in Table 7.1. The investigation of infants with suspected congenital infections should include:
1 review of maternal history for immunization and exposure to infectious agents;

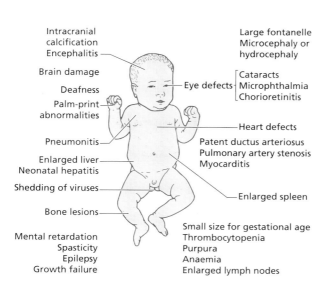

Intracranial calcification
Encephalitis

Brain damage

Deafness

Palm-print abnormalities

Pneumonitis

Enlarged liver
Neonatal hepatitis

Shedding of viruses

Bone lesions

Mental retardation
Spasticity
Epilepsy
Growth failure

Large fontanelle
Microcephaly or hydrocephaly

Eye defects { Cataracts
Microphthalmia
Chorioretinitis

Heart defects
Patent ductus arteriosus
Pulmonary artery stenosis
Myocarditis

Enlarged spleen

Small size for gestational age
Thrombocytopenia
Purpura
Anaemia
Enlarged lymph nodes

Fig. 7.1 Schematic representation of the clinical features of prenatal TORCH infections.

Table 7.1 Relative clinical features of prenatal rubella, cytomegalovirus and toxoplasmosis

	Rubella	Cytomegalovirus	Toxoplasmosis
Eye involvement	++	++	+++
Microphthalmia	+	+	+
Chorioretinitis	+	++	++
Cataracts	++	–	–
Intrauterine growth retardation	+++	+	+
Brain	++	++	+++
Hydrocephaly	–	–	++
Microcephaly	+	++	+
Calcification	++	++	++
Deafness	+++	+++	++
Hepatosplenomegaly	++	++	++
Cardiac	++	–	+ –
Purpura	++	++	–
Pneumonitis	+	++	+
Bony involvement	++	+	–

2 serological tests, including quantitative IgM and specific antibody serology for TORCH infections and polymerase chain reaction (PCR) to amplify DNA particles;
3 urine for CMV inclusions and viral culture;
4 throat and nose swabs, cerebrospinal fluid (CSF) and faeces for viral culture;
5 X-ray and ultrasound to detect intracranial calcification in toxoplasmosis, CMV and rubella, and X-rays of long bones to show periostitis in syphilis and viral osteopathy in rubella and CMV;
6 ophthalmological examination to detect chorioretinitis in toxoplasmosis and cataracts, retinitis and microphthalmia in rubella.

Rubella

Congenital rubella syndrome currently affects less than 50 children each year in the UK as a result of high immunization rates. If maternal infection occurs before 8 weeks of pregnancy, 85% of infants will have symptoms, falling to 52% if infection occurs at 9–12 weeks and 16% at 13–20 weeks. Congenital infection does not occur after 20 weeks of gestation. The risk of a fetus being damaged as a result of inadvertent rubella vaccination given to a pregnant woman is very small.

Cytomegalovirus

This is the commonest congenital infection in the UK and occurs in 3–4 per 1000 live births, but only 15–20% of congenitally infected infants develop symptoms. Serious symptomatic infection may occur with exposure after 28 weeks' gestation. Diagnosis is made by identifying the virus in urinary squames or from a throat swab in the first week of life. Viral embryopathy predominantly occurs with primary maternal CMV infection, with maternal reinfection or reactivation occasionally resulting in neonatal CMV viruria.

Toxoplasmosis

This protozoal organism is a rare cause of congenital infection in the UK and Australia. It is considerably more common in France. Fetal infection after maternal seroconversion may be diagnosed by PCR or serological testing on fetal blood obtained by cordocentesis. Maternal treatment with either spiramycin or pyrimethamine and sulphadiazine is an option. Symptoms may not appear for several years. Symptomatic infants may present with the triad of chorioretinitis, porencephaly and periventricular calcification, and antimicrobial treatment is recommended (Couvreur & Desmonts 1983). This comprises pyrimethamine 1 mg/kg/day plus sulphadiazine (70–120 mg/kg/day) orally until 1 year of age. Folinic acid 5–10 mg intramuscularly (i.m.) every 2–4 days prevents the side-effects of pyrimethamine. Spiramycin (100 mg/kg/day orally) is recommended in addition. Steroids have been used in the presence of active inflammatory disease.

Syphilis

Congenital infection is seen if maternal infection occurs after the fourth month of gestation. Penicillin is effective treatment for mother and fetus. Classically the infant at birth is found to have persistent snuffles, skin eruptions and widespread metaphyseal bony lesions.

Interstitial keratitis is the commonest feature of congenital infection, and hepatomegaly is present in almost all cases. Treatment of maternal syphilis in pregnancy usually eradicates infection in the infant. The mother will have positive VDRL (venereal disease research laboratory) and TPHA (*Treponema pallidum* haemagglutination assay) tests and the infant will also be positive owing to passive transfer of IgG to the fetus. More specific investigations are necessary.

The fluorescent *Treponema* antibody absorption (FTA-ABS) test should be performed for both IgG and IgM. The IgG response will remain positive for several weeks but should be negative by 6 months. The IgM response should be negative at birth. If positive, the infant should be treated for congenital syphilis with parenteral penicillin for 10 days. Prior to treatment the CSF should be examined. It is recommended that all neonates born with a positive VDRL test should be treated at birth.

Hepatitis B

Mothers who develop acute hepatitis B infection in the third trimester of pregnancy have a 70% risk of the infant developing the disease, but the neonatal disease is rarely severe or fatal. It is more common that mothers who are chronically hepatitis B 'surface antigen' positive pass the infection vertically to their baby via the placenta. In chronically infected mothers the risk of neonatal hepatitis is low, but it is believed to be a very important factor in the development of hepatocellular carcinoma later in the life of the child.

All women should be screened for hepatitis B at booking, with serological tests for surface antigen (HBsAg), but are at greatest risk of infecting their babies if they are also HBe antigen (HBeAg) positive. If a woman has antibody to HBe (antiHBe), then the risk of serious disease to her infants is very small. Therefore, women who are HBsAg positive and negative for HBeAg and have antiHBe are at low risk of their infants developing severe disease, but the infants may become chronic carriers of HBsAg and at risk of developing carcinoma of the liver.

Prevention of transmission is possible by immunizing infants born to women with acute hepatitis B in the last trimester of pregnancy, or where the mother is HBsAg positive, hepatitis B Ig (500 mg or 100 iu) must be given as soon after birth as possible. In addition, active immunization with hepatitis B vaccine should be given at birth, and at 1 and 6 months of age.

Hepatitis C

Perinatal transmission of hepatitis C virus (HCV) occurs in pregnant women with anti-HCV-positive tests. Pregnant women who are anti-HCV positive should have HCV RNA testing with PCR or recombinant immunoblot assay (RIBA). Infants born to pregnant women who are HCV RNA positive have a 6–8% risk of acquiring the infection, which is usually chronic. There is no evidence that breastfeeding increases the risk of perinatal transmission.

Either all pregnant women should be tested for HCV antibodies or at least those in high-risk groups, such as substance dependency, sex industry workers, hepatitis B or HIV positive.

Human immunodeficiency virus and AIDS

HIV is an important new perinatal pathogen. A recent screening programme in London has shown that 0.2–0.5% of all women attending an inner-city teaching hospital antenatal clinic are HIV positive. Although infection in the early 1980s was confined to homosexual men or intravenous drug abusers, it is now becoming increasingly common in the heterosexual population. In adults, the incubation period between infection and the development of acquired immunodeficiency syndrome (AIDS) or AIDS-related complex (ARC) is unknown, but is probably of the order of 5 years. The virus damages the immune system, causing frequent severe infections which eventually lead to death on average 2 years after AIDS is first diagnosed. Perinatally acquired infection may occur as the result of:

1 transplacental infection from the mother (this is the most common);
2 milk ingestion. HIV has been cultured from cell-free milk;
3 blood and blood products.

At present AIDS in the first year of life occurs rarely, but this is likely to increase. It is essential that women with high-risk behaviour for HIV infection should be recognized in the antenatal clinic and offered testing for HIV. Those refusing should be delivered as if they and their baby were at special risk of the condition, and extra precautions taken. A negative HIV test in pregnancy does not mean that the woman is not in the phase of having been infected, but as it takes up to 6 months for antibodies to be produced testing may give a misleading result.

The care of the at-risk woman and her baby must aim to enhance infection control measures in routine obstetric and neonatal practice. Special precautions relevant to the paediatrician include:

1 mouth-operated suction must *not* be used under any circumstances. This should apply to all deliveries, whether high risk or not. Wall suction or a mechanical pump must be available;
2 it is recommended that the baby should be bathed and dried before being handled without gloves;
3 the paediatrician called to attend the delivery should wear eye protection (spectacles or goggles), a full length gown, full protective footwear and surgical gloves;
4 all equipment used to resuscitate the newborn should be labelled as a biohazard and disposed of as appropriate. The resuscitaire should be disinfected with sodium hypochlorite. Great care must be taken when taking blood from the baby or from the umbilical cord.

The risk of breastfeeding the babies of HIV-positive women is not clear. HIV has been shown to be excreted in breast milk and it is possible that babies born to HIV-positive women who are not infected at birth may acquire infection through breast milk.

All babies will be HIV positive if born to mothers with an HIV-positive reaction, because of the passive transfer of IgG to the baby. It is now known that less than 30% of children born to HIV-positive women will themselves develop AIDS. AIDS in infancy rarely presents before 3 months. The early symptoms are repeated severe infection or interstitial pneumonitis due to unusual organisms (e.g. *Pneumocystis*). The infant usually has generalized lymphadenopathy and hepatosplenomegaly. In Britain it is recommended that women who are HIV positive and who intend to stay in the UK are discouraged from breastfeeding. HIV-positive women living in underdeveloped countries should be encouraged to breastfeed to minimize the risk of additional enteric infection (see Chapter 6). Zidovudine therapy in selected HIV-infected pregnant women and their newborn reduced the risk of perinatal transmission by approximately two-thirds.

Recommendations: Zidovudine at 14 and 34 weeks' gestation (100 mg five times daily orally), during labour 2 mg/kg intravenously (i.v.) and to newborn 2 mg/kg po four times a day for 6 weeks from 8 to 12 h after birth.

Parvovirus B19

This virus most commonly causes a mild illness known as erythema infectiosum, or fifth disease. It is characterized by mild systemic symptoms, including fever and a distinctive facial rash with a 'slapped cheek' appearance. Parvovirus B19 infection in pregnancy, which is often asymptomatic in the mother, can cause severe anaemia with resultant hydrops and fetal death, but the risk of death is less than 10% after proven maternal infection.

Varicella

Maternal chickenpox developing a week before or 5 days after birth predisposes the infant to a very high risk of potentially fatal varicella. Zoster immunoglobulin (ZIG) 2 mL should be given immediately to infants at high risk of congenital chickenpox. The infant is then carefully watched and, at the first sign of a vesicle, the antiviral agent acyclovir is given intravenously for 10 days. This treatment should prevent serious infections. Varicella in the first and second trimesters rarely causes congenital defects. If the pregnant woman is not immune to varicella zoster and the infection occurs before 20 weeks' gestation, then she should receive ZIG as soon as possible after contact.

General management

1 *Prevention*. Every effort should be made to prevent pregnant women from becoming infected. Infected infants should be isolated from pregnant nurses. Non-immunized women should be immunized against rubella before pregnancy.
2 *Specific*. There is no specific treatment for rubella, CMV and Coxsackie B infections.
3 *General supportive measures*. These include maintenance of normal temperature and intravenous fluids.

4 *Barrier nursing*. This is essential to prevent the spread of infection.
5 *Treatment of complications* such as convulsions, respiratory distress, congestive heart failure and hyperbilirubinaemia may be required.

INTRAPARTUM INFECTION

At birth it may be difficult to decide whether a baby is infected or not. The following factors should be considered:
1 maternal features of sepsis, e.g. fever, high white cell count, tender uterus, offensive or purulent liquor;
2 duration of rupture of membranes. If the membranes have been ruptured for more than 18 h, chorioamnionitis is expected;
3 duration of labour. A prolonged labour beyond 12 h carries an increased risk of systemic infection;
4 frequent vaginal examinations and instrumental delivery further increase the risk of infection;
5 the presence of fetal distress or birth asphyxia increases the likelihood of infection.

Critically ill infants with infection may exhibit respiratory distress, shock and renal failure. They may develop disseminated intravascular coagulation with internal and external bleeding.

Often congenital bacterial infections have a less dramatic clinical presentation, with lethargy, vomiting, diarrhoea, jaundice, apnoea or mild respiratory difficulty. The organisms detailed below may cause intrapartum infection.

Group B β-haemolytic streptococcus (GBS)

This is the commonest cause of serious intrapartum infection, and is fatal in 20% of cases. Vaginal colonization with GBS is found in 15–30% of pregnant women, and about 10% of infants born to colonized women will themselves be colonized. Only 0.5 in 1000 liveborn infants develop serious infection. Two forms of neonatal GBS sepsis are recognized: *early-*

onset disease presents with septicaemia, respiratory distress and septic shock, which if not suspected and treated early is rapidly fatal. The second form is *late onset*, characterized by meningitis which usually develops some time after 5–7 days. Serotype III GBS is often associated with late disease. The diagnosis may be made rapidly with a latex agglutination test or blood, urine or CSF. GBS is sensitive to high-dose penicillin and gentamicin. The possibility of early-onset GBS infection should be considered in any infant presenting with respiratory distress in the first 12 h of life.

PREVENTION

The widespread acceptance of intrapartum antibiotic prophylaxis based on bacteriological screening for genital carriage or risk factor analysis has resulted in a decline in incidence of early-onset disease from 1–2 to 0.5/1000 live births.

Escherichia coli

The K1 strain of *E. coli* is particularly associated with perinatal infection and may cause septicaemia or meningitis. The sensitivity of *E. coli* to antibiotics is variable.

Listeria monocytogenes

This is not an uncommon perinatal pathogen and may invade the fetus through intact membranes. Characteristically infected infants pass meconium *in utero*, and if this is seen in premature infants *Listeria* should be strongly suspected. The organism has a predilection for the lungs and brain. Hydrocephalus is a common sequel to *Listeria* meningitis. The organism is usually sensitive to ampicillin.

Herpes simplex

Neonatal herpes simplex infection is a rare but devastating condition. The herpes simplex virus can be classified as either type 1 or 2. Type 1 infection is generally limited to the lips and mouth (cold sores) and is very common.

Infection with type 2 virus is usually due to sexual contact and involves the genitalia. Up to a third of sexually active women have antibodies to herpes simplex type 2 virus. Infection of the newborn with type 2 virus occurs as the result of contact with an active lesion on passage through the genital tract. The virus enters through skin, eye or mouth and may disseminate to the brain or other organs.

The risk of an infant being infected from a parent, nurse or midwife with cold sores is very small. Careful hand-washing is all that is necessary to avoid this risk. Rarely, paronychia may be due to herpes virus, and staff with this type of active infection must not handle infants.

The presentation in the newborn may be mucocutaneous, disseminated or central nervous system (CNS). Signs usually occur after the first week, with skin vesicles, and the infection may rapidly disseminate with involvement of the CNS, in which case the mortality rate may be as high as 80%. If there are active genital lesions, prevention is possible by caesarean section. Treatment of suspected disease is with aciclovir or cytosine arabinoside.

Chlamydia trachomatis

Chlamydia is found in the vagina of 4% of pregnant women. Up to 70% of infants born through an infected cervix will acquire chlamydia, but most show no symptoms. Chlamydia conjunctivitis and, less commonly, pneumonia occur in a relatively small proportion of infants. The conjunctivitis is purulent and is clinically indistinguishable from that of gonococcal ophthalmia. Specific culture media are necessary for this organism. Infants should be treated with tetracycline eye ointment and oral erythromycin.

Others

Pneumococcus, *Haemophilus influenzae* and anaerobic organisms may cause significant perinatal infection. Anaerobes are contracted from the birth canal and require special culture media for their identification. The first two organisms are probably haematogenously spread from maternal septicaemia. They may cause profound shock in the infant, indistinguishable clinically from group B β-haemolytic streptococci.

Antibiotic policy

Many of these organisms cause severe and rapidly developing symptoms. Successful treatment depends on a high index of clinical suspicion, because in the most severe cases positive cultures may not be available until after the infant has died. Broad-spectrum antibiotic cover is required. Ampicillin will usually cover GBS, *Listeria*, pneumococcus and *Haemophilus*. Gentamicin is usually effective against coliforms. If anaerobes are suspected then metronidazole is the appropriate antibiotic. Ampicillin (100–200 mg/kg/day i.v.) and gentamicin (5 mg/kg/day i.v.) are recommended for cases of suspected intrapartum infection, and should be started as early as possible.

ACQUIRED (NOSOCOMIAL) INFECTION

It may be very difficult to differentiate infections acquired during delivery from those acquired postnatally. Generally bacterial infections developing after 48 h of life are more likely to be due to acquired neonatal infection. Almost every bacterium and virus known to infect humans may cause clinical infection in the newborn. *Staphylococcus* species are probably the most important group of infections infants acquire in the neonatal unit.

When a nosocomial infection is suspected, the following risk factors should be reviewed:
1 direct contamination by the hands of medical staff or parents due to faulty hand-washing techniques;
2 frequently performed procedures, such as intubation, insertion of catheters, humidification of oxygen, parenteral nutrition and exchange transfusions, all predispose sick babies to infection; and
3 cross-infection: the routes of neonatal cross-infection are illustrated in Fig. 7.2.

Clinical features

Symptoms of acquired infection are generally non-specific and include pyrexia, hypothermia, lethargy, hypotonia, irritability, poor feeding, weak cry, respiratory distress, apnoea, cyanosis, jaundice, hepatomegaly, abdominal distension, vomiting, diarrhoea, failure to thrive, rashes, purpura and a bulging fontanelle.

Investigations

If infection is suspected, the following investigations may be useful in finding the causative organism.

SUPERFICIAL SWABS

Throat, nose, umbilicus, rectum and auditory canal. A gastric aspirate specimen with pus cells and organisms on Gram staining may prove invaluable. The superficial swabs merely reflect contamination, but gastric aspirate and ear swabs probably reflect intrapartum

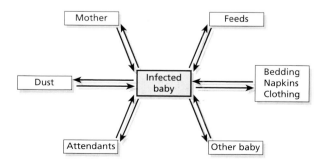

Fig. 7.2 Routes of neonatal cross-infection.

exposure to organisms. The gastric aspirate is useful because it provides early information about the infecting organisms and may therefore influence the initial choice of antibiotics.

DEEP CULTURES

Blood, urine, CSF and tracheal aspirate are sent to the microbiology laboratory for culture and antibiotic sensitivity testing.

FULL BLOOD COUNT AND FILM

Leukocytosis, leukopenia and thrombocytopenia may occur. Changes suggestive of infection may be seen in the cell morphology of the blood film, and include toxic granulations, vacuolations of neutrophils and Döhle bodies. There is frequently a left shift towards the more primitive cells in the neutrophil series. A computer-generated haematological score based on a 7-point scoring system markedly improves predictive accuracy in the diagnosis of sepsis (Rodwell *et al*. 1988).

Ancillary investigations

Because infection is often insidious in its presentation, attempts have been made to use screening tests to predict whether infection is likely to be the cause of illness or not. The best evaluated of these are:
1 C-reactive protein. This is an acute-phase protein released at times of stress, including infection. The test is weakly positive if the level is 10–20 mg/L and strongly positive if > 20 mg/L. It has been shown to be 62% sensitive for infection (Kite *et al*. 1988);
2 nitroblue tetrazolium (NBT) test. This examines neutrophils for uptake of the nitroblue dye, which indicates bacterial activation. If more than 13 of 100 neutrophils take up the dye the test is considered to be positive. This test has a 77% sensitivity;
3 plasma elastase α1-proteinase inhibition. Testing provides a sensitive but non-specific index of infection in the first 24 h after birth. Sequential testing serves as a guide to the

cessation of antibiotic treatment (Rodwell *et al*. 1992).

Common acute acquired infections

SEPTICAEMIA

Apart from perinatally acquired GBS and *E. coli*, the most common organisms to cause septicaemia in the newborn unit are coagulase-negative staphylococci. This is often dismissed as a contaminant, but if it is both cultured from blood culture bottles and the infant is unwell, it must be treated as a pathogen. It is particularly likely to occur when total parenteral nutrition is administered, especially if a silastic catheter 'long-line' is *in situ*. The 'long-line' should be removed when antibiotics are started if the infant is ill. Preservation of the long-line with successful antibiotic therapy is possible in some less ill patients.

Other organisms include *Staphylococcus aureus*, *Pseudomonas* sp., *Proteus* sp., *Klebsiella*, *Serratia* and *Candida albicans*. Disseminated intravascular coagulation (DIC) syndrome may occur and meningitis may also be associated with septicaemia.

MENINGITIS

Neonatal meningitis is more common, and mortality and morbidity rates higher, in the first month of life than at any other age. The organisms most usually encountered are *E. coli* and group B β-haemolytic streptococci. In addition to the other organisms seen with septicaemia, epidemics of *Listeria monocytogenes* occur.

Many of the early clinical manifestations are non-specific. Coma, convulsions, opisthotonus, increasing head size and a bulging fontanelle are late signs of meningitis.

Investigations for suspected septicaemia and meningitis

1 The CSF is often turbid and cloudy, with an elevated white cell count, low sugar and high protein. Positive cultures on CSF are obtained

in about 50% of cases of suspected bacterial meningitis.

2 Blood cultures are positive in about 50% of neonates with bacterial meningitis.

3 A full blood count may reveal variable pictures of neutropenia, neutrophilia and toxic changes.

4 Counterimmune electrophoresis: this technique can provide a rapid diagnosis of some bacterial pathogens.

5 If candida septicaemia is suspected the urine should be examined for budding hyphae. This is the most sensitive investigation for systemic candidiasis. If the infant has thrush in the groin this may contaminate the urine sample, and in such cases a suprapubic aspiration should be performed. *Candida* antigen may help in confirming the diagnosis.

Treatment of septicaemia

General supportive measures. Intravenous fluids, incubator care, heart rate/respiratory/blood pressure monitoring of vital signs.

Specific therapy. The clinical dilemma is whether to treat blindly without knowing which organism is causing the infection. A best-guess policy is required, but review of all cultures taken over the previous few weeks is helpful to establish whether the infant has been colonized by potentially pathogenic organisms. Knowledge of the sensitivities of 'local' pathogens is also important in order to choose the best antibiotics.

It is usual to commence with two or three antibiotics until bacteriological culture and sensitivity results are obtained. Flucloxacillin or vancomycin and gentamicin are a good combination, but for severe infection a combination of ampicillin, chloramphenicol and gentamicin may be valuable. More recently cephalosporins have been used in this context, but it is probably better to reserve these antibiotics for second-line choice once the sensitivities of the organisms are known. Once the organism and sensitivity have been identified, the appropriate antibiotic should be administered for 2–3 weeks.

Treatment of meningitis

When meningitis is suspected, antibiotics which penetrate into the CSF should be used. We recommend penicillin (100 mg/kg/24 h), gentamicin (2.5 mg/kg every 12–24 h depending on maturity of the infant) and cefotaxime (100 mg/kg/24 h). Once antibiotic sensitivities are available, antibiotics can be rationalized. Chloramphenicol (50 mg/kg/24 h) is still widely used, but resistance to it is relatively common.

Meningitis due to group B streptococcus should be treated with both gentamicin and penicillin for at least 2 weeks. Listeria is best treated with ampicillin and gentamicin.

Meningitis due to Gram-negative organisms has a 20% mortality and about 40% of the survivors are severely neurologically disabled. Cefotaxime is the antibiotic of choice for *E. coli* meningitis and ceftazidime for *Pseudomonas* infection. The choice of appropriate antibiotic depends on the organism's sensitivity and should be discussed with the microbiologist.

The use of intrathecal antibiotics for Gram-negative meningitis remains controversial. If in doubt, ventricular fluid may be sampled and intrathecal treatment instituted for persistent ventriculitis following initial systemic antibiotic treatment.

Progressive assessment of the infant is necessary, including head circumference measurement, regular ultrasound scan for the early detection of ventriculomegaly, subdural effusions and brain abscess. High mortality and morbidity rates, particularly associated with neurological sequelae and deafness, occur with bacterial meningitis in the newborn. Early diagnosis and effective treatment may prevent these complications.

SYSTEMIC CANDIDIASIS

Diagnosis of this condition depends on a high clinical suspicion for the organism. It may rarely be congenital, associated with maternal vaginitis, or acquired in a baby receiving neonatal intensive care. The best method of diagnosis is to identify budding hyphae in urine from a suprapubic stab. The organism may also be isolated from arterial and/or venous blood cultures. This may be treated with the imidazole antifungal agents such as miconazole (30 mg/kg/day) and/or ketoconazole (3 mg/kg/day). Alternatively, amphotericin B (0.5 mg/kg/day) and 5-flucytosine (100–150 mg/kg/day) is an effective combination and should be given for 2 weeks. A recent, expensive addition to the therapeutic options is liposomal amphotericin (0.5 mg/kg/day), which has markedly reduced toxicity with a shorter infusion time.

LOWER RESPIRATORY TRACT INFECTIONS

In the newborn, pneumonia is relatively common and is usually bacterial. Particular organisms involved are Gram-negative bacilli (for example *E. coli, Klebsiella, Pseudomonas*), group B streptococcus and *Staphylococcus* species. Rarer bacterial pathogens include *Listeria monocytogenes* and anaerobic bacilli. Non-bacterial pathogens include *Chlamydia trachomatis, Mycoplasma pneumoniae, Ureaplasma urealyticum, Candida albicans*, CMV and *Pneumocystis carinii*. Pneumonia may be contracted *in utero* and be present at birth (congenital), or acquired after birth (nosocomial). Congenital pneumonia may be due to ascending infection associated with prolonged rupture of the membranes, or less frequently to a transplacental infection. Viral pneumonitis is rare but may occur with CMV, Coxsackie virus, respiratory syncytial virus and rubella infection. The clinical picture may mimic that of the respiratory distress syndrome (RDS). Staphylococcal infections may be associated with pneumatocoeles, empyema, abscesses and pneumothoraces. Treatment consists of antibiotics and respiratory support (see p. 101).

URINARY TRACT INFECTION

The incidence of urinary tract infection is approximately 3 per 1000 live births. Symptoms and signs are non-specific, and therefore this condition must be constantly borne in mind. The main problem is that it is difficult to obtain uncontaminated urine. Ideally this should be with a clean-catch midstream specimen after cleansing the external genitalia with sterile water. Suprapubic aspiration of the bladder may be used to obtain uncontaminated urine, but care is necessary with this method to avoid complications. Often urethral catheterization is necessary to obtain a satisfactory collection (see p. 323).

Treatment should be with an appropriate antibacterial agent for 10–14 days. With all proven urinary tract infections in the newborn it is mandatory to follow the child for the first year of life, carrying out monthly cultures of urine. In addition, creatinine estimations at regular intervals, ultrasound examination of the kidneys and micturating cystourethrography to detect underlying anatomical abnormalities of the urinary tract should be performed. For details see Chapter 22.

CONJUNCTIVITIS ('STICKY EYES')

Mild eye infections are very common and are referred to as 'sticky eyes'. Purulent conjunctivitis may be either a congenital or an acquired infection. Conjunctivitis is sometimes secondary to a blocked nasolacrimal duct. Usually the organisms involved are *Staphylococcus aureus, E. coli, Pseudomonas* sp., *Chlamydia trachomatis* and *Neisseria gonorrhoeae*. Reddened swelling in the region of the lacrimal sac (dacrocystitis) may occur following infection of a blocked nasolacrimal duct. The term ophthalmia neonatorum is reserved for infection with *N. gonorrhoeae*.

Management

Conjunctival swabs should be taken and sent promptly to the laboratory. If ophthalmia neonatorum or *C. trachomatis* are suspected, swabs need to be taken by laboratory staff and applied to culture plates in the ward. Conjunctival scrapings need to be taken for Giemsa staining and cell culture. If maternal gonorrhoea is suspected, prophylactic treatment of the newborn's eyes with 1% silver nitrate eyedrops may prevent purulent conjunctivitis.

With mild conjunctivitis or 'sticky eyes', frequent eye toilet with normal saline may be all that is required. More florid infections will need the frequent instillation of antibiotic drops (e.g. chloramphenicol or sulphacetamide) after cultures have been taken and eye toilet carried out. After the conjunctivitis has settled somewhat, antibiotic ointment may be used.

Treatment of gonococcal ophthalmia involves local irrigation with crystalline penicillin in normal saline solution and systemic penicillin for 10 days. In severe ophthalmia the drops must initially be instilled every 10 min for an hour, then hourly for 4–6 h depending on the response. For the treatment of chlamydia, see p. 69.

OMPHALITIS AND FUNISITIS

Infections of the umbilical cord (funisitis) and umbilical stump (omphalitis) are usually due to *E. coli*, other Gram-negative bacteria or *Staphylococcus aureus*. Because of the potential seriousness of the spread of infection to the portal vein and subsequent portal hypertension, infection in this area must be treated promptly. If there are signs of spread with surrounding cellulitis, parenteral antibiotics such as flu-cloxacillin and gentamicin are necessary after appropriate swabs and cultures have been taken. Topical treatment with an antibiotic is also necessary. Routine cord care has evolved over recent years from cleansing with methylated spirits, to the use of normal saline and, currently, tapwater.

INFECTION OF THE SKIN AND SUBCUTANEOUS TISSUES

Paronychia

Reddening of the skin in the nailfold is common and may proceed to pus formation when staphylococcal infection is present. Topical treatment consists of applications of 1% aqueous gentian violet and is usually all that is necessary to eradicate *Candida albicans* and other minor bacterial infections.

Parenteral and topical antibiotics are indicated if systemic spread is suspected with bacterial infection.

Pustules

These may be single or in crops and must be distinguished from toxic erythema (see p. 276). Treatment consists of 1% chlorhexidine washes and sometimes systemic antibiotics. *Staphylococcus aureus* is the most frequently found pathogen.

Thrush

Infection with this yeast is common, particularly if there has been *Candida albicans* colonization of the maternal genital tract. It is also likely to occur in association with the use of broad-spectrum antibiotics and in debilitated neonates receiving total parenteral nutrition. It commonly occurs in the mouth and looks like milk curds that cannot be removed with a swab stick. The infection usually occurs towards the end of the first week of life. In the napkin area it appears as a spreading centrifugal rash. It sometimes occurs as a secondary infection following ammoniacal dermatitis. Napkin psoriasis is a rare condition which starts in the napkin area and may become widespread, usually secondary to thrush. The treatment of oral candidiasis consists of the use of nystatin or acyclovir mouth drops or gel instilled every 6 h for 1 week. For the napkin area, nystatin cream applied four times daily is usually sufficient. One per cent aqueous gentian violet may be used in both of these sites, but tends to cause staining of clothes. Treatment of systemic candidiasis is discussed on p. 73.

GASTROENTERITIS

Gastroenteritis usually occurs in epidemic form in neonatal nurseries. Outbreaks have in the past been associated with enteropathogenic *E. coli*, occasionally *Salmonella* sp., and *Shigella* sp., but currently the most frequent nursery pathogen is human rotavirus.

Because the neonate withstands salt and water loss poorly, dehydration may rapidly occur. The infant shows signs such as loss of skin turgor, sunken eyes and fontanelle, dry mouth and oliguria.

Treatment consists of isolation from non-infected infants and replacement of electrolytes and water. Antibiotics are of no value unless there is evidence of systemic bacterial infection.

Prevention of acquired infections

The procedures detailed below will help to reduce and control infections.

LABOUR WARD

1 Fastidious care in hand-washing.
2 The use of gloves for vaginal examinations, insertion of scalp electrodes and instrumental deliveries.

NURSERY

1 Careful hand-washing with the use of an antiseptic such as iodine or chlorhexidine before and after handling infants.
2 Cleansing of incubators and equipment.
3 Routine baths for babies using hygienic soap solutions.
4 Aseptic surgical techniques for procedures such as intubation, umbilical catheterization, intravenous cannulation and lumbar punctures.
5 Isolation techniques for infectious babies.
6 Avoidance of overcrowding and restriction of nursery 'traffic' to a minimum.

Immunoglobulin therapy

The prophylactic intravenous administration of pooled IgG for very low birthweight infants who are relatively immunoincompetent has not proved to be efficacious in a large random-ized control trial (Farnaroff *et al.* 1994) and the practice cannot be recommended.

REFERENCES

Couvreur, J. & Desmonts, C. (1983) Treatment of toxoplasmosis acquired during pregnancy with spiramycin. *Zentralblatt für Gynäkologie* **105**, 1104–1107.

Farnaroff, A.A., Korones, S.B., Wright, L.L. *et al.* (1994) A controlled trial of intravenous immune globulin to reduce nosocomial infections in very low birth weight infants. *New England Journal of Medicine* **330**, 1107–1113.

Kite, P., Millar, M.R., Gorham, P. & Congdon, P. (1988) Comparison of five tests used in diagnosis of neonatal bacteraemia. *Archives of Disease in Childhood* **63**, 639–643.

Rodwell, R.L., Leslie, A.L. & Tudehope, D.I. (1988) Early diagnosis of neonatal sepsis using a haematological scoring system. *Journal of Pediatrics* **112**, 761–767.

Rodwell, R.L., Taylor, K.M., Tudehope, D.I. & Gray, P.H. (1992) Capillary plasma elastase L1-proteinase inhibitor in infected and non infected neonates. *Archives of Disease in Childhood* **67**, 436–439.

FURTHER READING

Avery, G.B., Fletcher, M.A. & MacDonald, M.G. (eds) (1994) *Neonatology: Pathophysiology and Management of the Newborn*, 4th edn. Lippincott-Raven, Philadelphia.

Gilbert, G.L. (1991) *Infectious Disease in Pregnancy and the Newborn Infant*. Harwood Academic Publishers, Chur.

Isaacs, D. & Moxon, R.E. (1999) *Handbook of Neonatal Infections. A Practical Guide*. W.B. Saunders, London.

1997 Red Book. Report of the Committee on Infectious Diseases, 24th edn. American Academy of Pediatrics.

Remington, J.S. & Klein, J.O. (eds) (1995) *Infectious Diseases of the Fetus and Newborn Infant*. W.B. Saunders, Philadelphia.

8 The low birthweight infant

Newborn infants may be classified according to birthweight, gestational age or size (large or small) for gestational age (Table 8.1). A low birthweight infant may be either preterm or small for gestational age, or both (Table 8.1). The problems these infants develop depend on whether they have been born too early or are born too small for the duration of gestation. The paediatrician therefore needs an objective test for the assessment of gestational age and the Dubowitz examination (Dubowitz *et al.* 1970), or its abbreviated version the new Ballard examination (Ballard *et al.* 1991), is recommended. The Ballard examination quantifies six neurological and six physical parameters and should be performed with the baby fully exposed under a radiant heat warmer (Fig. 8.1).

The expanded New Ballard Score includes extremely premature infants and has been refined to improve accuracy in more mature infants.

THE PRETERM INFANT (PREMATURITY)

Clinical management of preterm labour

Premature birth has become the foremost problem of obstetric practice today. Although the high mortality and morbidity associated with preterm delivery have prompted a great deal of research into ways of predicting preterm birth with the hope of prevention, only limited benefits have resulted. Where possible, the woman in preterm labour should be transferred to a perinatal intensive care unit where optimal delivery, resuscitation and subsequent management of her infant can be carried out. *In utero* transfer should only be attempted when the preterm labour is not advanced or can be safely and effectively suppressed with tocolytic agents, at least for a few days. Obstetric management of preterm labour is rarely clearcut, and is a balanced decision

Table 8.1 Classification of newborn infants according to birthweight, gestational age or size for gestational age

		Incidence
(1) Birthweight		
< 2500 g	= low birthweight (LBW)	6.5%
< 1500 g	= very low birthweight (VLBW)	1.3%
< 1000 g	= extremely low birthweight (ELBW)	0.6%
(2) Gestational age (completed weeks after last normal menstrual period)		
< 37 weeks	= preterm	7%
> 41 weeks	= post-term	1%
(3) Size for gestational age		
weight between + 2 SD and − 2 SD from mean	= appropriate for gestational age (AGA)	95%
weight < − 2 SD from mean	= small for gestational age (SGA)	2.5%
weight > + 2 SD from mean	= large for gestational age (LGA)	2.5%

SD, standard deviation.

Maturity rating	
Score	Weeks
-10	20
-5	22
0	24
5	26
10	28
15	30
20	32
25	34
30	36
35	38
40	40
45	42
50	44

Skin	Sticky friable transparent	Gelatinous red, translucent	Smooth pink, visible veins	Superficial peeling &/or rash, few veins	Cracking pale areas, rare veins	Parching deep cracking no vessels	Leathery cracked wrinkled
Lanugo	None	Sparse	Abundant	Thinning	Bald areas	Mostly bald	
Plantar surface	Heel–toe 40–50mm:–1 <40mm: –2	>50 mm no crease	Faint red marks	Anterior transverse crease only	Creases ant. 2/3	Creases over entire sole	
Breast	Imperceptible	Barely perceptible	Flat areola no bud	Stippled areola 1–2 mm bud	Raised areola 3–4 mm bud	Full areola 5–10 mm bud	
Eye/ear	Lids fused loosely: –1 tightly: –2	Lids open pinna flat stays folded	Slightly curved pinna; soft; slow recoil	Well-curved pinna; soft but ready recoil	Formed & firm instant recoil	Thick cartilage ear stiff	
Genitals male	Scrotum flat, smooth	Scrotum empty Faint rugae	Testes in upper canal Rare rugae	Testes descending Few rugae	Testes down Good rugae	Testes pendulous Deep rugae	
Genitals female	Clitoris prominent Labia flat	Prominent clitoris Small labia minora	Prominent clitoris Enlarging minora	Majora & minora equally prominent	Majora large Minora small	Majora cover clitoris & minora	

Fig. 8.1 The expanded New Ballard Score. (From Ballard *et al.* 1991, reproduced with permission.) (*Cont'd on p. 78*)

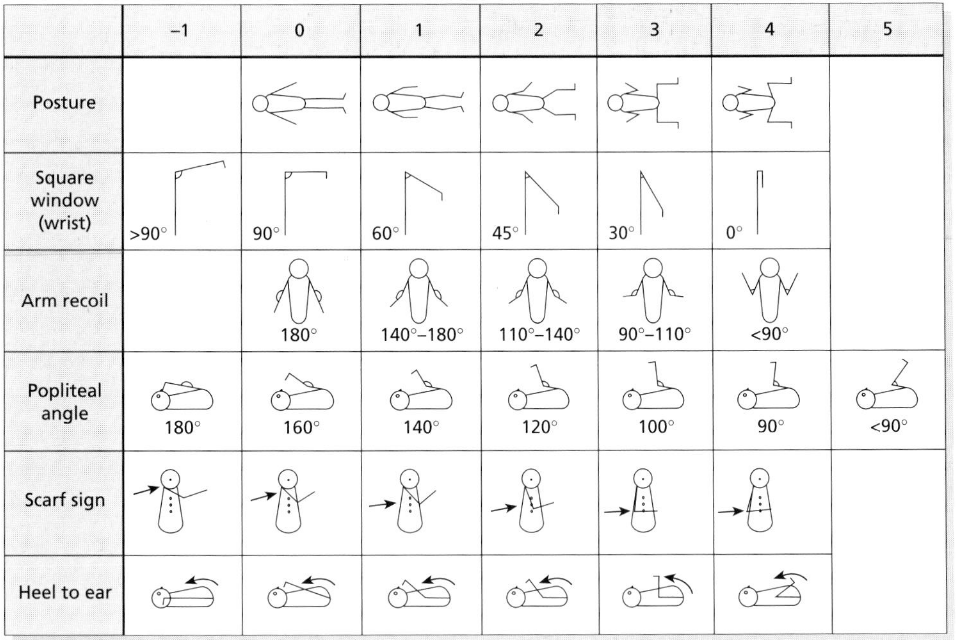

Maturity rating	
Score	Weeks
–10	20
–5	22
0	24
5	26
10	28
15	30
20	32
25	34
30	36
35	38
40	40
45	42
50	44

	–1	0	1	2	3	4	5
Posture							
Square window (wrist)	>90°	90°	60°	45°	30°	0°	
Arm recoil		180°	140°–180°	110°–140°	90°–110°	<90°	
Popliteal angle	180°	160°	140°	120°	100°	90°	<90°
Scarf sign							
Heel to ear							

Fig. 8.1 (cont'd)

between the relative risks to mother and fetus of continuing the pregnancy versus those of a preterm birth.

When a patient is admitted with a diagnosis of possible 'premature labour', the management plan depends on the following criteria.

1 Is the patient in active premature labour?

2 Is there an underlying cause for the onset of labour?

3 Should steroids be given to the mother to enhance fetal lung maturity?

4 Should drugs be used to reduce uterine activity?

5 Are the mother and fetus at risk of infection?

6 Where is the baby to be delivered?

7 How is the baby to be delivered?

In general, there are few clearcut answers to these questions.

Suppression of preterm labour is sometimes possible and desirable with tocolytic agents such as β_2 receptor agonists, magnesium sulphate, prostaglandin synthetase inhibitors and calcium channel blockers. Temporary suppression may enable *in utero* transport to a tertiary perinatal centre or the acceleration of fetal lung maturity with glucocorticoids. Suppression of labour is contraindicated in the presence of intrauterine infection, congenital abnormality, signs of fetal compromise and significant antepartum haemorrhage.

PRETERM BREECH PRESENTATION

The preferred mode of delivery for the preterm breech fetus has been the subject of considerable controversy. The hazards to the fetus of vaginal breech delivery include difficulty with delivery of the head and, rarely, entrapment of the aftercoming head. Although caesarean section in the preterm breech may be associated with some difficulties, it is probably the preferred method of delivery beyond 26 weeks' gestation.

Outcome for the preterm infant

The process of decision making in the management of preterm delivery has become increasingly difficult as short- and long-term outcomes have improved with rapid advances in perinatal care. Aggressive obstetric management and intervention for fetal reasons in late second-trimester deliveries are practised in many tertiary perinatal centres, and these attitudes are partly responsible for the improved outcomes obtained. Practitioners in perinatal units should develop their own guidelines for the management of extremely preterm labour.

Published survival rates vary markedly from centre to centre, but also depend on the inclusion or exclusion of the following infants:

1 those with lethal congenital abnormalities;

2 birthweight < 500 g;

3 born alive but not resuscitated or not resuscitable;

4 considered previable and not admitted to intensive care;

5 those dying after the neonatal period (day 28).

Representative figures are shown in Table 8.2.

The neurological and physical outcome of these infants depends on many factors. Units that admit a large number of high-risk babies, especially if born outside the hospital, have

Table 8.2 Representative survival figures in the mid-1990s by birthweight and gestational age

Birthweight (g)	Survival (%)	Gestational age (weeks)	Survival (%)
500–749	35	24–25	60
750–999	85	26–27	80
1000–1499	96	28–29	90
1500–1999	97	30–31	97
2000–2499	98	32–33	98

considerably higher morbidity figures than others (Levene & Dubowitz 1982). In the average referral intensive care unit approximately 10–15% of very low birthweight (VLBW) infants will have significant intellectual/neurological or physical handicap. Surviving infants with birthweight below 1000 g have rates of disability of 30% (10–15% severe) and cerebral palsy of 12%. Nevertheless, the vast majority of survivors can be expected to enjoy a good quality of life. (See Chapter 27 for details of physical and neurological morbidities.)

Transportation

The transportation of premature infants to regional intensive care units presents special problems and it is recommended that high-risk preterm infants be transferred *in utero* where possible. Women in preterm labour < 32 weeks' gestation should be delivered in a tertiary perinatal centre. When this is not feasible, consideration should be given to transportation of infants of less than 1500 g birthweight. This decision will be influenced by the expertise and facilities of the referring hospital, as well as the safety and availability of transportation.

If an infant is to be transferred to an intensive care unit, then the unit with the best transport facilities should undertake the transfer. This usually means a team from the referral unit going out with a specially equipped transport incubator to retrieve the baby. It is essential that the infant be carefully assessed and completely stabilized before transportation. Procedures such as the insertion of an intravenous line, intubation and the initiation of mechanical ventilation are performed prior to transport if indicated. Trying to intubate in an ambulance is an uncomfortable experience! Neonatal transport is fully discussed in Chapter 26.

Specific problems of the preterm infant

During the last 3 months of intrauterine life most organ systems are undergoing continued structural and functional development. Premature birth requires rapid adaptation to extrauterine life before these organ systems are adequately developed. The main problems are:

1 birth asphyxia;
2 thermal instability;
3 lack of primitive survival reflexes—suck, swallow and gag—which may predispose the infant to milk aspiration;
4 jaundice;
5 pulmonary diseases—apnoea, hyaline membrane disease, transient tachypnoea of the newborn, pneumothorax, pneumonia, Wilson–Mikity syndrome and bronchopulmonary dysplasia;
6 metabolic disturbances—hypoglycaemia, hypocalcaemia, hypomagnesaemia, hyponatraemia, hypernatraemia, hyperkalaemia;
7 patent ductus arteriosus—congestive heart failure;
8 neurological problems—intracranial haemorrhage, especially intraventricular haemorrhage/periventricular leukomalacia/ventricular dilatation;
9 susceptibility to infection;
10 gastrointestinal intolerance and necrotizing enterocolitis (NEC);
11 ophthalmic problems—retinopathy of prematurity, myopia, strabismus;
12 surgical lesions, undescended testes, inguinal and umbilical herniae;
13 haematological problems—haemorrhagic disease of prematurity, disseminated intravascular coagulation, iron deficiency anaemia;
14 renal immaturity—inability to concentrate urine, and inability to excrete an acid load with a low renal bicarbonate threshold, resulting in late metabolic acidosis. Late metabolic acidosis may be associated with failure to gain weight satisfactorily. Treatment with sodium bicarbonate and a more appropriate formula or expressed breast milk should result in a satisfactory response.

The specific problems of prematurity are discussed in the appropriate chapters.

Supportive care of the preterm infant

RESUSCITATION

Perinatal consultation should occur between all clinical staff to optimize care of mother and preterm infant. Perinatal asphyxia is a major risk of preterm delivery, and personnel competent in neonatal resuscitation should always be present. Immediate intubation or airway stabilization with continuous positive airway pressure has been advocated in infants below 30 weeks' gestation.

MONITORING

Heart rate, respiratory rate and temperature must be monitored continuously, with appropriate alarm signals, if cardiopulmonary disease is present.

OXYGEN THERAPY

Many sick preterm infants require oxygen therapy to relieve hypoxia. Oxygen is a toxic substance in the preterm infant, and may cause retinopathy of prematurity. It must therefore be administered with the utmost care. It is essential that regular estimates of Pao_2 are made in all premature infants requiring extra oxygen in order to prevent blindness. It is dangerous to treat ill premature infants where adequate blood-gas oxygen monitoring is not available. The arterial oxygen tension should probably be maintained between 50 and 80 mmHg (6.2–10 kPa). Whether it is administered directly into the incubator, via a head-box, nasal prongs, continuous positive airway pressure tube or endotracheal tube, its use must be monitored very carefully. Oxygen should be warmed to 35–37°C, humidified to 28–38 mg H_2O/L, and the inspired concentration continuously recorded with high and low alarms set.

CONTINUOUS OXYGEN MONITORING

1 Transcutaneous oxygen monitors (± trans-

cutaneous carbon dioxide monitor). These devices utilize a small heating element to heat the skin to 43–44°C and induce hyperaemia to arterialize the capillary blood and oxygen (± CO_2) diffusing through the skin, which is monitored continuously.
2 Pulse oximetry utilizes analysis of light transmitted through tissues to measure haemoglobin oxygen saturation in arterial blood.
3 An oxygen-sensitive probe attached to the tip of an umbilical arterial catheter provides a continuous readout of arterial oxygen tension.

INTERMITTENT OXYGEN MONITORING

Blood gases may be measured or arterial blood obtained from sampling an arterial catheter or peripheral arterial stab, or from heel-stick capillary blood.

BLOOD PRESSURE

Arterial blood pressure is an important variable to measure. If an indwelling arterial catheter is *in situ*, it can be attached to an electronic pressure transducer to measure blood pressure. Alternatively, a mechanical oscillometric device can be used, attached to a blood pressure cuff (e.g. Dinamap, Sentron). Normal blood pressure ranges are shown on p. 186. Blood pressure normally increases over the first 24 h of life, after which time mean blood pressure should be kept above 30 mmHg with the aid of plasma, blood or pressor agents such as dopamine. There is increasing clinical and experimental evidence that the maintenance of an adequate and stable cerebral blood flow is important to avoid cerebral ischaemic and haemorrhagic damage.

THERMOREGULATION

Body temperature must be maintained in the normal range (36.5–37.0°C per axilla) by nursing the preterm infant under an open radiant heat source or in a closed incubator (see Chapter 9).

FEEDING

Caucasian infants of less than 34 weeks' postmenstrual age do not have a good suck or swallow reflex and should be fed via an orogastric or nasogastric tube. Premature infants with small gastric capacity require frequent feeding (sometimes every 1–2 h) and should be started on 1–2 mL/kg per feed, increasing at each feed in increments of 1–2 mL/kg, as tolerated. Gastric aspirate must be checked before the next feed. Occasionally, this regimen is not tolerated and a continuous infusion of milk via an orogastric or nasojejunal tube will be necessary. This feeding technique is particularly applicable to infants of birthweight < 1000 g or < 29 weeks' gestational age (see Chapter 6).

PARENTERAL FLUIDS

Sick babies and infants of less than 1750 g may need parenteral feeding with 10% dextrose infusion into the umbilical or a peripheral vein. Sometimes intravenous alimentation with dextrose, crystalline L-amino acid solution and fat emulsion will be necessary (see Chapter 6).

The fluid requirements of ill preterm infants depend on a variety of factors, including postnatal age, renal function and transepidermal water loss. Consequently, the fluid intake is estimated on the basis of urine output, weight, serum electrolytes and urinary concentration. Water requirements will be increased for phototherapy (approximately an extra 20 mL/kg/day) and open radiant incubators (approximately an extra 20 mL/kg/day). Sick preterm infants, especially those with respiratory distress syndrome (RDS) and patent ductus arteriosus, should receive restricted fluid volumes.

In addition, the electrolyte requirement for premature infants is increased owing to the poor conservation by the immature kidneys. Close monitoring of serum electrolytes, including calcium, is necessary in order to replace losses adequately. Infants with severe late metabolic acidosis should have their maintenance sodium as sodium bicarbonate.

JAUNDICE

This is extremely common in the preterm infant and must be followed with frequent bilirubin estimations. Jaundice of prematurity is a diagnosis of exclusion after other causes have been eliminated. Preterm infants are more prone to bilirubin encephalopathy than term infants, and factors that affect the entry of free bilirubin into the brain include low albumin levels, acidosis, hypoxia, hypoglycaemia, hypothermia, certain drugs and starvation. Guidelines for the management of hyperbilirubinaemia are shown on p. 140.

RESPIRATORY DISTRESS SYNDROME (see Chapter 10)

Even with the advent of the lecithin/sphingomyelin (L/S) ratio estimation on amniotic fluid and steroid treatment, RDS remains the major problem of prematurity today. Most preterm infants who die have hyaline membranes demonstrated at autopsy, but may also have evidence of intraventricular haemorrhage, patent ductus arteriosus, pneumothorax, NEC and bronchopulmonary dysplasia.

For infants of birthweight < 1000 g or < 28 weeks' gestation it may be desirable to intubate and ventilate from birth to provide initial airway stabilization. Exogenous surfactant should be administered via the endotracheal tube prior to 2 h of age. Babies of birthweight less than 2000 g with RDS are best managed in an intensive care nursery.

VITAMINS

A single intramuscular dose of 0.5–1.0 mg of vitamin K is adequate unless the baby is receiving broad-spectrum antibiotics, when twice-weekly injections are necessary to compensate for loss of the endogenous vitamin K normally produced by bowel flora. Sick preterm infants requiring intravenous alimentation should receive additional multivitamins.

Preterm infants require additional vitamins from days 7–14 of life. These may be given as a multivitamin preparation such as Pentavite

0.5 mL daily or Abidec 0.6 mL daily. In addition, some VLBW infants may require extra vitamin D to prevent neonatal rickets (see p. 46).

ANAEMIA

Some sick preterm infants will be anaemic at birth or develop anaemia in the first week of life as a result of frequent blood sampling, and will require a transfusion with packed red blood cells cross-matched against mother and baby. The venous haematocrit should be maintained at more than 36% (haemoglobin 12 g/dL) in all sick babies. However, during the physiological trough of anaemia preterm infants may tolerate a haemoglobin concentration of 7 g/dL, especially if there is an adequate reticulocyte response (> 5%). To prevent iron deficiency anaemia, so prevalent after 3 months of age, all preterm infants less than 2.5 kg or 34 weeks' gestation should receive supplemental iron in a dose of 30 mg daily from the age of 3 weeks.

Preparation for discharge

The transition from hospital to home is a crucial step in the future wellbeing of the family. Once the requirements for intensive care are over, the baby will still need monitoring, incubator care and gavage feedings. This can be a very frustrating time for the parents, who have already experienced so much. Early discharge for low birthweight infants can be safely practised and may promote attachment. The baby may be discharged at 1900–2300 g, provided feeding is progressing well, weight gain is steady, the mother is handling her baby competently and the home situation is good.

SMALL FOR GESTATIONAL AGE INFANT

Although several synonyms have been used to describe the growth-restricted infant, including Clifford syndrome, dysmaturity, light for dates, small for dates and intrauterine growth retardation, the preferred term, based on common usage, is now 'small for gestational age' (SGA). There has been no such uniformity in the definition of SGA. From a statistical viewpoint, infants born at any gestational age and weighing more than two standard deviations below the mean can be defined as SGA. However, because they share common clinical problems, infants of birthweight at or below the 10th centile for gestational age are often regarded as SGA. Furthermore, many neonates with birthweights above the 10th centile will demonstrate evidence of acute or chronic weight loss, and should therefore fall into the spectrum of the growth-restricted infant. Variables such as fetal sex, race and altitude should be considered when determining growth curves for a given population, as a birthweight below the 10th centile in one population may not fall below the 10th centile growth curve in another, even though growth retardation may be present in both instances. Table 8.3 lists important factors which determine birthweight.

Table 8.3 Determinants of birthweight

Maternal factors before conception:
  Stature
  Weight
  Genotype
  Race
  Age
  Parity
  Socioeconomic status (occupation, education, income)

Factors at or around conception:
  Fetal genotype
  Singleton or multiple conception
  Fetal sex
  Genetic anomaly (chromosomal or major gene locus)

Factors between conception and birth:
  Altitude
  Fetal or maternal infection (rubella, malaria)
  Maternal work
  Maternal cigarette smoking
  Maternal diet
  Maternal alcohol, drugs, medications

Classification of SGA infants

Subdividing the heterogeneous SGA population into more homogeneous groups offers
the potential to establish a better understanding of the underlying cause of the problem, and
therefore more accurate prognoses and more
appropriate plans for postnatal management.

It is important to attempt to define the
neonate 'starved' as a result of intrauterine
growth restriction (IUGR). These babies show
growth failure greatest for weight, then length;
head circumference is the least affected. There
is little subcutaneous fat, the skin may be loose
and thin, muscle mass is decreased, especially
buttocks and thighs, and the infant often
exhibits wide-eyed, anxious facies. This type
can be distinguished from the uniformly
growth-retarded type, which implies either a
fetal cause (e.g. chromosomal) or a very early
insult.

Subcutaneous fat can be objectively assessed
by measuring the circumference of the
mid-upper arm or by measuring skinfold
thickness with special calipers. A simpler
measurement is the Ponderal Index. This is
derived from accurate measurements of the
infant's length and weight and calculated from
the formula:

Ponderal Index (PI) = Birthweight (g) × 100
Length (cm)^3

A normal PI is ≥ 2.41 and a low PI is < 2.41.
Table 8.4 shows the major differences between
the proportionate and the disproportionate
SGA infant.

Table 8.4 Classification of the growth-restricted fetus
and the SGA infant

Proportionate (type I IUGR)	vs.	Disproportionate (type II IUGR)
Symmetrical	vs.	Asymmetrical
Normal Ponderal Index	vs.	Low Ponderal Index
Intrinsic cause	vs.	Extrinsic cause
Hypoplastic	vs.	Hypotrophic

Many growth-restricted infants exhibit a mixture of
classifications.

Causes of IUGR

The causes of IUGR can be classified according
to whether they are fetal, placental or maternal
(Table 8.5). The growth failure can be classified
as 'intrinsic', which implies an abnormality at the
time of conception or within the first trimester
(fetal and some maternal causes), or 'extrinsic',
implying a later onset of growth retardation
(placental and some maternal causes).

INTRINSIC FETAL GROWTH RESTRICTION

Early-onset growth restriction, which tends to
give rise to an SGA infant who is proportionate, symmetrical, hypoplastic and has a normal
PI, is more likely to have an intrinsic cause
of growth failure. During the first trimester,
global insults include chromosomal anomalies
(e.g. trisomy syndromes), perinatal infections
(e.g. toxoplasmosis, other, rubella, cytome-

Table 8.5 Cause of intrauterine growth restriction

Fetal	Placental	Maternal
Chromosomal abnormalities	Toxaemia of pregnancy	Maternal disease
Prenatal viral infection	Multiple pregnancy	Alcohol
Dysmorphic syndromes	Small placental size	Smoking
X-rays	Site of implantation	Malnutrition
	Vascular transfusion in monochorial twin placentas	Altitude

galovirus, herpes simplex type II: TORCH), dwarfing syndromes (e.g. achondroplasia, chondrodystrophic dwarfism, Russell–Silver syndrome), maternal recreational drug abuse (e.g. alcohol, narcotics, cocaine) and exposure to teratogenic drugs and ionizing radiation. Constitutional growth retardation relates to parental stature and racial and ethnic factors. These infants, often referred to as having type I growth retardation, show symmetrical growth retardation, with similar growth reductions in weight, length and head circumference. They do not exhibit a head-sparing effect and, because of a decreased number of cells, as well as decreased cell size, do not have the potential for normal growth. Fortunately, this group comprises only about 10–30% of all SGA babies in modern western societies, but if they are evaluated after the first trimester by ultrasound assessment of biparietal diameter, an inappropriately low assessment of gestational age may result.

EXTRINSIC FETAL GROWTH RESTRICTION

Later onset of fetal growth restriction results from disorders of the placenta or from maternal problems. Extrinsic mechanisms operate during the latter half of pregnancy and are associated with impaired delivery of oxygen and nutrients from the placenta. These factors may become operative at different times during pregnancy, resulting in less predictable effects on fetal growth. Maternal factors include hypertension (e.g. essential, pregnancy-induced, renal), diabetes mellitus with vascular complications, renal disease, cardiac disease, sickle cell disease and collagen disorders. Maternal smoking, alcohol and narcotic abuse and maternal hypoxia (e.g. cardiac disease, pulmonary disease, residence at high altitude) may also cause IUGR.

PLACENTAL FACTORS

These all have the common feature of diminished placental blood flow, which may become more severe later in pregnancy. Twins will show a normal rate of intrauterine growth until the demands of the two fetuses outstrip the placental blood supply. This usually occurs at about 32 weeks' gestation, and fetal growth rates fall off from this time. Placental disorders associated with IUGR include chronic villitis, haemorrhagic endovasculitis, chorioangioma, chronic abruptio placentae, hydatidiform degeneration, single umbilical artery and twin–twin transfusion syndrome.

Specific problems of the growth-restricted fetus and SGA infant

When considering the problems of SGA babies, it seems more appropriate to compare them with their gestational age peers rather than with babies of similar birthweight.

When IUGR results from restricted nutrient supply, the fetus adapts to maximize the prospect of good outcome by sparing brain growth, accelerating pulmonary maturity and increasing the red cell mass (polycythaemia). These features may initially represent important adaptational strategies, but they later become pathological when deprivation is more extreme and fetal distress supervenes. Table 8.6 summarizes the problems that these fetuses and babies may face.

NEONATAL PERIOD

Perinatal asphyxia. Fetuses with chronic distress do not tolerate the additional hypoxic stress of delivery well, and readily develop hypoxia and acidosis.

Congenital malformations. There is a 20-fold increased incidence of congenital malformation in SGA babies compared to their normal birthweight peers.

Infection. There is a ninefold increased incidence of infection. This is partly explained by the greater incidence of TORCH infections, but also relates to a greater incidence of acquired infection.

Table 8.6 Anticipated problems in the fetus/neonate who is SGA

Fetus	Newborn	Subsequent outcome
Stillbirth	Asphyxia	Impaired growth
Fetal distress	Hypoglycaemia	Intellectual deficit
Meconium aspiration	Meconium aspiration syndrome	Cerebral palsy (due to asphyxia)
Oligohydramnios	Polycythaemia	
Congenital malformation	Hyperviscosity	
Deformations	Hypothermia	
Cord compression	Hypocalcaemia	
Premature rupture of membranes	Infection (impaired immune system)	
Preterm delivery	Pulmonary haemorrhage	
	Transient neonatal hyperglycaemia	

Hypoglycaemia. SGA infants have deficient hepatic and cardiac muscle glycogen stores and a limited capacity for gluconeogenesis. Hypoglycaemia is usually asymptomatic, but minor or major symptoms may develop if appropriate treatment is not instituted.

Hypocalcaemia. The increased incidence of hypocalcaemia relates to the birth asphyxia and not to SGA infants *per se.*

Polycythaemia. This is a common problem, especially when there has been prolonged intrauterine hypoxia resulting in elevated levels of erythropoietin.

Thermal instability. Maintenance of body temperature is a problem to the SGA infant, but less so than for the preterm infant. This probably relates to the large surface area to body weight ratio.

Respiratory distress. Respiratory distress in the SGA infant may be due to meconium aspiration, polycythaemia, massive pulmonary haemorrhage or pneumonia, but is not usually due to RDS. Growth restriction in extremely preterm infants does not protect them against RDS or subsequent chronic neonatal lung disease.

INFANCY AND CHILDHOOD

Growth

In the neonatal period the infant loses little weight and begins to gain weight rapidly after birth. However, this growth spurt is often not maintained and a permanent deficit in somatic growth may persist into childhood.

Full-term growth-retarded infants stand a good chance of catching up, particularly if growth restriction is due to maternal factors. Infants who are both severely preterm and growth restricted are much less likely to reach average size than infants of the same degree of prematurity but who are normally grown. If catch-up growth is going to occur, it usually does so by 6 months.

Development

A number of follow-up studies have shown that SGA infants born at term are prone to more developmental, behavioural and learning problems than infants born mildly preterm, and males are more vulnerable than females. If the baby is both SGA and premature he is predisposed to a greater risk of serious neurological abnormalities than if he were only premature or only SGA. If catch-up in head growth occurs, then the eventual IQ score is higher than in those infants whose head remains small.

Management

The appreciation that a fetus is growth restricted or that a baby is SGA will greatly influence management.

If IUGR is suspected, careful monitoring of fetal and uteroplacental function will be necessary with tests such as serial ultrasound scans, Doppler assessment of umbilical flow, cardiotocography and L/S ratio on amniotic fluid prior to early delivery.

A considered decision regarding the best method and timing of delivery will need to be made. If it is elected to deliver vaginally, then continuous intrapartum fetal heart rate monitoring should be undertaken. A paediatrician or other skilled resuscitationist should attend the delivery and suction the trachea under direct vision, if necessary, to prevent meconium aspiration.

If severely growth restricted, the baby should be transferred to a special care nursery for observation for signs of respiratory distress, hypoglycaemia and temperature instability. Usually incubator care will be necessary.

If catch-up growth is to occur and the child is to reach his full growth and intellectual potential, adequate and early feeding is essential. The SGA infant should commence feeds at 2 h of age, if possible, and initially feeding should be every 2 h with dextrose. Estimates of blood glucose should be made before each feed. The first feed should be 10% dextrose followed by full-strength breast milk or formula. Feeding regimens are discussed in Chapter 6. The expected weight of the SGA infant should be calculated by estimating the 50th percentile weight for the infant's gestation and then feeding the infant to a weight halfway between that weight and the actual weight. The infant should receive at least 60 mL/kg on day 1, and increase up to 200 mL/kg of expected weight.

If the infant develops hypoglycaemia (heelprick estimate less than 2.5 mmol/L despite early feeding), 10% dextrose is given by uninterrupted intravenous infusion, in addition to the oral feed.

A capillary haematocrit should be performed at 4–6 h of age. If this is greater than 70%, a venous haematocrit is indicated. If the venous haematocrit is greater than 70%, or if the baby has symptoms of polycythaemia, an isovolaemic, dilutional exchange transfusion with plasma (30 mL/kg) is indicated.

A careful examination for congenital malformations should always be made. The most common anomaly is a single umbilical artery. The baby should be examined for features suggestive of intrauterine infection, such as hepatosplenomegaly, petechiae, cataracts and microcephaly. If an intrauterine infection is likely, or even if there is no obvious cause for growth retardation, a cord blood immunoglobulin M (IgM) level and appropriate TORCH serology should be performed. If it is likely that the infant is infected, he should be isolated and barrier nursed.

When two or more dysmorphic features are present, chromosome analysis should be undertaken.

REFERENCES

Ballard, J.L., Khoury, J.C., Wedig, K., Wang, L., Eilers-Wlashman, B.L. & Lipp, R. (1991) New Ballard Score, expanded to include extremely premature infants. *Journal of Pediatrics* **119**, 417–423.

Dubowitz, L.M.S., Dubowitz, V. & Goldberg, C. (1970) Clinical assessment of gestational age in the newborn infant. *Journal of Pediatrics* 77, 1.

Levene, M.I. & Dubowitz, L.M.S. (1982) Low birth weight babies: long-term follow-up. *British Journal of Hospital Medicine* **November**, 487–493.

FURTHER READING

Avery, G.B., Fletcher, M.A., MacDonald, M.G.

(eds) (1994) *Neonatology: Pathophysiology and Management of the Newborn,* 4th edn. Lippincott-Raven, Philadelphia.

Roberton, N.R.C. (ed.) (1992) *Textbook of Neonatology,* 2nd edn. Churchill Livingstone, Edinburgh.

Spitzer, A.R. (1994) *Intensive Care of the Fetus and Neonate.* Mosby, St Louis.

9 Thermoregulation

The full-term infant is a homeotherm but his ability to regulate body temperature is not as effective as that of older children or adults. The small for gestational age (SGA) infant, and particularly the preterm infant, have greater problems than the normally grown full-term baby in maintaining body temperature.

An infant's temperature depends on the site at which the measurement is made. Central (or core) temperature should be maintained between 36.7 and 37.3°C, and is measured by a rectal thermometer. This is inserted 3 cm into the rectum in term infants and 2 cm for premature infants, and should be left for at least 30 s. Axillary temperature also approximates to core temperature, but the thermometer needs to be left for at least 2 min. Skin temperature is lower than core temperature and the skin of the trunk is warmer than the periphery. Skin temperature is recorded by taping a thermistor to the abdomen. Normal abdominal temperature is 35.5–36.5°C in a term infant and 36.2–37.2°C in small premature infants. If the difference between abdominal and peripheral (e.g. toe) temperature is large, then the infant is vasoconstricted to conserve heat (or because he is infected or shocked). If the difference is small, he is vasodilated and attempting to lose heat. This information is of value to distinguish infection from environmental overheating in mature infants who are pyrexial.

Mechanisms of heat loss

Heat is lost from the body to the environment via the classic physical mechanisms.

Evaporation. When a moist baby is exposed to room temperature there is conversion of liquid to vapour, with subsequent loss of heat.

Radiation. Heat is dissipated down a concentration gradient via the surrounding air.

Conduction. There is direct heat loss from the skin to cooler objects, such as a cold wrap, cold towel or wet nappy.

Convection. Heat loss occurs via a current of moving air.

Mechanisms to conserve heat

When exposed to cold the normal baby tries to conserve heat by a variety of means:
1 peripheral vasoconstriction;
2 increased heat production:
  (a) increased basal metabolism with increased oxygen consumption;
  (b) increased voluntary muscular activity;
  (c) involuntary muscular activity—shivering. Shivering is virtually non-existent in the preterm infant and his ability to increase muscular activity is limited;
3 non-shivering thermogenesis. Full-term infants are born with a layer of brown fat, mainly around the neck, between the scapulae and along the aorta. Brown fat can be rapidly metabolized to generate heat, and this is under the control of the sympathetic nervous system.

Why is the newborn prone to heat loss?

1 Large surface area to body weight ratio. A preterm infant's limited ability to flex limbs and trunk increases the exposed surface area for heat loss.
2 Limited ability to shiver.
3 Deficiency of subcutaneous fat tissue.
4 Relative deficiency of brown fat and glycogen.

5 The baby is often born covered in liquor, vernix, meconium or blood. Moist skin predisposes to loss of heat and fluid by evaporation.

Prevention of excessive heat loss

The provision of warmth is the first essential in resuscitation of the newborn. The baby must be dried completely with a prewarmed, sterile wrap. An overhead radiant heat warmer may be useful. The baby should be transported to the nursery wrapped in a warm blanket, in a preheated transport incubator. He should be weighed promptly, ideally under an infrared warmer. Handling by parents is desirable, but care must be taken to ensure the infant is properly wrapped.

NURSERY

1 Very low birthweight (VLBW) infants do not have a superficial layer of keratin, and consequently water and heat are lost through the permeable skin. Adequate ambient humidity in the incubator will prevent this.
2 Reduce radiant and convective heat loss by dressing the infant whenever possible.
3 Avoid positioning the infant near a cold window in order to prevent radiant heat loss. A

warm incubator (particularly if double walled) will also reduce radiant loss, and this is further limited by a perspex heat shield over the infant.
4 Avoid placing the infant in draughts. A perspex shield over the infant with the foot end blocked off will prevent draughts in the incubator.
5 Never place an infant on a cold surface or in a cold cot.
6 Whenever possible the infant should be clothed, especially with a bonnet, bootees and jacket, to reduce thermal gradients.

Thermoneutral environment

The thermoneutral environment is the ambient temperature at which oxygen consumption and energy expenditure are at a minimum to maintain vital activities.

If an infant is cold, he will attempt to keep warm via the mechanisms listed above, including shivering, vasoconstriction and increased activity. These are energy-requiring processes. Similarly, an infant who is too hot will vasodilate and sweat (also using extra energy) to stay cool. Infants who are either heat or cold stressed maintain a normal body temperature. The ambient temperature at which the infant uses the least energy to maintain his body temperature is referred to as the thermoneutral environmental temperature (Fig. 9.1).

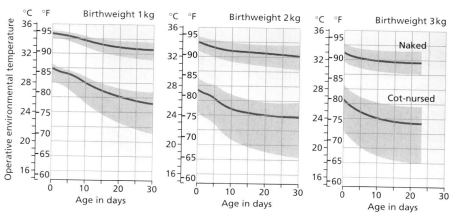

Fig. 9.1 The thermoneutral temperature range for three birthweight groups of healthy babies. The upper graph represents infants nursed naked and the lower is for clothed babies. (Hey 1971; reproduced with permission from Churchill Livingstone.)

Table 9.1 The mean temperature needed to provide thermal neutrality for a healthy baby nursed naked in draught-free surroundings of uniform temperature and moderate humidity. (Reproduced from Hey 1975, with permission)

Birthweight (kg)	Operative environmental temperature*			
	35°C	34°C	33°C	32°C
1.0	For 10 days →	After 10 days →	After 3 weeks →	After 5 weeks
1.5	—	For 10 days →	After 10 days →	After 4 weeks
2.0	—	For 2 days →	After 2 days →	After 3 weeks
> 2.5	—	—	For 2 days →	After 2 days

* To estimate operative temperature in a single-walled incubator, subtract 1°C from incubator air temperature for every 7°C by which this temperature exceeds room temperature. Clothed babies require lower incubator temperatures.

Unfortunately, it is not possible to guess the thermoneutral temperature in any one infant, as it depends on birthweight and postnatal age. Hey (1971) has devised charts to predict the appropriate incubator temperature for various groups of infants (Fig. 9.1). The thermoneutral temperature also varies depending on whether the infant is nursed dressed or undressed. These charts were devised by measuring the oxygen consumption of normal infants and may not be reliable for ill babies, but unfortunately there is no better guide to use. Table 9.1 summarizes this.

Incubator care

Ill or small infants are nursed in incubators, which are of two types.

CLOSED INCUBATOR

These are designed to reduce heat loss. The baby is enclosed in a perspex box with various ports and doors for access. A heater keeps the air warm, which is circulated by a fan. With modern incubators the infant can be nursed in either air mode or baby mode. In the former a thermistor within the incubator detects the environmental temperature and regulates the heater to maintain air at a constant preset temperature. The baby's temperature must be checked regularly. Baby mode (sensor-controlled) incubators rely on a thermistor attached to the baby, so the heater is regulated to keep the infant's temperature constant. Overheating can occur if the thermistor becomes detached from the baby.

Incubators usually have the facility to humidify the ambient air. This is valuable in infants of 1500 g and below to prevent excessive evaporative water and heat loss from the immature skin. All VLBW or cold infants (temperature < 35°C) should be nursed in humidified incubators. However, such incubators carry the risk of bacterial contamination with *Pseudomonas aeruginosa* or, less commonly, *Serratia* sp., which colonize the water reservoir and may lead to neonatal infection. The water should be changed every 24 h and cultured to detect these organisms. Normally humidification is only necessary during the first week of life in VLBW infants, as after this time a keratin layer has formed which waterproofs the skin.

OPEN INCUBATOR

The infant lies on a mattress under a heating element which delivers radiant heat energy. A thin, clear plastic blanket (bubblewrap or clingfilm) reduces insensible water loss. It works on a servo-controlled mechanism by means of a thermistor on the baby's abdominal wall, and the radiant heater is automatically switched on and off to maintain body temperature at a preset level (usually 36.5°C).

The great advantage of this device is that it gives easy access to the infant for surgical or nursing procedures. It is also useful for rapidly warming cold babies (see below). Its disadvantages are obvious in that heat loss is large and transepidermal water loss considerable, particularly in the most immature babies. Careful fluid and electrolyte balance is essential (see p. 43). In some units a perspex heat shield with one end closed is placed between the infant and the radiant heater to reduce water loss and prevent draughts. In general closed incubators are associated with fewer complications than open radiant incubators.

Neonatal cold injury

Prolonged exposure to a cold environment increases oxygen consumption and glucose utilization, and consequently the baby readily becomes hypoxic and hypoglycaemic. There is peripheral cyanosis with redness of the face, refusal to feed and lethargy, followed by oedema and sclerema (localized hardening of the subcutaneous tissue). Babies often have apnoeic spells, worsening of their respiratory distress syndrome, severe metabolic acidosis, pulmonary haemorrhage and finally intracranial haemorrhage.

Hypoglycaemia and metabolic acidosis are most likely to occur when the infant is being warmed. Restoration of metabolic processes creates a demand for glucose and this should be anticipated. Regular stick tests for glucose must be performed. As blood pressure and perfusion improve the products of anaerobic metabolism are washed out into the circulation, causing a severe metabolic acidosis.

Therapeutic hypothermia (see also p. 20)

Controlled mild-to-moderate hypothermia (33–35°C) has been proposed as treatment for potentially brain-injured babies. Although this technique shows beneficial effects in experimental animal models, there are currently no data in human infants. At the present time, deliberately maintaining a baby hypothermic is to be avoided, as the adverse effects of controlled hypothermia on organs other than the brain have not been sufficiently studied and may be detrimental.

REFERENCES

Hey, E.N. (1971) The care of babies in incubators. In: *Recent Advances in Paediatrics* (eds D. Gairdner & D. Hull), pp. 171–216. Churchill, London.
Hey, E.N. (1975) Thermal neutrality. *British Medical Bulletin* 31, 69–74.

FURTHER READING

Sinclair, J.C. (ed.) (1972) Thermal control in premature infants. *Annual Review of Medicine*, **23**, 129–148.
Sinclair, J.C. (ed.) (1978) *Temperature Regulation and Energy Metabolism in the Newborn*. Grune & Stratton, London.

10 Respiratory disorders

At birth major cardiopulmonary changes take place in order to prepare the baby for extrauterine existence. The fluid in the fetal lung is rapidly replaced by air. Associated with lung inflation and increased oxygenation there is a marked decrease in the pulmonary vascular resistance, with consequent increased pulmonary blood flow and closure of the ductus arteriosus, foramen ovale and ductus venosus. As a result the lungs take over the respiratory function previously carried out by the placenta. Many pathological processes can interfere with this normal sequence of events. Respiratory disorders in the newborn present in three different ways:

1 respiratory distress;
2 apnoea and bradycardia (see Chapter 12); and
3 upper airway obstruction (see Chapter 12).

RESPIRATORY DISTRESS

Respiratory distress is a general term used to describe respiratory symptoms and is not synonymous with respiratory distress syndrome (RDS) or hyaline membrane disease. It is assessed clinically by the following signs:

1 tachypnoea—a respiratory rate greater than 60/min;
2 expiratory grunt—the infant expires against a closed glottis, which maintains a higher residual lung volume, thus preventing alveoli from collapsing and thereby improving gaseous exchange. It occurs particularly in preterm infants with RDS;
3 chest retraction or recession—this may be intercostal, lower costal, sternal or substernal;
4 flaring of the ala nasae—this represents the infant's use of accessory respiratory muscles;
5 cyanosis in air—the cyanosis is central

and should be differentiated from peripheral cyanosis associated with poor circulation due to chilling, polycythaemia or shock.

Diagnosis

The presence of two or more of the above signs persisting for 4 h or more suggests respiratory distress. There are many causes of respiratory distress in the newborn (Table 10.1). A critical evaluation of the cause of respiratory distress should always be undertaken. Diagnosis will be made by a full clinical history, physical examination and appropriate investigation, including a chest X-ray. Perinatal history should include gestational age, the presence of polyoligohydramnios, anomalies on ultrasound, risk factors for sepsis, the passage of meconium, depression at birth and duration of membrane rupture. Physical examination includes observation, vital signs, palpation of dextrocardia and hepatomegaly, and auscultation of the lungs for air entry, symmetry and adventitial breath sounds.

Investigations for respiratory distress

1 Bacteriological cultures on blood, urine, cerebrospinal fluid (CSF) and gastric aspirate.
2 Viral cultures and rapid-yield immunodiagnostic tests.
3 Haematocrit and full blood count.
4 Lecithin/sphingomyelin (L/S) ratio or 'shake test' on gastric or tracheal aspirates (or on amniotic fluid when available; see p. 97).
5 Chest transillumination with a cold light source if pneumothorax suspected.
6 Passage of nasogastric catheters for choanal and oesophageal atresias.
7 The nitrogen washout test to differentiate from cyanotic congenital heart disease (see p. 191).

Table 10.1 Common causes of acute respiratory distress

Primary respiratory

Transient tachypnoea of the newborn (or retained fetal lung fluid)

RDS (hyaline membrane disease)

Pneumonia

Pneumothorax; pneumomediastinum; pulmonary interstitial emphysema

Aspiration syndromes, e.g. meconium, milk, blood

Pulmonary hypoplasia, e.g. Potter's syndrome, oligohydramnios

Surgical conditions, e.g. choanal atresia, Pierre Robin sequence, diaphragmatic hernia, lobar emphysema, oesophageal atresia with tracheo-oesophageal fistula

Massive pulmonary haemorrhage

Chronic neonatal lung disease, e.g. bronchopulmonary dysplasia, Wilson–Mikity syndrome, chronic pulmonary insufficiency of prematurity

Secondary to extrapulmonary pathology

Following birth asphyxia

Persistence of fetal circulation (or persistent pulmonary hypertension)

Congenital heart disease

Anaemia

Polycythaemia

Cerebral damage

Infection

Metabolic disease

Treatment of respiratory distress

Supportive care

The supportive care of the infant with respiratory distress is similar regardless of aetiology. Infants with mild respiratory distress require frequent observations of respiratory and heart rates, temperature, blood pressure and signs of respiratory distress, whereas infants with more severe respiratory distress require continuous monitoring of these parameters with appropriate alarm signals. Accurate fluid balance charts are essential. Adequate thermoregulation may be obtained in a closed incubator or in an open, radiant heat source incubator.

Oxygen

Oxygen is a useful and life-saving therapeutic agent, but is potentially dangerous, particu-larly in the preterm baby, when it may damage the eyes (retinopathy of prematurity) and the lungs (bronchopulmonary dysplasia). When administered, it should be warmed to 34–37°C and 90–100% humidified. Oxygen therapy is discussed in Chapter 8.

Fluids

Infants with respiratory distress should not be breast- or bottle fed. With mild respiratory distress gavage feeding may be adequate, but with severe respiratory distress fluids via intravenous and/or arterial routes will be required. Usually a 10% dextrose solution is used and other electrolytes added after 24 h, depending on serum levels.

Acid–base studies

With moderate or severe respiratory distress

assessment of the arterial acid–base status, with samples from an intra-arterial catheter, or intermittent puncture of the radial or brachial arteries, is necessary. Continuous transcutaneous monitoring of Po_2 and Pco_2 decreases the requirement for blood sampling and enables rapid detection of fluctuations in clinical status. If respiratory acidosis is severe (pH less than 7.20 with Pco_2 greater than 60 mmHg, 8 kPa), assisted ventilation may be necessary. For a severe metabolic acidosis an infusion of sodium bicarbonate may be indicated. Arterial catheterization is indicated when there is a need for frequent sampling for gas analysis, and is used for direct aortic blood pressure monitoring (see p. 186).

Assisted ventilation

In more severe cases respiratory support may be necessary, but the further management depends on the size of the infant.

MILD RESPIRATORY DISTRESS

1 Colour—presence of central cyanosis.
2 Chest recession.
3 Grunt and flaring of the ala nasae.
4 Heart rate—hourly recordings.
5 Respiratory rate—hourly recordings.
6 Temperature—4-hourly measurements.
7 Blood pressure—4-hourly. If there is deterioration with an increasing respiratory rate, onset of cyanosis or falling blood pressure, then more intensive monitoring is necessary.

MODERATE TO SEVERE RESPIRATORY DISTRESS

1 Heart rate monitoring with alarm system for bradycardia.
2 Respiratory monitoring with alarm system for apnoea.
3 Transcutaneous Po_2 and Pco_2 or pulse oximetry.
4 Regular arterial blood-gas monitoring (4-hourly).

5 Hourly blood pressure monitoring.
6 24-h fluid balance chart.

UMBILICAL ARTERY CATHETERIZATION

This is a useful technique in infants who require regular blood-gas estimations and it can also be used for direct aortic blood pressure monitoring. Indications for the insertion of an umbilical artery catheter (UAC) include:
1 infants < 1000 g;
2 infants requiring intensive care or ventilatory support;
3 infants with increasing respiratory distress;
4 infants with severe recurrent apnoea.

The technique for insertion of a UAC is described on p. 314.

OXYGEN THERAPY

Oxygen is a vital therapeutic agent but may cause severe retinal changes, leading to retinopathy of prematurity (see p. 240) if not carefully monitored. Oxygen therapy is discussed fully in Chapter 8.

INCUBATOR THERAPY

See Chapter 9.

FLUID BALANCE AND FEEDING

See Chapter 6.

BLOOD PRESSURE MONITORING

See Chapter 17.

TRANSIENT TACHYPNOEA OF THE NEWBORN (RETAINED FETAL LUNG FLUID)

This occurs in approximately 1–2% of all newborn infants. Tachypnoea is generally the outstanding feature. Transient tachypnoea of the newborn (TTN) is usually benign and self-limiting, with symptoms rarely persisting beyond 48 h.

Pathogenesis

Most of the fetal lung fluid is squeezed out during descent through the birth canal or within the first few breaths after birth, but some is reabsorbed into the pulmonary capillaries and lymphatics. Occasionally, there is an excess of fluid or the clearance mechanisms are inefficient. In these cases retained fluid causes respiratory distress.

Predisposing factors for TTN are prematurity (34–36 weeks), heavy maternal analgesia, birth asphyxia, caesarean section, breech presentation, male sex, hypoproteinaemia and excessive fluid administration to the mother in labour. Polycythaemia may produce a similar clinical picture resulting from hyperviscosity with resultant pulmonary plethora.

Diagnosis

The diagnosis of TTN is confirmed by chest X-ray and the clinical course. Resolution of the respiratory distress within 48 h confirms the clinical diagnosis retrospectively. Chest X-ray shows streakiness caused by interstitial fluid, fluid in the lung fissures and perihilar cuffing. Pleural effusions and cardiomegaly may also sometimes be seen.

Treatment

TTN does not usually require respiratory support, other than extra inspired oxygen. Regular blood-gas measurements should be performed in the first hours of the illness. In more severe cases continuous positive airway pressure may aid resolution. If the blood gases deteriorate, the diagnosis should be reconsidered or complications such as pulmonary hypertension or pneumothorax may have developed. Sometimes the typical picture of TTN evolves over several days into one of RDS.

RESPIRATORY DISTRESS SYNDROME (HYALINE MEMBRANE DISEASE)

RDS is a specific clinical entity occurring predominantly in preterm infants owing to a lack of surfactant (a surface tension-lowering agent) in the alveoli. It has a characteristic clinical course and specific X-ray changes.

Incidence

This condition occurs in 1% of all births. Although there have been a number of recent advances in the management of premature delivery, including suppression of labour, estimation of L/S ratios and the use of steroids, the incidence of this condition has remained remarkably static. It is related to the degree of prematurity and is unusual in full-term infants (Fig. 10.1).

Predisposing factors

1 Prematurity.
2 Infant of a diabetic mother.
3 Antepartum haemorrhage.
4 Second twin.
5 Hypoxia, acidosis, shock.
6 Male sex.
7 Possibly caesarean section (many factors involved).

Historical background

This important condition was first described in 1903 when hyaline membranes were demonstrated in the lungs of dead premature infants (Comroe 1977). Further important landmarks in the understanding of the disease have

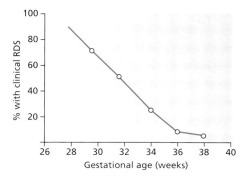

Fig. 10.1 Incidence of RDS related to gestational age.

included the demonstration in the 1950s that this condition was associated with the deficiency of a substance which prevented alveolar collapse (called surfactant). In the 1970s a method for detecting a deficiency of surfactant became available, and cortico-steroids were used to accelerate lung maturity. In the 1980s exogenous surfactant became available for administration into the lung in affected infants.

Aetiology and pathogenesis

The lack of surfactant results in alveoli remaining unexpanded (atelectatic) and gaseous exchange is impaired. Surfactant is a phospholipid secreted by the type II alveolar cells of the lung and is stored in lamellar bodies. The major active component is lecithin, but other phospholipids and protein must be present for full activity. These surface-active agents are released into alveoli, reducing the surface tension and helping to keep the alveoli open.

Lung maturity is assessed by measuring the L/S ratio either on amniotic fluid obtained by amniocentesis or on gastric aspirate, which reflects the L/S ratio of the swallowed liquor. An L/S ratio < 1.5 predicts a high risk of RDS (70% incidence); a ratio of 1.5–2.0 predicts a 40% risk of developing RDS; and a mature ratio > 2 indicates a very small risk unless the mother is diabetic (Roberton 1981). In diabetic pregnancies the presence of phosphatidylglycerol (PG) in the liquor suggests that the infant will not develop RDS.

Surfactant is secreted into the fetal lung at 30–32 weeks' gestation. It forms a surface film over the alveolus and because of its molecular structure is poorly compressible, thereby preventing the alveolus from collapsing down to its unexpanded state. The action of surfactant can be understood by the LaPlace equation:

$$P = 2\,\sigma/r$$

where P = pressure required to inflate a sphere, σ = surface tension and r = radius (Fig. 10.2).

The equation explains why, in the presence of high surface tension, large alveoli tend to

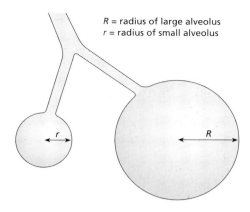

R = radius of large alveolus
r = radius of small alveolus

Fig. 10.2 Schematic representation of two alveoli demonstrating LaPlace's law (see text for details).

become larger and small ones remain collapsed. Assuming that both small and large alveoli receive equal perfusion with blood, there will be a ventilation/perfusion (V/Q) imbalance. This results in severe biochemical disturbances with hypoxia and acidosis which give rise to a deterioration in pulmonary perfusion, thus causing further deterioration in V/Q. This may become progressively more severe and lead to persistent pulmonary hypertension (see p. 199).

When the lungs of an infant who has survived for several hours after birth are examined at autopsy, hyaline membranes may be demonstrated lining the respiratory bronchioles and alveolar ducts. The term hyaline membrane disease is derived from the examination of pathological material.

Clinical features

The signs of RDS start immediately after birth or become obvious in the first 6 h of life. In the absence of surfactant each breath the infant takes is like the first breath in an effort to expand the alveoli. Respiratory failure is contributed to by fatigue. The clinical course is usually associated with worsening of the symptoms, with a peak severity at 48–72 h, although occasionally maximum severity may occur in infants less than 12 h old. In the early stages the infant lies in a 'frog-like' position,

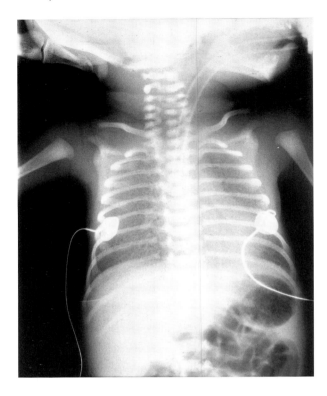

Fig. 10.3 Chest radiograph showing the characteristic 'ground glass' appearance of RDS.

and may have difficulty with copious pharyngeal secretions, which require suctioning for clearance. As the disease progresses the infant shows a need for increasing oxygen to abolish cyanosis, the expiratory grunt may diminish and prolonged apnoea may occur. Apnoea is a late sign of respiratory failure and, if it occurs in the first 6 h of life, infection (particularly due to group B β-haemolytic streptococcus) is a likely cause. The breath sounds are decreased and there may be a fall in blood pressure. The infant is oliguric initially and has evidence of increasing peripheral oedema. At about 48 h a diuresis often occurs, with a concomitant clinical improvement in less severely affected infants.

Radiology

The X-ray is usually characteristic, showing underaeration and a fine reticular or granuloreticular pattern, often referred to as 'ground glass'. In addition, air bronchograms are seen in the lung fields (Fig. 10.3). The appearance of the chest X-ray may not correlate well with the clinical severity of RDS.

Treatment

OXYGEN

The aim of treatment is to maintain the Pao_2 within the normal range. This is done in mild cases by increasing the inspired oxygen concentration (Fio_2). In more severe cases respiratory support may be necessary, but the further management depends on the size of the infant.

Infants < 1500 g. Although continuous positive airway pressure (CPAP) may be administered shortly after birth, most infants will require mechanical ventilation. Indications for mechanical ventilation are as follows:

1 Fio_2 exceeds 60% to maintain Pao_2 > 60 mmHg (8 kPa);

2 apnoea;

3 rising $Paco_2$ which exceeds 60 mmHg (8 kPa), particularly if there is a falling pH (< 7.25).

Infants > 1500 g. CPAP is indicated if Fio_2 exceeds 60% to maintain Pao_2 > 60 mmHg (8 kPa). Mechanical ventilation is recommended if:
1 Fio_2 exceeds 80% to maintain Pao_2 > 60 mmHg (8 kPa) while on CPAP;
2 severe or recurrent apnoea;
3 rising $Paco_2$ which exceeds 60 mmHg (8 kPa), particularly if there is a falling pH (< 7.25).

Details of CPAP and mechanical ventilation are described in Chapter 11.

CHEST PHYSIOTHERAPY

Infants receive regular position changes and airway suctioning to reduce the risk of mucus retention, airway plugging and pulmonary collapse. Active chest percussion and cupping is only practised for problematic secretions and collapse/consolidation demonstrated on chest X-ray. Physiotherapy should not be employed for at least 24 h after surfactant instillation.

ANTIBIOTICS

Broad-spectrum antibiotics are usually administered to all babies with RDS after superficial and deep cultures have been taken. Antibiotics should be stopped once cultures, blood count and ancillary investigations for sepsis are reported as negative.

APPROPRIATE FLUID BALANCE

See p. 44.

BLOOD PRESSURE MONITORING

See p. 186.

MINIMAL HANDLING AND NURSING IN THE NEUTRAL ENVIRONMENTAL TEMPERATURE

See Chapter 9.

SURFACTANT REPLACEMENT THERAPY

Various types of exogenous surfactant (homologous, heterologous, partially synthetic, synthetic) have been studied since 1980, in both prophylactic and rescue modes. Mortality is reduced by about 40% when exogenous surfactant is administered via the endotracheal tube either to infants with established RDS (rescue mode) or as a prophylaxis in high-risk preterm infants. Pulmonary air leaks are less common, but there is no clear effect on the incidence of bronchopulmonary dysplasia, intraventricular haemorrhage or patent ductus arteriosus. It is general practice to give at least one dose of surfactant down the endotracheal tube as soon as RDS is diagnosed clinically and confirmed on chest X-ray. The role of surfactant in other lung diseases, such as meconium aspiration, diaphragmatic hernia and pneumonia, awaits further clinical trials.

Complications

In general, the risk of complications is related to the severity of the underlying RDS. Table 10.2 lists the commoner short- and long-term complications.

Prognosis

Most infants do not die of RDS but rather of a related complication (intraventricular haemorrhage, infection, chronic lung disease). Those weighing 1250 g or below are most at risk. More mature infants, even with severe RDS, are unlikely to die but may require mechanical ventilation for some weeks. Survival figures by birthweight are shown in Table 10.3.

PNEUMONIA

Pneumonia in the newborn infant is relatively common and may be due to viral, bacterial or other agents. Pneumonia may be contracted *in utero* and be present at birth (congenital) or acquired after birth (nosocomial). Congenital pneumonia may be due to ascending infection

Table 10.2 Short- and long-term complications of RDS

Acute	Subacute	Chronic
Respiratory		
Perinatal asphyxia	Convulsions	Cerebral palsy
Pulmonary air leak	Collapse/consolidation	Bronchopulmonary dysplasia
	Pulmonary haemorrhage	SIDS
	Prolonged intubation	Subglottic stenosis
Cardiac		
Patent ductus arteriosus	Lung oedema	Chronic neonatal lung disease
Pulmonary hypertension	Cor pulmonale	
Cerebral		
Cerebroventricular haemorrhage	Ventricular dilatation	Hydrocephalus
	Convulsions	Porencephaly
Periventricular leukomalacia	Cysts	Cerebral palsy
Gastrointestinal		
Necrotizing enterocolitis	Bowel obstruction	Malabsorption
	Gut perforation	
Special senses		
	Retinopathy of prematurity	Visual impairment
	Airway secretions	Conductive/sensorineural hearing loss

Table 10.3 Typical incidence and survival rates for infants of different birthweight groups with a diagnosis of RDS

	Birthweight categories (g)	Incidence (%)	Survival (%)
	< 500	100	10
	500–999	80	80
	1000–1499	55	95
	> 1499	20	100
Total	500–5000	N/A	94

with prolonged rupture of membranes, or less frequently due to a transplacental infection (see Chapter 7). The diagnosis is suspected on maternal history, clinical examination and chest radiograph, and confirmed by bacteriological cultures from blood and tracheal aspirate.

Aetiology

Pneumonia in the newborn is usually bacterial, and the most frequent bacterial pathogens causing congenital and acquired pneumonias are the Gram-negative bacilli (*Escherichia coli, Klebsiella, Pseudomonas, Serratia* sp.), group B β-haemolytic streptococcus and *Staphylococcus* sp.

Rarer bacterial infections include *Listeria monocytogenes* and anaerobic bacilli. Occasionally, pneumonia is due to *Chlamydia trachomatis, Mycoplasma pneumoniae* or opportunistic pathogens such as *Candida albicans* and *Pneumocystis carinii*. Viral pneumonitis is rare but occurs with cytomegalovirus (CMV), Coxsackie virus, respiratory syncytial virus and rubella.

Clinical features

The early clinical signs and symptoms are often non-specific and may include lethargy, apnoea, bradycardia, temperature instability and intolerance of feeds. At birth it may be difficult to distinguish pneumonia from other forms of lung disease. In other cases the typical signs of respiratory distress may be present from birth. The maternal and birth histories may reveal predisposing factors for neonatal infection.

Auscultation of the chest may reveal diminished air entry over areas of consolidation or effusion. Adventitial breath sounds may be heard on inspiration.

Radiology

The appearances are non-specific and pneumonia may be difficult to distinguish radiologically from aspiration syndromes and even TTN. There are usually patchy opacities or more confluent areas of radiodensity through the lung. Lobar pneumonia is rarely seen in the newborn.

Treatment

1 *Antibiotics*. Broad spectrum after deep and superficial cultures have been taken.
2 *Physiotherapy*. Positioning for postural drainage and active chest physiotherapy for areas of consolidation.
3 *Respiratory support* (see Chapter 11).

PULMONARY AIR LEAKS

These are common in newborn infants and are of several types.
1 Pneumothorax—air in the pleural space (Fig. 10.4).
2 Pneumomediastinum—air in the anterior mediastinum (Fig. 10.5).

3 Pneumopericardium—air in the pericardial sac.
4 Pulmonary interstitial emphysema (PIE)— air in interstitial lung spaces (Fig. 10.6).
5 Pneumoperitoneum—air in the peritoneal cavity.
6 Air embolus—air dissecting into pulmonary veins and disseminating throughout the bloodstream.

The pathophysiology of these conditions is similar in that the alveoli become hyperinflated and rupture. Air then escapes into the lung interstitium (PIE) and tracks along the perivascular spaces into the mediastinum (pneumomediastinum) through the visceral pleura (pneumothorax), or rarely into the pericardium (pneumopericardium).

Spontaneous pneumothorax occurs in approximately 1% of vaginal deliveries and 1.5% of caesarean sections. Many of these have only minor symptoms and are discovered unexpectedly on a chest X-ray.

Resuscitation with positive-pressure ventilation makes the occurrence of a pneumothorax far more likely. Surfactant therapy has markedly reduced the incidence of pulmonary air leaks in ventilated infants.

Pneumothoraces commonly occur in the following conditions:
1 stiff lungs, e.g. hyaline membrane disease;
2 hyperinflated lungs, e.g. meconium aspiration;
3 hypoplastic lungs, e.g. Potter's syndrome, diaphragmatic hernia;
4 mechanical ventilation or CPAP predisposes to pulmonary air leaks in about 10% of ventilated infants. Prolonged inspiratory time and high end-expiratory pressures are particularly likely to cause pneumothorax. Active expiration against a ventilator 'breath' is also a probable cause (see p. 122).

Clinical features

Infants with a tension pneumothorax exhibit signs of severe respiratory distress. Frequently a pulmonary air leak occurs in a baby who already has respiratory distress and there may be sudden deterioration, with cyanosis, poor

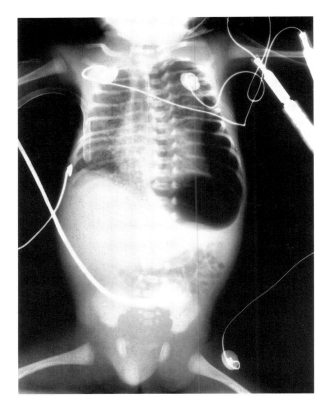

Fig. 10.4 Chest radiograph showing left-sided tension pneumothorax.

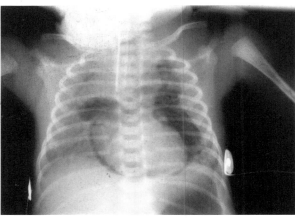

Fig. 10.5 Chest radiograph showing pneumomediastinum. The heart and thymus are outlined by gas.

peripheral perfusion and bradycardia. Specific signs of a tension pneumothorax are a shift of the mediastinum to the opposite side, asymmetrical chest expansion, asymmetrical air entry and weak peripheral pulses. A prominent sternum may suggest a pneumomediastinum.

Occasionally, unilateral PIE develops as a result of a ball-valve effect in a main bronchus. The emphysematous lung may cause compression of the more normal lung, thereby further embarrassing ventilation (Fig. 10.7).

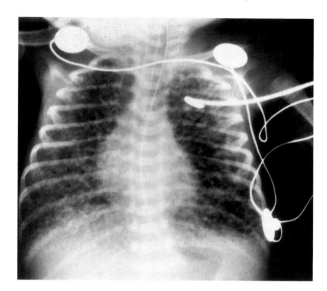

Fig. 10.6 Chest radiograph showing extensive PIE. Note the overinflated chest with flattened diaphragm.

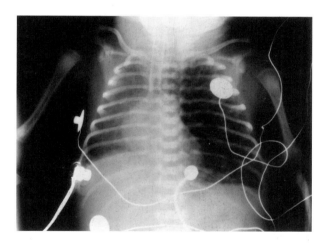

Fig. 10.7 Chest radiograph showing left-sided PIE. The mediastinum and right lung are compressed by the overinflated left lung.

Diagnosis

The definitive diagnosis is made by an anteroposterior chest X-ray. To detect a small pneumothorax, an erect film will be required, whereas a lateral film will be necessary to diagnose air in the anterior mediastinum. When a pneumomediastinum is present, the chest X-ray reveals the sail or spinnaker sign. In the critically ill infant who has a tension pneumothorax, chest transillumination may be used to make the diagnosis. Occasionally, the insertion of a 21G butterfly needle with stopcock and syringes may be life-saving in suspected tension pneumothoraces. This is an emergency diagnostic and therapeutic procedure undertaken when there may be delay in obtaining an X-ray in a critically ill infant. Blind needling of the chest may create a pneumothorax and should not be attempted except in an emergency.

Management

A tension pneumothorax will need to be released by an intercostal catheter inserted into the second intercostal space in the mid-clavicular line and connected to underwater seal drainage or a Heimlich one-way flutter valve (see p. 312). Occasionally, evacuation of the pneumothorax will be incomplete with this catheter, and a catheter sited more posteriorly in the sixth intercostal space in the midaxillary line will be necessary. For non-tension pneumothoraces in full-term infants, nursing in 100% oxygen for up to 12 h may accelerate reabsorption of the pneumothorax. The rare pleural effusion or chylous effusion in the newborn may require thoracocentesis if large.

PIE is best managed with fast-rate ventilation (see p. 124) or high-frequency oscillation ventilation. Severe unilateral PIE with compression of the other lung can be treated by selectively intubating the more normal lung, thereby allowing the emphysematous lung to collapse (Brooks *et al.* 1977). After 24–48 h, and when radiological improvement has occurred, the tube is withdrawn.

MECONIUM ASPIRATION SYNDROME

Meconium aspiration syndrome is a serious and potentially preventable cause of respiratory distress in the newborn. Meconium staining of the amniotic fluid occurs almost always in full-term or post-term infants and is seen in about 13% of deliveries. The passage of meconium often indicates fetal distress, but in the breech presentation may be normal. Whether it is a sign of fetal distress or not, the possibility of aspiration into the lungs must be taken seriously. Meconium aspiration may occur during labour or at the onset of neonatal respiration. The response of the infant to intrapartum asphyxia is to gasp, and if meconium is present it will be aspirated deep into the bronchi. Once respiration begins, distal migration of the meconium into small airways occurs.

Clinical features

There is a wide spectrum of presentations, ranging from severe birth asphyxia requiring active resuscitation through early onset of respiratory distress to a vigorous baby with no major problems. Typically the infant is born covered in meconium-stained liquor and has meconium staining of the umbilical cord, skin and nails. The chest appears to be hyperinflated and there may be a prominent sternum. Respiratory distress may be mild initially, becoming rapidly more severe after several hours. The baby may also show signs of cerebral irritability.

Pathogenesis and aetiology

Meconium causes plugging of the airways, with consequent atelectasis. It also causes a 'ball-valve' obstruction with hyperinflation of the lungs and a high risk of pulmonary air leaks. Meconium is irritating to the airways, causing a chemical pneumonitis. Sometimes secondary bacterial infection occurs. A proportion of infants with severe aspiration syndrome develop marked ventilation/perfusion inequality leading to a right to left shunt and pulmonary hypertension (see p. 199).

Radiology

Chest X-rays show hyperinflation (flat diaphragms, widening of rib spaces) with diffuse patchy opacities throughout both lung fields (Fig. 10.8). Pneumothorax or pneumomediastinum may also be seen.

Prophylactic management

Morbidity and mortality from meconium aspiration syndrome can be prevented or minimized by optimal perinatal management. There is controversy as to whether a neonatal paediatrician should attend every delivery where there is meconium staining of the liquor. It is important, however, that an experienced neonatal paediatrician be present for the delivery if *thick* meconium is present. Under these circumstances the following should be undertaken:

1 once the head crowns, and before the shoulders are delivered, the oropharynx should be

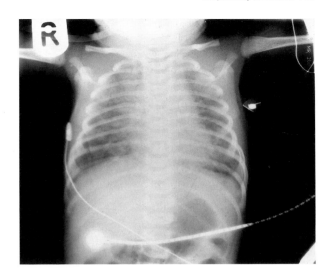

Fig. 10.8 Chest radiograph showing meconium aspiration syndrome. There is extensive discrete shadowing throughout both lung fields.

quickly and efficiently suctioned by the obstetrician. The umbilical cord should be doubly clamped for arterial gas analysis;

2 after delivery the baby should be transferred to the resuscitation trolley, where the resuscitationist sucks out the oropharynx under direct laryngoscopic vision with a suction catheter;

3 in a depressed infant, if meconium is seen in the posterior pharynx, at or below the vocal cords, the baby is intubated with a wide-bore endotracheal tube and the trachea is suctioned clear. Suctioning is facilitated by the use of a meconium aspirator. Mouth to endotracheal tube suctioning must not be practised. Further suction is applied directly to the endotracheal tube as it is being removed. If a large quantity of meconium is present in the endotracheal tube after extubation, the baby should be reintubated and further tracheal suction applied. The stomach should be aspirated following intubation and, if there is a moderate or large volume of meconium in the stomach, the gastric tube should be left *in situ* for lavage to be performed later;

4 if the baby is vigorous and in good condition and only thin meconium is suctioned from the posterior pharynx, then tracheal intubation is not necessary;

5 all babies who are born with thick meconium in the liquor should be carefully assessed and regularly monitored for signs of meconium aspiration syndrome.

Treatment of established meconium aspiration syndrome

The treatment will be the same as for respiratory distress (see Chapter 12). Particular emphasis should be given to:

1 humidification of inspired oxygen;

2 postural drainage positioning, suctioning of airways and chest percussion;

3 antibiotics: usually given, although efficacy has not been established.

PULMONARY HYPOPLASIA

For adequate fetal lung development the fetus must be able to make breathing movements and move a column of amniotic fluid up and down the trachea and main bronchi. Hypoplasia may therefore be due to:

1 failure of fetal breathing (neuromuscular disorders);

2 inability to expand the lungs (diaphragmatic hernia, pleural effusions);

3 lack of liquor (oligohydramnios) due to

renal or bladder neck abnormalities or prolonged rupture of the membranes.

Infants with pulmonary hypoplasia may have associated facial abnormalities and limb contractures. The fetal side of the placenta should be examined for amnion nodosum, which is suggestive of severe oligohydramnios, especially Potter's syndrome.

Clinical features

The infant develops severe respiratory distress from birth, with marked hypoxia, hypercapnia and metabolic acidosis. Pneumothorax is a common complication. The lungs are very stiff and there is little chest movement with mechanical ventilation. It may be difficult to diagnose lung hypoplasia on chest X-ray. Severe lung hypoplasia is incompatible with life, and less severe forms contribute towards chronic ventilator dependency and bronchopulmonary dysplasia.

MASSIVE PULMONARY HAEMORRHAGE

Massive pulmonary haemorrhage has a characteristic clinical presentation in newborn infants, with cardiovascular collapse associated with an outpouring of bloodstained fluid from the trachea and mouth. The condition is usually fatal and occurs in about 1/1000 births. It has been described in association with severe birth asphyxia, hypothermia, small for gestational age (SGA) infants, coagulation disturbances and congenital heart disease. Pulmonary haemorrhage has also been reported following exogenous surfactant therapy. Haemorrhagic pulmonary oedema has been suggested as the probable cause in the majority of cases.

Treatment

The treatment will be that of respiratory distress (see Chapter 11). However, particular emphasis must be given to:

1 resuscitation of cardiovascular collapse with volume expanders such as plasma protein fraction, blood and sodium bicarbonate;
2 treatment of pulmonary oedema with frusemide and perhaps morphine;
3 correction of coagulation disturbances;
4 if mechanical ventilation is required, high positive end-expiratory pressures should be used to decrease bleeding.

CONGENITAL DIAPHRAGMATIC HERNIA

The hernia is usually a posterolateral (Bochdalek) type; 80% occur on the left side. This occurs through a defect in the diaphragm as a result of a persistent pleuroperitoneal canal caused by failure of the muscular components to develop. The defect in the diaphragm permits herniation of the abdominal contents into the thorax. Consequently, there is hypoplasia or compression of the lung on the side of the hernia, with displacement of mediastinum to the contralateral side. Sometimes there is hypoplasia of the contralateral lung. Babies with a large diaphragmatic hernia have rapidly progressive respiratory failure after birth, with persistent cyanosis. A less acute diaphragmatic hernia may present in the nursery, with respiratory distress, or occasionally on routine examination a 'dextrocardia' or scaphoid abdomen will be found. On auscultation of the lungs, bowel sounds may be heard on the side of the lesion if gas has entered the gastrointestinal tract. The lungs will not inflate adequately with normal pressure.

Diagnosis

Most cases are now diagnosed *in utero* by routine obstetric ultrasound at 17–19 weeks' gestation or following investigation of polyhydramnios. The diagnosis of a diaphragmatic hernia is confirmed by chest X-ray, which shows bowel loops in the thorax (Fig. 10.9). If the X-ray is taken shortly after birth, there

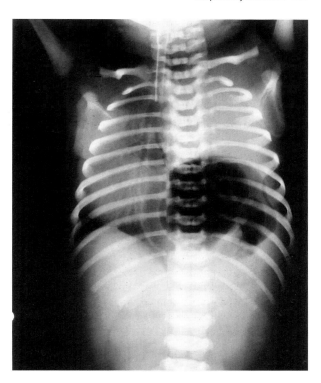

Fig. 10.9 Chest radiograph showing a left-sided diaphragmatic hernia.

may be some difficulty in determining whether the bowel is in the chest, especially if there is little air in the gastrointestinal tract. The X-ray should be taken with a radio-opaque catheter in the stomach and should include the abdomen, to show a paucity of abdominal gas pattern. A rarer form of diaphragmatic hernia is through an anteromedial defect beneath the sternum (Morgagni type). This typically contains part of the colon. It is usually symptomless and often detected on a lateral chest X-ray.

Treatment

If a congenital diaphragmatic hernia is suspected, an orogastric tube should be inserted and the abdominal contents in the chest aspirated free of gas and secretions. If the baby requires assisted ventilation, it should be via an endotracheal tube and never by bag and mask, because of the increasing gaseous distension of the bowel within the chest. Care must be taken

to prevent rupture of the contralateral lung, as the baby is almost exclusively dependent on this lung for ventilation. Following initial diagnosis the baby should be stabilized and referred to a paediatric surgeon for operative treatment. Surgery for the more severe cases is often delayed for 3–7 days to enable maximum stabilization, often with high-frequency oscillation ventilation. Surgery consists of reduction of the abdominal contents, closure of the diaphragmatic defect and correction of any bowel malrotation.

Pulmonary hypertension is a common complication of severe diaphragmatic hernia and usually develops after a postoperative 'honeymoon' period of 24–48 h. The infant then develops severe hypoxia with a right to left shunt. Elective hyperventilation and infusion of sodium bicarbonate to induce alkalosis (pH > 7.5) have been recommended to reduce the risk of this complication. Magnesium sulphate, prostacycline or tolazoline may be of value, but inhaled nitric oxide has no long-term benefits (see p. 200). The continuation of post-operative anaesthesia with muscle paralysis may be necessary on return from the operating theatre in the more severe cases. Extra-corporeal membrane oxygenation (ECMO) for this condition is of minimal benefit at best. The role of fetal surgery is being reinvestigated, with procedures to plug the trachea being performed typically at 23 weeks' gestation.

Prognosis

This depends on the degree of pulmonary hypoplasia and the age at presentation. Infants with respiratory distress in the first 6 h have a high mortality (about 70%), and those presenting between 6 and 24 h a much better prognosis (mortality rates 10–15%). Later presentation is not likely to be associated with pulmonary hypoplasia and the prognosis is very good. Bad prognostic features include polyhydramnios, persistently elevated P_{CO_2} levels with mean airway pressure > 20 cmH$_2$O, and hypoxia requiring pulmonary vasodilators.

OESOPHAGEAL ATRESIA AND TRACHEO-OESOPHAGEAL FISTULA

Oesophageal atresia is a congenital anomaly in which there is usually complete interruption of the lumen of the oesophagus, in the form of a blind upper pouch. This is commonly associated with a tracheo-oesophageal fistula. The commonest variety of this condition is a blind-ending upper oesophageal pouch, with the lower oesophagus arising from the trachea above the carina (Fig. 10.10c). A variety of other patterns occur much less commonly (Fig. 10.10).

Clinical features

Maternal hydramnios occurs in 60% of cases and is largely responsible for the high frequency of premature births. The oesophageal atresia is associated with excessive saliva and mucus production, with a high incidence of aspiration pneumonia. If the infant is fed, milk accumulates in the upper pouch and spills over into the trachea. The aspiration of gastric contents and bile into the bronchial tree via the fistula results in pulmonary complications, with collapse and pneumonia. Abdominal distension is due to air passing down the fistula into the stomach, and may develop rapidly.

Coexistent congenital anomalies may be present and may be either major or minor. Major anomalies consist of cardiac disease, intestinal atresia, imperforate anus, skeletal anomalies and renal anomalies. VACTERL association is the term often used to describe these anomalies. This stands for Vertebral, Anal, Cardiac, Tracheal, 'Esophagus', Renal and Limb. The most important aspect of oesophageal atresia is that it should be recognized as soon as possible after birth, preferably prior to the first feed, so that pulmonary complications are less likely to occur. All babies should have a size 5 nasogastric tube passed down each nostril in turn and into the

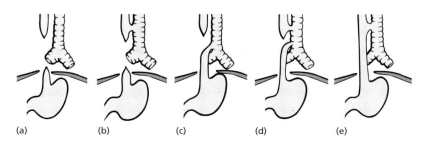

(a) (b) (c) (d) (e)

Fig. 10.10 Variants of tracheo-oesphageal fistula with or without oesophageal atresia. Type c accounts for 85% of cases, the others being equally uncommon.

stomach shortly after birth. In this way most cases of oesophageal atresia and choanal atresia can be diagnosed before feeding. If this is not practised, oesophageal atresia is generally diagnosed by excessive secretions or cyanosis and coughing with feeds. The definitive diagnosis is made by the inability to pass a firm radio-opaque no. 10 catheter into the stomach, as it arrests about 10 cm from the lips. Once the catheter has been passed as far as possible, an X-ray of the neck and upper chest should be taken to confirm that it has become obstructed at this level. The abdominal X-ray should be inspected for gas in the stomach and the chest X-ray assessed for areas of collapse. Air is a useful contrast medium in the upper pouch. It is not usually necessary to put radio-opaque contrast medium into the upper pouch to confirm the diagnosis, but if this is done a non-irritant substance such as metrizimide should be used. For an H-type fistula, which presents with recurrent aspiration or infections, radiological diagnosis may be difficult. A cine contrast swallow will usually confirm the diagnosis.

Treatment

A baby with oesophageal atresia and tracheo-oesophageal fistula should be nursed supine and propped head-up 60° to avoid gastric contents spilling into the lung through the fistula. An intravenous infusion should be commenced and the baby rehydrated with correction of electrolytes and blood glucose disturbances in preparation for surgery. Surgery should be performed by a paediatric surgeon as soon as the baby has been adequately resuscitated and stabilized. Antibiotics will be required if there has been significant aspiration pneumonia. Surgery consists of division of the tracheo-oesophageal fistula and anastomosis of the two segments of the oesophagus if possible. Occasionally, the atretic segment is too long to enable primary anastomosis, and exteriorization of the cervical oesophagus as an oesophagostomy and the stomach as a gastrostomy will be necessary. A definitive operation will be undertaken at a later date.

With a cervical oesophagostomy the baby should be encouraged to practise sucking on a dummy during gastrostomy feedings. Complications and sequelae from surgery are frequent and include a brassy cough, associated with co-existent tracheomalacia, oesophageal stricture, breakdown of the anastomosis with mediastinitis, recurrence of the tracheo-oesophageal fistula and gastro-oesophageal reflux.

LOBAR EMPHYSEMA

Congenital lobar emphysema is a rare anomaly due to a cartilaginous deficiency of the lobar bronchus, most commonly involving the left upper lobe (50%), the right middle lobe (24%) or the right upper lobe (18%), and is frequently associated with congenital heart disease (30%), such as tetralogy of Fallot, ventricular septal disease (VSD) or total anomalous pulmonary venous drainage. The onset of respiratory distress is frequently insidious, usually taking 2–3 weeks to develop, and is caused by lung collapse around the hyperinflated lobe. The mediastinum becomes displaced and the chest wall is prominent over the affected area. Breath sounds are diminished and the percussion note is hyperresonant. Once a definitive diagnosis is made, a lobectomy is generally required. Acquired lobar emphysema may be secondary to an extrinsic or intrinsic bronchial obstruction, such as a mucous plug. This type should be treated conservatively with physiotherapy and postural drainage.

CYSTIC ADENOMATOID MALFORMATION

Cystic adenomatoid malformation (CAM) is a rare cystic lesion found more often in males and is often diagnosed on antenatal ultrasound. This haematomatous lesion may be associated with polyhydramnios, hydrops fetalis, prematurity and stillbirth. There are three distinct types. Type I CAM (70%) presents as single or multiple large cyst(s) confined to one lobe; type II (18%) is composed of multiple medium sized cysts and 50% have other anomalies; type III (10%) is a large bulky lesion with evenly distributed small cysts. This is one of the few conditions which is treatable by fetal surgery in selected cases.

CHRONIC NEONATAL LUNG DISEASE

Chronic neonatal lung disease is usually defined as occurring in preterm infants with evidence of pulmonary parenchymal disease on chest radiography who require increased inspired oxygen for more than 28 days to maintain oxygen tension > 60 mmHg. Shennan *et al.* (1988) have suggested that for very low birthweight (VLBW) infants the need for oxygen beyond 36 weeks' postmenstrual age is a better predictor of abnormal pulmonary outcome than oxygen requirement beyond 28 days.

The classification of the various types of chronic neonatal lung disease is confusing. There are distinct entities such as bronchopulmonary dysplasia (BPD), but many of the varieties described overlap and some preterm infants exhibit lung changes that do not adhere

Table 10.4 Classification of chronic neonatal lung disease

Bronchopulmonary dysplasia

Wilson–Mikity syndrome

Chronic pulmonary insufficiency of prematurity

Recurrent aspiration:
  Pharyngeal incoordination
  Gastro-oesophageal reflux
  Tracheo-oesophageal fistula

Interstitial pneumonitis:
  Cytomegalovirus
  Candida albicans
  Chlamydia
  Pneumocystis carinii
  Ureaplasma urealyticum

Chronic pulmonary oedema due to a left to right shunt

Rickets of prematurity

to any of the described patterns. Table 10.4 lists a classification of chronic neonatal lung disease.

Previously, chronic lung disease in infancy was rare, but with increasing survival rates of extremely preterm infants it is becoming more frequent. Approximately 80% of babies with birthweights of 501–750 g are oxygen dependent on day 28; this falls to 40% for infants of birthweights 751–1000 g, and 13% for those weighing 1001–1500 g.

Bronchopulmonary dysplasia

This is usually associated with the healing phase of severe RDS, but occasionally complicates meconium aspiration, pulmonary haemorrhage, severe neonatal pneumonia or even recurrent apnoea. It has also been called respirator lung, oxygen-toxic lung and Northway's disease (Northway *et al.* 1967).

AETIOLOGY

BPD occurs in about 5% of VLBW infants and the aetiological factors are numerous. The incidence relates to the severity of RDS and the degree of prematurity. It has only been described in infants who have received positive-pressure ventilation, and probably relates to barotrauma as measured by the mean airway pressure (this term is used to include inspiratory pressure, expiratory pressure, inspiratory/expiratory ratio and rate) and volume trauma to the lung. Inspired oxygen tension more than 60% for prolonged periods of time appears to be necessary for its development, but is not the cause of the condition. Other probable associations are pulmonary interstitial emphysema and pulmonary oedema. The roles of gastro-oesophageal reflux with recurrent aspiration and infectious agents such as *Ureaplasma urealyticum* are not clear.

CLINICAL FEATURES

Infants who develop BPD have persistent chest retractions, crepitations and rhonchi on chest auscultation, gross hyperinflation of the lungs and an increased anteroposterior chest

Table 10.5 Radiological classification of bronchopulmonary dysplasia

Stage	Days of life	Description	X-ray appearances
1	2–3	Acute RDS	Generalized granuloreticular pattern, air bronchograms or 'white out'
2	4–10	Period of regeneration	Near or total opacification
3	10–20	Period of transition	Small cystic infiltrates, chronic disease
4	> 4 weeks	Period of chronic disease	Hyperlucency, strand-like infiltrates, enlargement of cysts

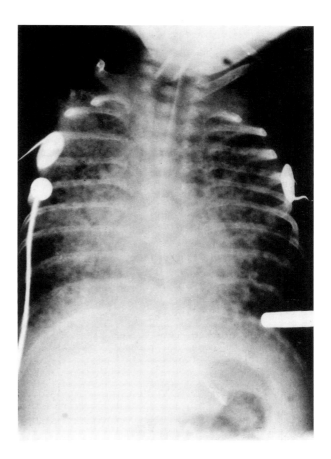

Fig. 10.11 Chest radiograph showing severe bronchopulmonary dysplasia.

diameter. Most of these infants also have a patent ductus arteriosus, and after a period of time may develop right heart failure (cor pulmonale).

RADIOLOGY

The original description of BPD by Northway et al. (1967) staged the radiological appearances in four grades (Table 10.5). The first two are indistinguishable from RDS and are not helpful for descriptive purposes. In the most severe form there is an irregular honeycomb appearance to the lung, with overinflated lung fields, extensive fibrosis and multiple cysts of irregular size (Fig. 10.11).

The majority of infants with BPD do not develop these gross radiological signs but exhibit a finer, more homogeneous pattern of abnormality, with some dense streaks on chest X-ray.

MANAGEMENT

The prevention of BPD requires careful management of infants receiving mechanical ventilation. Pulmonary interstitial emphysema, pulmonary oedema and patent ductus arteriosus and overhydration appear to increase the risk of BPD developing. Early closure of a patent ductus arteriosus which is producing congestive heart failure, either medically with indomethacin or surgically, is desirable. Established BPD is often associated with congestive cardiac failure or cor pulmonale, and under these circumstances fluid restriction, diuretics and digitalis are used. The following methods of treatment are thought to be of some benefit:

1 *dexamethasone*. Studies have shown that dexamethasone reduces the oxygen requirements of babies with BPD. Courses of this drug have varied between 5 and 42 days, but the optimal duration or timing of the start of the course is unclear;

2 *diuretics*. Diuretic therapy reduces interstitial lung fluid and has been shown to reduce oxygen requirements;

3 *therapy directed at reducing oxygen toxicity*. Antioxidants such as vitamin E appear to be of no benefit, but other substances, such as vitamin A and superoxide dismutase, are currently being assessed;

4 *negative-pressure ventilation*. Placing the baby in a tank which provides intermittent negative thoracic pressure appears to reduce oxygen requirements, but is not fully evaluated as a reliable form of therapy.

Adequate oxygenation throughout all daily activities (O_2 saturation 92–96%) minimizes progressive pulmonary vascular disease. Additional nutritional requirements are necessary to obtain optimal growth in the presence of high energy consumption due to the work of breathing.

PROGNOSIS

Mortality figures vary from 0 to 75%, depending on when the diagnosis is made. If stage 4 BPD is diagnosed while the baby is still requiring ventilation, the chance of 'weaning' him or her off the ventilator is unlikely. Most infants with resolving BPD have episodes of wheezing, often associated with a viral infection. The healing stage is associated with continued lung growth and may take 2–3 years. The majority of surviving infants are asymptomatic by 2 years, and chest X-rays are normal by 2–3 years. Respiratory function tests are abnormal for many years, although the child is usually asymptomatic. Many infants with severe BPD are discharged home on continuous low-flow intranasal oxygen, with intermittent monitoring of oxygen requirement by pulse oximetry.

Children with BPD have been shown to have increased airway resistance and are more likely to wheeze. They also have increased airway reactivity. Episodic wheezing is commonly seen in infants and children who had BPD in the newborn period. The wheeze may be resistant to sympathomimetic and xanthine drugs, but steroids may be of benefit.

Lower airway infection in the first year of life is a particular risk to children who had BPD in the neonatal period. They appear to be particularly likely to develop respiratory syncytial virus (RSV)-positive bronchiolitis, which may cause very severe respiratory failure. The antiviral agent, ribaviron (Respigam) and anti-RSV γ-globulin are effective prophylactic agents. Advice must be given to the parents to avoid exposing the baby to the risk of viral infection in the first year or two of life.

Wilson–Mikity syndrome (pulmonary dysmaturity) (Northway *et al*. 1967)

This condition usually occurs in preterm infants of less than 32 weeks' gestation who did not have RDS. The onset is insidious, in most cases in the second or third week, and progresses with increasing dyspnoea, chest

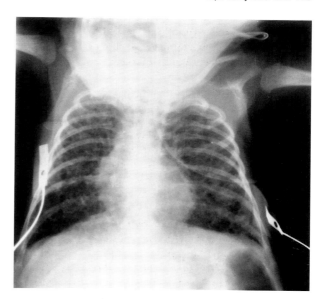

Fig. 10.12 Chest radiograph showing the fine reticulation seen in Wilson–Mikity syndrome.

retractions, apnoea and increasing oxygen requirements.

The chest X-ray is usually normal initially, but bilateral coarse streaky infiltrates with small cysts begin to appear in the second or third weeks. The cysts enlarge and the lungs become overinflated. Osteopenia of the bones and sometimes rib fractures are seen on the X-ray.

AETIOLOGY

The aetiology of this condition in preterm infants is unknown and may be due to a variety of insults, including viruses, chronic aspiration of milk and retention of bronchial secretions. There is an increasingly abnormal air distribution with a V/Q imbalance. The incidence of the disease has declined over the last decade at the same time that the incidence of BPD has been increasing. It is possible that the decline in Wilson–Mikity syndrome is associated with the increasing use of xanthine derivatives to prevent recurrent apnoea of prematurity.

RADIOLOGY

Diffuse bilateral shadows are seen forming a uniform lace-like appearance with multiple small cysts throughout both lung fields (Fig. 10.12).

PROGNOSIS

Most infants survive and usually make a complete clinical and radiological recovery. Affected infants may require additional oxygen for months before the condition resolves. Survivors are prone to recurrent wheezing episodes associated with viral infections in the first 2 years of life.

Chronic pulmonary insufficiency of prematurity

This is a clinical entity caused by a variety of pathological processes. Chronic pulmonary insufficiency of prematurity (CPIP) describes the premature infant who continues to require oxygen, or develops the need for extra oxygen, and has a typical hazy chest X-ray appearance. It is usually due to microatelectasis associated with stiff lungs (slow resolution of RDS), diaphragmatic weakness or a floppy chest wall. The commonest cause of the latter is neonatal rickets (see p. 46). The poorly ossified ribs, together with a degree of muscle weakness, allow the lungs to progressively collapse. Viral infections may cause a similar picture.

MANAGEMENT

This includes recognition and treatment of rickets if this is present. Xanthines may be effective in improving respiratory muscle tone, and a short course of CPAP has been used to reinflate the collapsed alveoli. The infant may require additional oxygen for some weeks, but eventually recovers completely.

REFERENCES

Brooks, J.G., Bustanente, S.A., Koops, B.L., Hiton, S., Cooper, D., Wesenberg, R.L. & Simmons, M.A. (1977) Selective bronchial intubation for the treatment of localised PIE in newborn infants. *Journal of Pediatrics* **91**, 648.

Comroe, J.H. (1977) *The Retrospectoscope: Insights Into Medical Discovery.* Von Gehr, California.

Northway, W.H., Rosan, R.C. & Porter, D.Y. (1967) Pulmonary disease following respirator therapy of hyaline membrane disease; broncho-pulmonary dysplasia. *New England Journal of Medicine* **276**, 357–368.

Roberton, N.R.C. (1981) Developments in neonatal paediatric practice. In: *Recent Advances in Paediatrics* 6 (ed. D. Hull), pp. 13–50. Churchill Livingstone, Edinburgh.

Shennan, A.T., Dunn, M.S. & Ohlsson, A. (1988) Abnormal pulmonary outcome in premature infants: prediction from oxygen requirement in the neonatal period. *Pediatrics* **82**, 527–532.

FURTHER READING

Avery, G.B., Fletcher, M.A., MacDonald, M.G. (eds) (1994) *Neonatology: Pathophysiology and Management of the Newborn*, 4th edn. Lippincott-Raven, Philadelphia.

Rennie, J.M. & Roberton, N.R.C. (1998) *Textbook of Neonatology*, 3rd edn. Churchill Livingstone, Edinburgh.

Spitzer, A.R. (1994) *Intensive Care of the Fetus and Neonate.* Mosby, St Louis.

Yu, V.Y.H. (1986) *Respiratory Disorders in the Newborn.* Churchill Livingstone, Edinburgh.

11 Respiratory physiology, respiratory failure and mechanical ventilation

Respiratory distress is a non-specific term referring to a group of clinical signs with multiple causes. The management of infants with respiratory disorders involves careful clinical assessment as well as the evaluation of radiological and biochemical data. The decision to give respiratory support by means of continuous positive airway pressure (CPAP) or mechanical ventilation depends on a number of variables, which are discussed below. Respiratory failure is used to describe the endpoint of a variety of respiratory, neurological and cardiac conditions. If respiratory failure occurs, respiratory support is necessary. This chapter outlines the methods and indications for such support, and aspects of relevant respiratory physiology are reviewed.

RESPIRATORY PHYSIOLOGY

Oxygen transport

Oxygen is essential for the production of adenosine triphosphate (ATP), a molecule which stores and releases energy. Severe hypoxaemia greatly reduces the production of ATP and the resultant anaerobic metabolism produces lactic acid. Lactic acid accumulation significantly contributes to the development of metabolic acidosis.

Oxygen diffuses across the alveolar membrane from a higher to a lower concentration. It is carried in the blood attached to haemoglobin, or to a lesser degree dissolved in plasma. The partial pressure of oxygen (P_{O_2}) refers to the amount dissolved in plasma. Delivery of oxygen to the tissues depends on oxygen concentration and tissue perfusion. Oxygen combines with haemoglobin to be transported as oxyhaemoglobin. The saturation of the haemoglobin refers to the percentage of it that carries oxygen. There is not a constant relationship between the oxygen saturation and the P_{O_2}, so that at a relatively low tissue P_{O_2} larger amounts of oxygen are released than when the P_{O_2} is higher. Fetal haemoglobin (HbF) has a different oxygen dissociation curve from adult haemoglobin (HbA) in that it is shifted to the left (Fig. 11.1). The fetus lives in a relatively hypoxic environment and the oxyhaemoglobin saturation is greater at lower partial oxygen pressures. This is of benefit to the fetus but is disadvantageous to the newborn infant, who at any given P_{O_2} level gives up less oxygen to the tissues than older children with HbA. Table 11.1 lists the factors responsible for a shift in the oxygen dissociation curve.

Carbon dioxide transport

Carbon dioxide may be transported dissolved in the blood, but is mainly present as bicarbonate ions (HCO_3^-). Carbon dioxide is produced as a byproduct of cellular respiration and is liberated into the blood. It diffuses through the

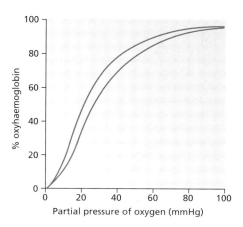

Fig. 11.1 Oxygen dissociation curve for fetal haemoglobin (upper line) and adult haemoglobin (lower line).

Table 11.1 Factors that influence the oxygen dissociation curve

Factors producing (L) shift	Factors producing (R) shift
↓ Temperature	↑ Temperature
↓ Basal metabolic rate	↑ Basal metabolic rate
↓ $Paco_2$	↑ $Paco_2$
↑ pH	↓ pH
↓ 2,3-DPG	↑ 2,3-DPG
↑ Fetal haemoglobin	↓ Fetal haemoglobin

2,3-DPG, 2,3-diphosphoglycerate.

alveoli to be excreted in the expired air. The CO_2 content of the blood is referred to as the partial pressure of CO_2, or Pco_2.

Acid–base balance

In the presence of the enzyme carbonic anhydrase (CA), carbon dioxide dissolved in plasma forms carbonic acid, which in turn dissociates to H^+ and HCO_3^- ions. This is described in the Henderson–Hasselbach equation:

$$H_2O + CO_2 \overset{CA}{\rightleftharpoons} H_2CO_3 \rightleftharpoons HCO_3^- + H^+$$

As a result of this dissociation carbonic acid can be indirectly excreted through the lungs. Lactic acid must be excreted through the kidneys, and this occurs more slowly.

Buffer systems exist in the body to prevent rapid pH changes. The HCO_3^-/CO_2 relationship is an important buffer system; other buffers include haemoglobin and, to a lesser extent, plasma proteins. Disturbance of the acid–base balance can produce either acidosis or alkalosis, which may be due to either metabolic or respiratory causes.

During aerobic metabolism CO_2 is produced and in the presence of respiratory disease is less effectively excreted, causing the $Paco_2$ to rise. As a result the infant becomes acidotic—respiratory acidosis. If the infant with relatively normal lungs breathes or is ventilated rapidly, more CO_2 is excreted and the reaction moves in the other direction to produce a respiratory alkalosis.

Lactic acid, the product of anaerobic metabolism, can only be excreted by the kidneys and, if in excess, the H^+ ions are buffered by haemoglobin, proteins and H_2CO_3. The HCO_3^- can be excreted through the lungs to compensate, thereby leaving an excess of H^+ causing a metabolic acidosis. Persistent vomiting causes loss of H^+, resulting in an excess of HCO_3^- with consequent metabolic alkalosis.

Thus, to keep the blood pH stable, the Pco_2 will fall in both metabolic acidosis and respiratory alkalosis, and the Pco_2 will rise in metabolic alkalosis and respiratory acidosis. In practice a simple respiratory acidosis rarely occurs, and in neonatal lung disease there is likely to be impairment of CO_2 excretion, together with production of lactic acid as a result of anaerobic metabolism, leading to a mixed respiratory and metabolic acidosis.

The base excess is derived from the relationship between pH and Pco_2 using the Siggaard Anderson nomogram. It is the amount of buffer base added to blood, assuming that Pco_2 is 40 mmHg, to correct the pH to 7.40. Thus, it is a direct measurement of the metabolic component of acidosis or alkalosis. Positive values represent excess of base and negative values excess of acid. The base excess is therefore valuable in assigning a predominant metabolic or respiratory component to acidosis or alkalosis.

The acid–base status of the infant can be derived from the blood gases. Normal biochemical ranges for arterial blood in term and preterm infants are shown in Table 11.2.

Specific treatments for various abnormalities of acid–base balance are described below.

METABOLIC ACIDOSIS

Metabolic acidosis arises when there is tissue hypoxia (inadequate perfusion, hypoxaemia), excessive acid intake (total parenteral nutrition (TPN) or cows' milk feeding), the production of excessive or abnormal acids (inborn errors of metabolism) or renal inability to excrete the acid load (tubular acidosis). In the presence of normal lungs the pH may be normal but the Pco_2 is low, and the base excess may be

Table 11.2 Normal biochemical range for arterial blood in term and preterm infants

	Term	Preterm
P_{O_2} mmHg (kPa)	60–90 (8–12)	50–80 (6.7–10.7)
P_{CO_2} mmHg (kPa)	35–42 (4.7–5.6)	30–40 (4–5.3)
pH	7.35–7.42	7.32–7.40
Base excess (BE) (mmol/L)	–2–0	–4–0
Bicarbonate (mmol/L)	22–26	19–24

–8 mmol/L or more. Treatment is directed at the underlying problem.

In addition, metabolic acidosis may be treated by infusion of a molar (8.4%) solution of sodium bicarbonate. 8.4% $NaHCO_3$ has 1 mmol of $NaHCO_3$ in 1 mL of solution and is usually infused slowly as a half-strength solution. The dose is calculated as follows:

Vol. of 8.4% $NaHCO_3$ (mL) = base excess × weight in kg × 0.5

The factor 0.5 represents the proportion of extracellular fluid to body weight in infants. The usual dose is 2–5 mmol/kg.

Sodium bicarbonate combines with excess hydrogen ions to produce unstable carbonic acid, which in turn is hydrolysed to CO_2 and H_2O. The CO_2 is excreted by the lungs. For this reason, bicarbonate must not be given in the presence of high P_{CO_2}. Under these circumstances trishydroxyaminomethane (THAM) is preferable to bicarbonate, and this is described in the section on respiratory acidosis.

METABOLIC ALKALOSIS

This metabolic derangement usually occurs following excessive vomiting or the overuse of sodium bicarbonate. The pH may be normal or high. The P_{CO_2} is usually raised and the base excess is positive. Treatment is by infusion of normal saline.

RESPIRATORY ACIDOSIS

This is due to lung disease and is usually aggravated by a metabolic acidosis as a result of anaerobic metabolism and poor tissue perfu-

sion. If there is a mixed acidosis the pH is low, P_{aCO_2} high and base excess strongly negative. Treatment depends on the severity of the lung disease, but if the pH is below 7.25 the infant will usually require mechanical ventilation. Sodium bicarbonate should not be given if the P_{aCO_2} is more than 45 mmHg (6 kPa). If the base excess is more than –10 mmol/L and the P_{aCO_2} exceeds 45 mmHg (6 kPa), then THAM can be used. The dose is 0.3 M strength, 7 mL/kg infused over 30–60 min. THAM buffers H^+ and binds CO_2, thus lowering the P_{aCO_2}. It may cause apnoea and should only be used in infants being mechanically ventilated.

RESPIRATORY ALKALOSIS

This is due to overventilation and if it occurs while an infant is receiving mechanical ventilation it is simply treated by reducing the ventilator rate or inspiratory pressure.

Typical examples of acid–base derangements in the newborn, with interpretation and possible causes, are shown in Table 11.3.

Respiratory failure

This can be defined clinically as occurring when a baby fails to maintain adequate ventilation because of apnoea, on the basis of blood-gas estimations. Hypoxia may be due to either respiratory or cardiac abnormalities and, as an isolated factor, is not of great value in predicting the need for respiratory support. Hypercapnia is a much better indicator of respiratory failure. A rising P_{aCO_2}, particularly in the presence of a falling pH (respiratory

Table 11.3 Examples of abnormal arterial blood-gas results and their interpretation

F_{IO_2}	P_aO_2 mmHg (kPa)	pH	P_aCO_2 mmHg (kPa)	BE	Bicarbonate (mmol/L)	Interpretation	Possible cause
0.21	75 (10)	7.13	60 (8)	−10	13	Mixed acidosis	Severe birth asphyxia
0.65	53 (7)	7.18	60 (8)	−8	15	Mixed acidosis. Hypoxia	Acute RDS
0.35	53 (7)	7.33	68 (9)	+8	34	Chronic resp. acidosis with renal compensation	Bronchopulmonary dysplasia
0.21	83 (11)	7.53	53 (7)	+15	44	Metabolic alkalosis with mild respiratory compensation	Vomiting. Pyloric stenosis

Table 11.4 Causes of respiratory failure in the neonate

Poor respiratory effort	Extreme immaturity, CNS depression, postoperative infections, metabolic, neuromuscular disease
Abnormal lungs	Surfactant deficiency—RDS Retained fetal lung fluid—TTN Pulmonary oedema—hydrops, CCF
Abnormal airways	Infections—pneumonia Obstructed airways—meconium, pneumothorax
Hypoplastic lungs	Obstructive uropathy Diaphragmatic hernia
Small thoracic volume	Bowel obstruction, exomphalos/gastroschisis repair, ascites, chondrodystrophic dwarfism

acidosis), is an ominous sign. A $Paco_2$ above 60 mmHg (8 kPa), with a respiratory acidosis (pH < 7.25), indicates the need for mechanical ventilation. Some infants, particularly if very small, may require ventilation before these criteria are met, and this may be important in the prevention of intracranial haemorrhage. Hypercapnia and acidosis are strongly associated with the development of intraventricular haemorrhage in premature infants see p. 227. The causes of respiratory failure are listed in Table 11.4.

Assisted ventilation

The methods of conventional ventilation for infants with respiratory distress are:

1 continuous distending airway pressure by either CPAP or continuous negative pressure to the chest wall. CPAP is the technique usually employed, and this may be administered via a face mask, a single nasal prong, twin nasal cannulae or an endotracheal tube; and

2 positive-pressure ventilation by means of a continuous-flow, pressure-limited, time-cycled mechanical ventilator.

CONTINUOUS POSITIVE AIRWAY PRESSURE

Mechanisms of CPAP

The first published report of the use of CPAP in the treatment of respiratory distress syndrome (RDS) was in 1971 (Gregory *et al.* 1971), and since then the technique has been widely used in the treatment of this condition. Infants with RDS often grunt on expiration because of their own attempts to apply an end-expiratory distending pressure. Exhalation against a closed glottis produces a grunt and maintains a larger functional residual capacity. CPAP mimics and augments this expiratory grunt. Continuous distending pressure maintains expansion of the alveoli and terminal bronchioles on expiration. This ensures a reasonable lung volume with more even ventilation and reduces surfactant consumption. In addition, the better expanded alveoli excite pulmonary stretch receptors (Herring–Breuer reflex), which stimulate central respiratory drive. CPAP results in increased Pao_2 in surfactant-deficient 'stiff' lungs, but has a variable effect on $Paco_2$.

The introduction of CPAP to a preterm infant with RDS results in a decrease in respiratory rate, expiratory grunt, chest retractions and apnoea, and improves oxygenation, regularity of breathing and, from a physiological viewpoint, dynamic compliance, tidal volume and functional residual capacity.

Applying CPAP

CPAP may be administered by:

1 *face mask*. A soft-rimmed face mask (Bennett or Laerdal) is attached over the mouth and nose by Netelast tubing around the infant's head. In the past the mask was applied

by a tight Velcro band and this caused significant compression of the occipital bone, which damaged the cerebellum. The mask must not be too tightly applied in an attempt to produce an airtight seal.

The disadvantages of this method are difficulty in securing it in active babies, inability to suction the mouth and nose and the production of gastric distension. It obviates the need for cannulation of the nostril or trachea;

2 *nasal prong(s)*. A lubricated straight silastic or PVC cannula is inserted into one or both nostrils. Alternatively, a short tube may be positioned in the anterior nares or a slightly longer catheter situated in the nasopharynx. A 2.5 or 3.0 mm soft, opaque endotracheal tube cut short is ideal. This leaves the mouth and airway available for suction.

A recent advance in the delivery of nasal CPAP is the CPAP Driver, which utilizes the concept of coandal effect and fluidic flip to decrease the work of breathing and produce more even pressure throughout the respiratory cycle.

The disadvantages of nasal prongs include obstruction of the narrow-bore tube, gastric distension and pressure necrosis of the nares. Increased nasal secretions and mucus plugs lead to obstructive and mixed apnoea, often delaying the successful removal of CPAP; and

3 *endotracheal tube*. This method is of value when a baby is being weaned from the ventilator. It has the disadvantages of tracheal intubation (see p. 308) but protects the airway and allows nasogastric feeding.

The circuit is set up so that there is a continuous flow of well-humidified gas across the tube or face mask. A pressure valve on the distal side of the circuit measures CPAP. The pressure is varied by altering the flow rate of the air and oxygen mixture or by a limiting valve. It is usually administered through a pressure-limited mechanical ventilator set to CPAP mode.

Indications for CPAP

1 *RDS*. This is the classic indication in spontaneously breathing babies. For infants less than 1500 g birthweight CPAP is indicated if inspired O_2 exceeds 60%, to maintain $Po_2 > 60$ mmHg (8 kPa). For many infants CPAP will be adequate, but mechanical ventilation is indicated if Fio_2 exceeds 0.8–0.9. For infants of 800–1500 g birthweight who are vigorous at birth, CPAP may be commenced to maintain airway stabilization and allow time to assess the presence and severity of RDS. Mechanical ventilation is required if Fio_2 exceeds 0.6, $Paco_2$ exceeds 55 mmHg (7.3 kPa) (particularly if pH < 7.25) or the baby has apnoea. CPAP has proved beneficial in facilitating successful extubation in very low birthweight (VLBW) infants in many randomized trials.

The optimal pressure is difficult to predict. Generally CPAP of 4–8 cmH$_2$O is appropriate, but some infants benefit from higher pressures. This can be assessed by increasing the CPAP to 10 cmH$_2$O while watching a continuous readout of Pao_2. The lowest pressure that produces the best arterial oxygenation is the optimal CPAP pressure.

Regular evaluation of $Paco_2$ and arterial pH is necessary to assess the infant's response to CPAP, and mechanical ventilation may be necessary if deterioration occurs.

2 *Apnoea*. Stimulation of the Herring–Breuer reflex by CPAP at 2–3 cmH$_2$O may be effective in treating recurrent apnoea in some babies. Methyl xanthine treatment is usually tried before resorting to CPAP (see p. 329).

3 *Neuromuscular disorders*. In conditions where there is reduced lung volume owing to poor fetal breathing movements, CPAP may be of some value.

4 *Skeletal disorders*. In certain conditions, such as neonatal rickets, where there is a highly compliant chest wall, CPAP of 4 cmH$_2$O may be beneficial by increasing functional residual capacity and thereby reducing the work of breathing.

5 *Chronic pulmonary insufficiency of prematurity*. See p. 113.

6 *Pulmonary oedema*. This may be due to congestive cardiac failure, fluid overload or patent ductus arteriosus.

Complications

1 Pneumothorax or pulmonary interstitial emphysema due to overdistension of alveoli.
2 Gastric distension and vomiting with face mask and nasal prongs.
3 Hypercapnia.
4 Pressure necrosis owing to a tight nasal tube.
5 Cerebellar haemorrhage and skull deformities with a tight face mask.
6 Nasal secretion, mucus plugs.

Ventilation techniques

There is no agreement as to the best method for ventilating ill neonates, and the ventilator settings will vary with the indication for mechanical ventilation. Babies with RDS have stiff lungs (low compliance) and relatively fast rates are usually used. These vary between 60 and 100 cycles/min. Larger babies (> 1800 g) with severe RDS can be successfully ventilated at considerably slower rates (approximately 30 cycles/min). Clearly the rate will to some extent dictate the choice of inspiratory and expiratory times. Babies with pulmonary interstitial emphysema (PIE) or persistent pulmonary hypertension are usually ventilated fast (80–120 cycles/min) with very short inspiratory times (0.2–0.3 s), and this allows lower peak inspiratory pressures to be used. High-frequency oscillatory ventilation is being used more frequently for severe lung disease (p. 124), although this technique has not been fully evaluated.

INSPIRATION

The appropriate inspiratory pressure also depends on the underlying disease process. Infants with normal lungs (apnoea, asphyxia, sedation) require low pressures (< 18 cmH_2O), whereas those with stiff lungs may require considerably higher pressures (up to 40 cmH_2O or above). Higher positive inspiratory pressure (PIP) will generally improve ventilation but may impair venous return, with resultant systemic hypotension.

EXPIRATION

Expiration is a passive process caused by relaxation of the chest wall and the lungs. The shorter the expiratory phase the less fully the lungs deflate, and hyperinflation may occur. Full expiration is generally 1.5 times the inspiratory time. Initial ventilator settings for an infant with RDS who has not yet received surfactant might be: rate 60 cycles/min, inspiratory time 0.4 s and expiratory time 0.6 s. After surfactant treatment, inspiratory time can be shortened to 0.25–0.3 s and inspiratory pressure reduced.

PEEP

Positive end-expiratory pressure (PEEP) is used in mechanically ventilated infants in a similar way to CPAP in spontaneously breathing infants. Levels of 4–8 cmH_2O may be appropriate. The PEEP may be altered by adjusting the rate of gas flow through the ventilator or by adjusting the expiratory relief valve.

INITIAL VENTILATOR SETTINGS

The initial intermittent positive-pressure ventilation (IPPV) settings for various indications are shown in Table 11.5.

Paralysis/sedation/analgesia

Infants requiring mechanical ventilation benefit from sedation with agents such as midazolam or lorazepam and/or analgesia with morphine or fentanyl. These drugs may be used as continuous infusions or intermittent dosing as required. The newer techniques, such as trigger ventilation, reduce the need for sedation or analgesia.

Large infants often struggle or 'fight' the ventilator, which makes adequate ventilation difficult. If a baby (large or small) makes vigorous expiratory efforts which coincide with the inspiratory phase of ventilation, there is a high risk of pneumothorax (Greenough *et al*. 1984). To prevent these problems neuromuscular paralysis with pancuronium has been recom-

Table 11.5 Ventilator settings when initiating ventilation for four different conditions. Changes are made on the basis of blood-gas data and non-invasive monitoring

	RDS (pre-surfactant)	PIE/pulmonary hypertension	Apnoea	Meconium aspiration
Rate	60/min	80/min	30/min	60/min
PIP (cmH$_2$O)	25–30	20–25	14–16	30
PEEP (cmH$_2$O)	5	4	3–5	5
I : E ratio	2 : 3	1 : 1	–	2 : 3
Inspiratory time (s)	0.4	0.4	0.4	0.4
Fio_2	0.8	1.0	0.21	1.0

I : E, inspiration: expiration.

mended. This is a non-depolarizing muscle relaxant with a variable duration of action. Inducing paralysis is dangerous if accidental extubation occurs. An experienced paediatrician should be nearby to reintubate any paralysed infant. After muscle paralysis ventilator settings may need to be increased to prevent hypoventilation associated with loss of spontaneous respiratory activity. Ileus is often induced by muscle relaxants and limb contractures may develop. Regular passive movement of all joints should be carried out throughout the duration of paralysis.

MECHANICAL VENTILATION

Since 1971 the standard method of mechanical ventilation has been intermittent mandatory ventilation (IMV), a technique combining mechanical and spontaneous breathing. From 1971 to 1995 a myriad of positive-pressure, continuous-flow, time-cycled ventilators were developed, most being pressure controlled, but some volume controlled. The 1990s has seen an explosion of more advanced forms of ventilatory support, such as patient-triggered ventilation, high-frequency oscillatory ventilation (HFOV), high-frequency jet ventilation and extracorporeal membrane oxygenation (ECMO).

Conventional ventilation

Positive-pressure ventilation applies a positive-

pressure breath directly to the lungs through an endo- or nasotracheal tube. Face masks may also be used, but a reliable seal between mask and face is difficult to maintain. Tracheal intubation is described in the procedure manual (see p. 308).

Conventional ventilators are of the pressure-cycled, time-limited variety. The ventilator delivers gases at a preset pressure and maintains this for a predetermined period of time, producing either a square-wave or a sine-wave pattern on inspiration and expiration (Fig. 11.2). In addition, there should be a continuous flow of gas throughout the respiratory cycle. This allows IMV or the ability to wean the baby by prolonging the expiratory time when the baby's own respiratory effort is improving. CPAP is a valuable method of treating RDS and its application in mechanical ventilation is referred to as PEEP. The ventilator must also have an integrated humidifier with a preset heater to control inspired gas temperature. Alarms which indicate gas supply failure or accidental disconnection are also essential. Advances in microprocessor technology and ventilation design have enabled the introduction of patient-triggered ventilation for achieving synchronization between spontaneous and mechanical breaths. Synchronized ventilation modes are characterized by the delivery of mechanical breaths in response to a signal delivered from the infant's spontaneous respiratory effort. Terminology varies, but collectively these modes are usually called 'patient-triggered ventilation' (PTV) and consist of synchronized

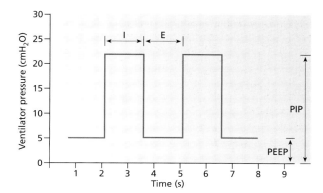

Fig. 11.2 Square-wave pattern of inspiration (I) and expiration (E) produced by a modern pressure-cycled, time-limited ventilator.

intermittent mandatory ventilation (SIMV), assist/control (also known as synchronized intermittent positive-pressure ventilation (SIPPV)) and pressure support ventilation.

Pulmonary vasodilators

In the presence of intrapulmonary shunting or pulmonary hypertension, pulmonary vasodilators such as magnesium sulphate, tolazoline, prostacyclin or nitroprusside are commonly used. These drugs are non-specific vasodilators and usually cause systemic hypotension, necessitating intravascular volume expansion and pressor agents. The response to these agents is unpredictable and often not sustained. Inhaled nitric oxide is a specific pulmonary vasodilator with a more predictable response and fewer unwanted side-effects. The treatment of persistent pulmonary hypertension is discussed fully on p. 199.

Endotracheal tube care

The endotracheal tube is the narrowest part of the entire ventilator circuit and is most likely to cause problems. The estimated length of the endotracheal tube is shown in Table 30.1 (see p. 309).

BLOCKAGE

Tube blockage with secretions or blood is common and should be anticipated if the infant deteriorates suddenly. Reintubation should

be performed if there is any doubt as to its patency. Blockage is best avoided by regular lavage and suction of the endotracheal tube. Normal saline (0.5–1 mL) is instilled into the tube and the infant ventilated for a further three to five cycles before suctioning of the endotracheal tube. This is not necessary on the first day of life but should be performed routinely 4-hourly after this time. In some infants with excessive secretions (e.g. meconium aspiration, or pneumonia postoperatively) more frequent suctioning is required.

MISPLACED TUBE

After intubation the position of the endotracheal tube tip should be checked radiologically. The tube may cause collapse due to blockage of the right upper lobe bronchus. If the tube is pushed down the right main bronchus, the entire left lung may collapse. Pulling the tube back and chest physiotherapy usually result in complete re-expansion.

General management of ventilated infants

1 Regular arterial blood-gas assessment, initially 4-hourly and less frequently as the infant stabilizes. Continuous monitoring of oxygenation with transcutaneous Po_2 monitor and/or pulse oximetry and CO_2 with transcutaneous Pco_2 monitor.
2 Regular or continuous blood pressure monitoring with vigorous treatment of hypotension

(see p. 185) by plasma, albumin solution or dopamine.

3 Regular bacteriological surveillance and appropriate use of antibiotics.

4 Chest physiotherapy.

5 Adequate humidification of inspired gases.

6 Nursing in a thermoneutral environment.

7 Careful assessment of fluid balance.

Assessment of ventilation

The effectiveness of mechanical ventilation is judged by the observation of symmetrical chest wall movement, auscultation of equal air entry to both lungs and arterial blood-gas measurements.

Troubleshooting

If sudden deterioration occurs during mechanical ventilation, then check ventilator failure, e.g. tube connection, tube blockage, accidental extubation into the oesophagus and tension pneumothorax.

When hypoxia or hypercapnia occur during ventilation it is essential to check whether a mechanical mishap or medical complication has occurred. If these factors are excluded, it may be appropriate to alter the ventilator settings.

Depending on the clinical circumstances hypoxia would generally be defined as a PaO_2 < 50 mmHg (6.7 kPa); the clinical response would depend on circumstances and ventilator settings, but would include:

↑Fio_2; ↑PIP; ↑PEEP; ↑Insp. time

The concept of permissive hypercapnia ($Paco_2$ = 45–60 mmHg) is widely accepted, but a $Paco_2$ > 60 mmHg would generally necessitate a change in ventilator settings, including:

↑rate; ↑PIP; ↓PEEP; ↓dead space if possible

Complications of mechanical ventilation

1 Pneumothorax and pulmonary air leak (see p. 101). Reversed I : E ratio and high levels of PEEP are most likely to cause this condition.

2 Intraventricular haemorrhage (see p. 227).

3 Patent ductus arteriosus (see p. 198).

4 Subglottic stenosis (see p. 132).

5 Bronchopulmonary dysplasia (see p. 110).

New strategies in mechanical ventilation

PATIENT-TRIGGERED VENTILATION

With this system the baby's spontaneous inspiratory efforts are detected and the ventilator responds by providing an inspiratory breath approximately 50 ms later. The rationale for the widespread introduction of PTV into clinical practice has been to reduce complications, decrease the need for sedation and facilitate earlier extubation.

HIGH-FREQUENCY OSCILLATORY VENTILATION

This technique uses very high frequency rates of 600–900 cycles/min (10–15 Hz) to maintain oxygenation, eliminate CO_2 and stabilize the circulation. High-frequency oscillators are essentially airway vibrators, usually piston pumps or vibratory diaphragms. During HFOV inspiration and expiration are both active, with little bulk gas delivery. Pressure oscillators within the airway produce tiny tidal volumes around a constant mean airway pressure, which maintains lung volume.

The amplitude of airway pressure oscillators (σP) is the prime determinant of CO_2 removal, with decreases in frequency occasionally required for hypercarbia. Inadequate oxygenation, atelectasis and poor lung expansion usually respond to increases in mean airway pressure. The multicentre trials provide conflicting results but the technique is gaining acceptance for the ventilation of infants with pulmonary air leaks, surfactant-resistant RDS, congenital diaphragmatic hernia and persistent pulmonary hypertension.

HIGH-FREQUENCY JET VENTILATION

Gas from a high-pressure source is delivered

into the trachea in very short bursts down a fine cannula within the endotracheal tube. These 'bullets' of gas entrain additional gas down the endotracheal tube. This technique may be particularly useful in infants with PIE as the PIP can be lowered.

EXTRACORPOREAL MEMBRANE OXYGENATION

This technique is widely used in the USA but has not become available in more than a few centres in Europe and Australia. The main indications appear to be severe respiratory failure and pulmonary hypertension due to conditions such as meconium aspiration. The technique requires access to both a central vein and a common carotid artery, which is ligated. More recently venovenous circuits have been used, thereby sparing the artery. The circuit oxygenates the blood and returns it to the baby. The criterion for considering ECMO is a > 80% predicted mortality from conventional ventilation. Because of the technical difficulties and the requirement for systemic heparinization, the technique is confined to babies weighing less than 2 kg. A multicentre controlled study of ECMO vs. traditional ventilation undertaken in Britain demonstrated a decreased death rate in infants allocated to ECMO irrespective of primary diagnosis, disease severity or type of referral centre. There was one extra survivor for every 3–4 infants allocated ECMO (UK Collaborative ECMO Trial Group, 1996).

LIQUID VENTILATION

It has been shown that babies can be ventilated using oxygenated inert fluorocarbon liquid at about 10 cycles/min, and this is the subject of considerable research interest.

REFERENCES

Greenough, A., Morley, C.J., Wood, S. & Davis, J.A. (1984) Pancuronium prevents pneumothoraces in ventilated premature babies who actively expire against positive pressure inflation. *Lancet* **1**, 1–3.

Gregory, G.A., Kitterman, J.A., Phibbs, R.H., Tooley, W.H. & Hamilton, W.K. (1971) Treatment of the idiopathic respiratory distress syndrome with continuous positive airway pressure. *New England Journal of Medicine* **284**, 1333–1339.

UK Collaborative ECMO Trial Group (1996) UK Collaborative randomised trial of neonatal ECMO. *Lancet* **348**, 75–82.

FURTHER READING

Avery, G.B., Fletcher, M.A. & MacDonald, M.G. (eds) (1994) *Neonatology: Pathophysiology and Management of the Newborn*, 4th edn. Lippincott-Raven, Philadelphia.

Spitzer, A.R. (1994) *Intensive Care of Fetus and Neonate*. C.V. Mosby, St Louis.

The Cochrane Collaboration Library: Pregnancy and Childbirth Database (CD-ROM), Update Software Ltd, Oxford.

12 Apnoea, bradycardia and upper airway obstruction

PHYSIOLOGY

The onset of breathing begins early in fetal life. It is intermittent, irregular and occurs only during periods of active (rapid eye movement, REM) sleep. The function of fetal breathing is not fully understood as it has no role in gas exchange. Lung growth is dependent at least in part on fetal breathing activity, and the fetus who does not breathe is at risk of lung hypoplasia (p. 106).

After birth there is a marked change from intermittent fetal breathing to continuous breathing, but the mechanism by which this happens is not known, although increased Pao_2 levels after birth are a factor. Although neonatal breathing is continuous it is irregular, and this is particularly the case in the preterm infant. Infants, particularly the preterm, have less well-developed chemoreceptor responses to hypoxia and hypercapnia. Hypercapnia increases respiratory activity and hypoxia causes an initial increase in respiratory activity lasting several minutes, followed by a decrease in ventilatory frequency.

Normal breathing patterns in the newborn can be divided into four different types.

1 *Regular*. This is infrequent, when there are nearly equal breath-to-breath intervals.

2 *Irregular*. Unequal breath-to-breath intervals; this is particularly common in preterm infants.

3 *Periodic breathing*. Cycles of hyperventilation alternating with periods of hypoventilation and eventual apnoea lasting about 3 s.

4 *'Apnoea'*. Episodes of respiratory pause lasting 6 s or more. With advancing gestation to term, the proportion of time the infant is breathing regularly increases and phases of irregular, periodic and apnoeic periods decline. Further maturation occurs in the months after birth.

APNOEA AND BRADYCARDIA

Clinically significant apnoea is defined as a cessation of breathing lasting for 20 s or more. Apnoea lasting for less than 20 s is also significant if accompanied by colour change, or bradycardia of less than 100 beats/min.

Apnoea is most common in more immature babies. It is seen in 25% of infants of birthweight < 2500 g and over 80% of infants with birthweight < 1000 g (Miller & Martin 1992). It is most common at the end of the first week of life, and then tends to become less frequent as the baby matures.

Aetiology of apnoea and bradycardia

In the term infant the aetiology is usually identified, whereas in the preterm infant it is unusual to find a cause. Recurrent apnoea of prematurity is presumed to be due to immaturity of the respiratory centre in the brainstem and immaturity of chemoreceptor response to hypoxia and acidosis.

Types of apnoea

CENTRAL APNOEA

Central apnoea accounts for 25% of all cases of neonatal apnoea. It is due to factors affecting the respiratory centre in the brainstem or the higher centres in the cerebral cortex. Causes include:

1 prematurity;

2 hypoxia/acidosis (e.g. in respiratory distress syndrome (RDS), pneumonia, pneumothorax);

3 drugs (e.g. maternal narcotics, trishydroxyaminonethane (THAM), prostacyclin, magnesium sulphate);

4 metabolic (e.g. hypoglycaemia, hypocalcaemia, hypomagnesaemia or hypermagnesaemia);
5 generalized sepsis or specific infection (meningitis, encephalitis). Apnoea occurring early in the course of respiratory distress must alert the medical attendant to the possibility of group B β-haemolytic streptococcal septicaemia;
6 intracranial haemorrhage;
7 polycythaemia with hyperviscosity;
8 necrotizing enterocolitis;
9 patent ductus arteriosus;
10 convulsions (see p. 230);
11 developmental anomalies of the brain;
12 temperature instability. Nursing an infant in too high an environmental incubator temperature is an important and common cause of apnoea. In addition, hypothermia, too rapid warming or too rapid cooling may be associated with apnoea.

OBSTRUCTIVE APNOEA

Babies are obligatory nose breathers and if their nares are obstructed, especially while sleeping, they are prone to severe apnoea. Obstructive apnoea accounts for 15% of cases and occurs with congenital malformations, such as choanal atresia and the Pierre Robin syndrome. Preterm infants with small upper airways may have apnoea when in the supine position, especially during active (REM) sleep. Apnoea of this type may be minimized by nursing the infant in the prone position. Babies with milk, mucus or meconium lodged in the upper airway are likely to have severe episodes of obstructive apnoea.

MIXED APNOEA

Mixed apnoea accounts for the majority (approximately 60%) of cases, but may be difficult to diagnose clinically. Superficially it resembles central apnoea initially, with cessation of respiration, but then the baby makes intermittent respiratory efforts without achieving gas exchange.

REFLEX APNOEA

Babies may develop reflex apnoea or vagally mediated apnoea due to suction of the pharynx or stomach, the passage of a nasogastric tube, physiotherapy, or sometimes even in response to defecation. Apnoea associated with gastro-oesophageal reflux may be reflex and/or obstructive.

Investigation of apnoea

All babies who suffer from apnoea must be carefully examined to exclude respiratory or remote disease. Investigations are carried out to determine treatable causes of apnoea and will depend on the prevailing clinical condition. Investigations include:
1 full blood count;
2 bacterial culture of blood, urine, cerebrospinal fluid (CSF), tracheal aspirate and other potential sites of infection;
3 chest X-ray;
4 blood glucose;
5 serum electrolytes, including calcium, magnesium and sodium;
6 arterial blood gases and continuous monitoring of oxygen saturation and perhaps P_{CO_2};
7 ultrasound examination of the head;
8 if gastro-oesophageal reflux is suspected, a number of further investigations may be undertaken, including an intra-oesophageal pH probe and/or contrast study (see p. 56);
9 in special circumstances further neurological investigations may be necessary, i.e. electroencephalogram (EEG), polygraphic sleep studies.

APNOEA MONITORING

A variety of respiratory monitors are available, including a pressure-sensitive pad on which the infant lies, an air-filled plastic blister attached to the abdomen (Graseby Medical) and impedance monitors using electrodes attached to the chest wall. None of these will detect obstructive apnoea until the infant stops fighting for breath. The use of an electrocardiogram (ECG) monitor together with an apnoea monitor is recommended in order to recognize bradycardia occurring with an obstructed airway.

Treatment of apnoea

GENERAL MANAGEMENT

Prevention and early detection

Apnoeic episodes should be prevented whenever possible. This involves careful handling of low birthweight infants and attention to feeding techniques, with avoidance of stomach distension and rapid feeding. The infant's temperature needs to be maintained in the thermoneutral range. Careful suctioning of the airway will minimize obstruction.

Treatment of an underlying cause

This depends on the results of the relevant investigations.

Acute episode

A suggested approach is shown in Fig. 12.1. The following procedures are recommended:
1 stimulation of the infant. If the episodes are brief and not associated with systemic features, this may be all that is necessary;
2 suction of the upper airways is indicated when obstruction is the likely cause;
3 manual ventilation with a face mask and bag;
4 intubation and intermittent positive-pressure ventilation will be necessary when the baby fails to respond to bag-and-mask ventilation, or when severe apnoeic attacks occur frequently.

Recurrent apnoea

This usually occurs in preterm infants and may be very difficult to manage. However, before embarking on extreme forms of treatment, the potential hazards of the therapy must be carefully balanced against the brain-damaging effects of the apnoeic episode. The following techniques are employed in the management of recurrent apnoea:
1 nurse in the prone position;
2 consider altering feeding regimen, i.e. a continuous milk infusion may be better tolerated than intermittent feeds or transpyloric feeding;
3 if anaemia is thought to be a cause, then it should be treated by blood transfusion, but the lowest acceptable level of haemoglobin may be difficult to determine (see p. 204);
4 increasing the inspired oxygen to 25% while monitoring the oxygen tension;
5 specific treatment includes drugs, continuous positive airway pressure (CPAP) and frequent stimulation.

STIMULATION

Tactile stimulation by regular stroking of the infant has been shown to reduce the number of apnoeic episodes, but this is not a feasible method for routine use. A variety of rocking mattresses have been devised which gently rock or undulate the baby and which appear to reduce the frequency of apnoeas in some infants.

DRUG TREATMENT

This is only indicated when specific causes of apnoea have been treated. Drugs for apnoea are usually continued until the baby is 35–37 weeks of postmenstrual age.

Methyl xanthines

Theophylline is given orally in a loading dose of 6 mg/kg and a daily maintenance dose of 3 mg/kg/day in two or three divided doses. The half-life of theophylline varies between 12 and 56 h. Serum levels of both aminophylline and theophylline should be maintained between 6 and 13 µg/mL. Levels up to 20 µg/mL may be acceptable if there is a poor clinical response to the lower range. Tachycardia and irritability are the first signs of overdosage.

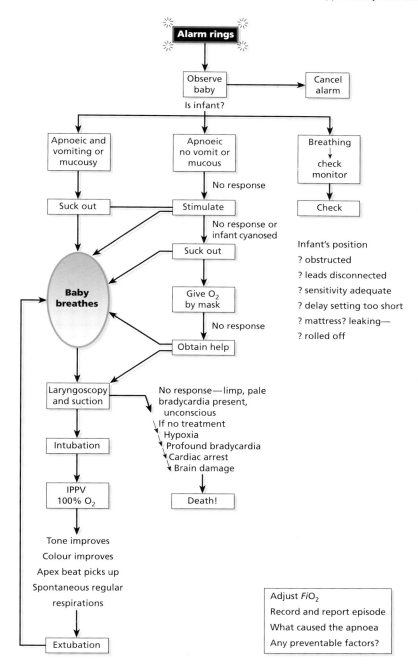

Fig. 12.1 Suggested protocol following an apnoea or bradycardia alarm.

Caffeine. The neonate methylates theophylline to caffeine and caffeine may be used to treat apnoea. The loading dose is 20 mg/kg orally followed by 2.5–5 mg/kg once daily. Serum levels of caffeine should be monitored and the therapeutic range is between 10 and 20 μg/mL.

Aminophylline is given intravenously, with a loading dose of 6 mg/kg followed by a maintenance dose of 4.5 mg/kg/day given in divided doses 8- or 12-hourly. Serum levels must be regularly monitored starting 48 h after the loading dose.

Doxapram is effective in infants in whom recurrent apnoea cannot be controlled by methyl xanthines. The dose is 0.5–2.0 mg/kg/h by continuous infusion. Extreme jitteriness is a well-recognized side-effect.

Ventilatory support

CPAP may be effective in treating or preventing apnoea. It probably acts in a number of ways, but mainly by splinting open the upper airway structures. It has little effect on central apnoea. The use of nasal prongs to administer CPAP (2–4 cmH$_2$O) may produce additional effects by local stimulation. The administration of CPAP is described in Chapter 11.

In a controlled study of aminophylline vs. CPAP in the treatment of recurrent apnoea of prematurity, aminophylline was found to be more effective and associated with fewer complications (Jones 1982), and is the recommended first-line treatment. Theophylline may be more effective for central apnoea and CPAP may be more effective in obstructive or mixed apnoea.

In infants who are resistant to CPAP and respiratory stimulants and who continue to have severe apnoeic attacks, intubation and mechanical ventilation are required to avoid major physiological changes associated with the apnoeic episodes. Only minimal pressures and rates are usually required.

Prognosis

It is important to distinguish the cause of the apnoea from its effect with respect to prognosis. There is an association between recurrent apnoea and later cerebral palsy, but this may reflect the common origin of the brain lesion that causes both the movement disorder, the prematurity and the resultant apnoea. In general, outcome is related to the underlying cause, and when correction is made for confounding factors, apnoea *per se* has no additional deleterious effect on outcome.

Recurrent apnoea of prematurity has usually resolved by 37 weeks' postmenstrual age, but in some infants apnoea may persist beyond the expected date of delivery and no cause can be found. In some cases discharge home on methyl xanthine drugs is recommended, and home apnoea monitors may be of benefit.

SUDDEN INFANT DEATH SYNDROME

Neonatologists must be aware of the risk of sudden infant death syndrome (SIDS) in survivors of neonatal care and give appropriate advice to reduce the risk once the baby has gone home. There are a number of risk factors for SIDS which are relevant to the neonatologist. These include:
1 maternal smoking or drug abuse;
2 prematurity;
3 low birthweight;
4 multiple births;
5 apparent life-threatening events in the neonatal unit (see below).

The incidence of SIDS has fallen in recent years by up to 75% in countries where risk reduction procedures have been widely adopted. These include:
1 putting babies to sleep on their backs;
2 avoiding exposing the baby to tobacco smoke;
3 avoidance of overwrapping the baby and prevention of overheating;

4 breastfeeding has been shown to have a protective effect in some countries;

5 additional factors which may be important include early advice about minor illnesses, and discouraging having the baby in the bed with the parents (cosleeping).

It is important for staff on neonatal units to recognize those babies at high risk and to discuss risk reduction procedures with the parents. Instruction on resuscitation (showing the parents an appropriate video followed by a question and answer session), and for a few the provision of an apnoea monitor for when the baby goes home, is part of this care.

HOME APNOEA MONITORS

The parents of prematurely born babies may request apnoea monitors for use at home. There is no evidence that home monitoring reduces the risk of a major life-threatening event occurring out of hospital, nor do they prevent death: babies have died despite being monitored.

The American National Institutes of Health published a Consensus Statement (1987) on home apnoea monitoring. The group agreed that there was no evidence that apnoea of prematurity is an independent risk factor for either apnoeic spells later in infancy or for SIDS. An apparent life-threatening event (an episode of apnoea with colour change and limpness that is frightening to the observer) is, however, a risk factor for later SIDS, and these babies should have home apnoea monitoring. The consensus view on indications for home apnoea monitoring includes:

1 one or more apparently life-threatening events associated with apnoea and requiring vigorous resuscitation;

2 symptomatic preterm infants;

3 siblings of two or more SIDS victims. The group felt that home apnoea monitoring of subsequent infants after a single case of SIDS could not be scientifically justified;

4 infants with hypoventilation conditions.

Most paediatricians believe that the use of monitors at home for less rigorous indications than those recommended by the consensus group is justified if it is felt that this will lead to significantly reduced parental anxiety. It is essential that the parents are shown how to apply basic resuscitation skills to their infant prior to giving them an apnoea monitor, in case the baby is found apnoeic or collapsed at home.

UPPER AIRWAY OBSTRUCTION

Upper airway obstruction frequently presents in the delivery room or nursery as a result of foreign material in the airway, and can readily be relived by suction. Upper airway obstruction not relieved by suction is unusual and may be mild, occurring only when the infant is distressed, crying or during feeds. Severe airway obstruction at birth due to anatomical abnormalities may be life threatening.

Clinical Features

The cardinal signs of upper airway obstruction are:

1 stridor. This will be inspiratory if the obstruction is extrathoracic. If the obstruction is intrathoracic, there will be an expiratory component to the stridor;

2 suprasternal retractions. Although chest retractions may be evident, the most marked retractions will be suprasternal;

3 croupy cough;

4 hoarse cry.

With severe increasing upper airway obstruction the baby may develop cyanosis followed by apnoea and bradycardia.

Aetiology

The causes of upper airway obstruction in the newborn may be conveniently classified according to the site of obstruction:

1 intraluminal: foreign material such as mucus, blood, meconium or milk. Vocal cord

prolapse is a rare complication of a traumatic birth, or of inexpert intubation;

2 intramural obstruction: subglottic stenosis, laryngeal web, diaphragm, papilloma or haemangioma. Following intubation the most common cause of stridor is subglottic oedema; and

3 extramural obstruction: goitre, vascular ring or cystic hygroma.

Causes of persistent stridor have been reported to be (Phelan *et al.* 1982):

1 supraglottic, 62% (laryngomalacia 56%, lingual cysts 6%);

2 vocal cord, 15% (nerve palsies, webs, papilloma, foreign body);

3 subglottic stenosis, 14%;

4 tracheomalacia, 9%.

Laryngomalacia (infantile larynx)

The larynx in children with this condition is unusually floppy and narrows on inspiration, with resultant stridor. The stridor is often only present on crying. It is a benign condition that improves with age, but the stridor may not disappear until 6–9 months from birth. Diagnosis is made at laryngoscopy and the parents should be reassured that the condition is self-limiting in the majority of cases, although if persistent a paediatric ear, nose and throat (ENT) opinion is valuable.

Choanal atresia

This is a developmental anomaly of the nasal airways. It is caused by failure of the embryonic bucconasal membrane to cannulate, resulting in a bony or membranous obstruction which is usually unilateral and rarely bilateral. In the latter case recurrent cyanotic and apnoeic spells are a major problem from birth.

MANAGEMENT

The condition is diagnosed by the inability to pass a catheter through the nasal passage. An infant with bilateral choanal atresia might develop acute upper airway obstruction while sleeping or during a feed, and experience severe apnoea. Treatment involves the provision of a patent airway using a pharyngeal (Guedel) airway until corrective surgery can be undertaken.

Subglottic stenosis

This is most commonly an acquired condition and in the rarer congenital cases the baby often presents early with stridor. Acquired subglottic stenosis is usually related to trauma of the glottic structures by vigorous suction or intubation. More commonly it is related to prolonged intermittent positive pressure-ventilation (IPPV) through an endotracheal tube. With modern endotracheal tubes the incidence of this condition has fallen, and it now occurs in only 1% of ventilated infants.

The mechanisms by which stenosis develops are multifactorial, but physical ulceration from the tube, together with the piston action of the ventilator, is a very important causative factor. In addition, poor humidification of inspired gases and local infection may be contributory. The duration of intubation is important, but stenosis has been reported not uncommonly in infants intubated for only a few days.

Most infants with stridor following extubation have some subglottic oedema. Those with stenosis usually do not present until after discharge, when an intercurrent upper respiratory tract infection precipitates serious upper airway obstruction. Tracheostomy should be avoided wherever possible as, in many of these children, later closure of the tracheostomy is difficult. Surgical procedures such as repeated dilatation, or cryo- or laser surgery to split the cricoid cartilage anteriorly, may be successful in managing the condition.

DIAGNOSIS

A full physical examination must be undertaken to exclude cutaneous haemangiomas and cardiovascular system disease. Palpation for lingual and pharyngeal cysts should be carried out.

Investigations include:

1 *X-ray*. To show the soft tissues of the neck (lateral and anteroposterior views);

2 *laryngoscopy*. Some infants will tolerate laryngeal examination with a neonatal laryngoscope without a general anaesthetic. More severe forms of upper airway obstruction will require direct laryngoscopy and bronchoscopy under general anaesthesia;

3 *ciné barium swallow*. This will be necessary to exclude a vascular ring;

4 *special investigations*. Tomography or angiography may on occasion be necessary.

TREATMENT

1 *Emergency*. In the acute, severe situation where intubation is impossible, insertion of an intravenous cannula between the first and second tracheal rings or tracheostomy may be lifesaving.

2 *Corticosteroids*. Mucosal damage and oedema may be transient but resolution can be accelerated by the use of corticosteroids. These are given as intramuscular or intravenous dexamethasone 0.5 mg/kg body weight 8-hourly for 48 h.

3 *Non-specific measures*. Humidification with ultrasonic mist may be useful. Further laryngeal trauma should be avoided.

4 *Nebulized adrenaline*. Inhalation of nebulized adrenaline (0.5 mL of 1/1000 adrenaline in 0.5 mL saline) for 20–30 s every 2 h may assist the resolution of subglottic oedema.

5 *Treatment of the specific cause*. This may be necessary after close consultation with a paediatric physician and an ENT surgeon. Treatment may include tracheostomy.

REFERENCES

Consensus Statement (1987) National Institutes of Health Consensus Development Conference on Infantile Apnoea and Home Monitoring. *Pediatrics* **79**, 292–299.

Jones, R.A.K. (1982) Apnoea of immaturity. 1. A controlled trial of theophylline and face mask continuous positive airway pressure. *Archives of Disease in Childhood* **57**, 761–765.

Miller, M.J. & Martin, R.J. (1992) Apnea of prematurity. *Clinics in Perinatology* **19**, 789–808.

Phelan, P.D., Landau, L.I. & Olinsky, A. (eds) (1982) *Respiratory Illness in Children*, 2nd edn. Blackwell Scientific Publications, Oxford.

FURTHER READING

Hunt, C.E. (1992) Apnea and SIDS. In: *Clinics in Perinatology*, 19, number 4. W.B. Saunders, Philadelphia.

Kattwinkel, J. (1980) Apnoea in the neonatal period. *Paediatric Review* **2**, 107.

13 Jaundice

Neonatal jaundice is the most common problem encountered in the newborn. About 50% of all full-term infants and 85% of preterm infants are visibly jaundiced within the first week of life.

Unconjugated bilirubin, which is elevated in the most common forms of neonatal jaundice, can pass through the blood–brain barrier and cause permanent brain damage with chronic disability (see Kernicterus, p. 144).

Physiology of bilirubin metabolism

FETAL

In the uterus, the fetal liver is relatively inactive. The placenta and maternal liver metabolize the bilirubin from worn-out red blood cells. If there is excessive fetal red cell haemolysis, for example in rhesus haemolytic disease, the placenta and maternal liver may not be able to deal with the excessive bilirubin load and the umbilical cord and amniotic fluid will be stained yellow by the bilirubin pigment produced. In addition, the bone marrow and extramedullary organs of erythropoiesis may not be able to keep up with the production of red cells, so that the fetus will become anaemic. Hydrops fetalis, a condition associated with generalized oedema, pleural effusions, ascites and hepatosplenomegaly, is due to a combination of anaemia, intrauterine hypoxia, hypoproteinaemia, a low colloid osmotic pressure and congestive heart failure.

The fetus is capable of conjugating bilirubin in small amounts and when haemolysis occurs *in utero*, as for example in severe rhesus isoimmunization, bilirubin conjugation increases and high levels of direct-reacting bilirubin may be measured in the umbilical cord blood.

NEWBORN

The metabolism of bilirubin in the newborn is summarized in Fig. 13.1. Each of the steps in the metabolism of bile will be discussed in turn.

Bilirubin production

Most of the daily bilirubin production comes from senescent red blood cells. The red cells are destroyed in the reticuloendothelial system and the haem is converted to unconjugated bilirubin. One gram of haemoglobin will produce 600 μmol (35 mg) of unconjugated bilirubin. Haemolysis may be increased by maternal drugs such as salicylates, sulphonamides, phenacetin and Furadantin. Twenty-five per cent of the daily production of bilirubin comes from sources other than the red cells, such as haem protein and free (tissue) haem.

Transport and liver uptake

Most of the unconjugated bilirubin in the blood is bound to serum albumin and is transported as a bound complex to the liver. This binding is extremely important and may be altered by many factors. Those that decrease albumin binding ability include low serum albumin, asphyxia, acidosis, infection, prematurity and hypoglycaemia.

In addition, there are many competitors for bilirubin binding sites, and these include:
1 non-esterified (free) fatty acids produced by starvation, cold stress or Intralipid therapy;
2 drugs (sulphonamides, cephalosporins, sodium benzoate (present in diazepam), frusemide and thiazide diuretics).

When bilirubin is bound to albumin it is probably non-toxic, but free, unbound,

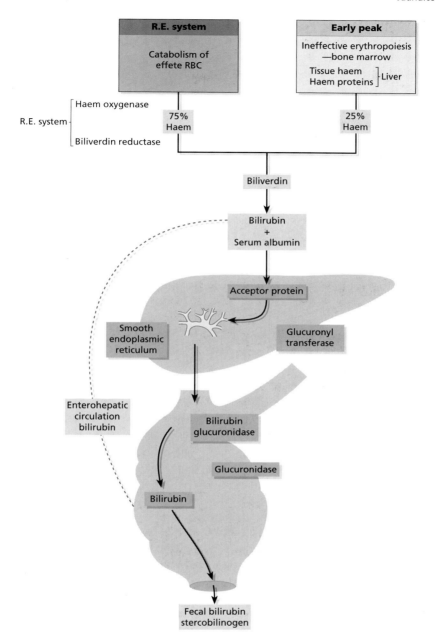

Fig. 13.1 Summary of neonatal bilirubin metabolism. (Redrawn from Maisels & Avery 1994, with permission.)

unconjugated bilirubin is fat soluble and can be transported across the blood–brain barrier and be deposited in certain neurons, causing kernicterus.

The hepatocytes lining the liver sinusoids are able to extract unconjugated bilirubin from the blood and this is then accepted in the liver cell by the Y and Z proteins (ligandins).

Conjugation and excretion

The unconjugated bilirubin is conjugated in the liver and the reaction involves the conversion of insoluble unconjugated bilirubin to direct-reacting bilirubin (water soluble). Each molecule of bilirubin is conjugated with two molecules of glucuronic acid and is catalysed by the enzyme glucuronyl transferase. The conjugated bilirubin is excreted into the bile and then into the duodenum and small intestine. In the older child the bilirubin is reduced to stercobilinogen by bacteria in the small bowel, but in the newborn with a relatively sterile bowel and poor peristalsis much of the conjugated bilirubin may be hydrolysed by glucuronidase to unconjugated bilirubin, which enters the enterohepatic circulation for further liver metabolism.

This may be important in pathological situations, and reinforcement of the enterohepatic circulation will increase unconjugated bilirubin levels in prematurity, small bowel obstruction, functional bowel obstruction and pyloric stenosis.

Clinical assessment of the jaundiced infant

Jaundice can be detected in the newborn period when the serum level is approximately 100 µmol/L. As jaundice is common it is essential to have a clinical method for determining its severity.

One clinical method of assessing the degree of jaundice present before investigations are undertaken is the use of Kramer's rule (Kramer 1969). This technique depends on the blanching of the infant's skin with the examiner's finger at standard zones (1–5) and observing the colour in the blanched area (Fig. 13.2). The zones of jaundice reflect the downward progression of dermal icterus.

In assessing the significance of jaundice in a newborn infant the following guidelines may be useful. Investigations should be carried out under the following circumstances:
1 any infant who is visibly jaundiced in the first 24 h of life;
2 any jaundiced infant whose mother has rhesus antibodies;
3 a preterm infant whose estimated serum bilirubin is greater than 150 µmol/L;
4 a term infant whose estimated serum bilirubin exceeds 200 µmol/L;
5 any infant who has the clinical signs of obstructive jaundice;
6 prolonged hyperbilirubinaemia beyond 1 week in term infants and 2 weeks in preterm infants.

When an infant is considered to have clinically significant jaundice, the assessment must include a thorough physical examination after careful history taking.

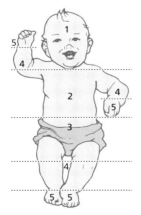

Kramer's rule	Serum indirect bilirubin (per µmol)	
Zone	Jaundice	Average
1	Limited to head and neck	100
2	Over upper trunk	150
3	Over lower trunk, thighs	200
4	Over arms, legs, below knee	250
5	Hands, feet	>250

Fig. 13.2 Kramer's rule for clinical assessment of neonatal jaundice. (Reproduced from Kramer 1969.)

The presence or absence of the following features should be noted:
1 extravascular blood, e.g. bruising, cephalhaematoma, purpura, petechiae;
2 plethora or pallor;
3 hepatosplenomegaly;
4 evidence of intrauterine infection: small for gestational age, cataracts, microcephaly;
5 infection: umbilicus, skin;
6 neurological signs: hypertonia, opisthotonus, fits, abnormal eye movements;
7 abdominal distension: associated with bowel obstruction, bowel stasis or hypothyroidism.

The routine physical examination of a jaundiced neonate should always include a urine test for bile and reducing substance and a description of the stools, i.e. whether they are pale. Bilirubin in the urine (tested by a 'stick' test) indicates that a component of the serum bilirubin is conjugated. This is an important factor in investigating the cause of jaundice.

Investigations

The investigation of a jaundiced newborn infant must take into consideration the history of the pregnancy, the gestational age and postnatal age of the infant and the initial physical examination. It is also important to note whether drugs or toxins may have been involved in its production, and the racial origins of the parents.

In any jaundiced infant two questions must be answered.
1 Is the unconjugated hyperbilirubinaemia likely to cause neurological damage?
2 Is the bilirubin conjugated?

Conjugated hyperbilirubinaemia is likely to be associated with a more serious cause, which in the case of biliary atresia must be rapidly diagnosed and early surgical treatment undertaken.

Repeated total serum bilirubin estimations should be performed in infants with a rapid and early rise of (unconjugated) bilirubin so that treatment for hyperbilirubinaemia can be instituted. Bilirubin in the urine indicates that the conjugated fraction of bilirubin should be estimated in the laboratory and causes of conjugated hyperbilirubinaemia considered. Table 13.1 lists the possible causes of jaundice

Table 13.1 Possible causes of jaundice presenting at different times in the neonatal period

Day	Unconjugated jaundice	Conjugated jaundice
1	Haemolytic disease assumed until proven otherwise	Neonatal hepatitis Rubella CMV Syphilis
2–5	Haemolysis Physiological Jaundice of prematurity Sepsis Extravascular blood Polycythaemia G-6-P dehydrogenase deficiency Spherocytosis	As above
5–10	Sepsis Breast milk jaundice Galactosaemia Hypothyroidism Drugs	As above
10 +	Sepsis Urinary tract infection	Biliary atresia Neonatal hepatitis Choledochal cyst Pyloric stenosis

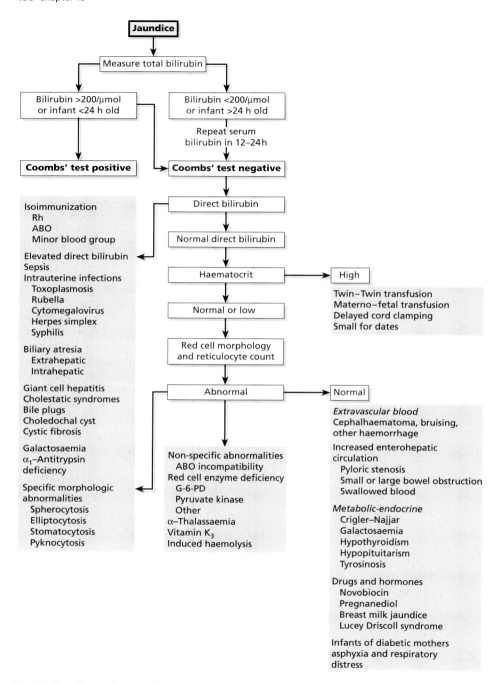

Fig. 13.3 Flow diagram showing a diagnostic approach to neonatal jaundice. (Modified from Maisels 1994.)

presenting at different times in the neonatal period.

A diagnostic approach to neonatal jaundice is shown in Fig. 13.3.

UNCONJUGATED HYPERBILIRUBINAEMIA

Causes

The causes of prolonged unconjugated hyperbilirubinaemia are shown in Table 13.2.

Investigations

Prolonged jaundice requires investigation when present for more than 10 days in a term infant, and 14 days in a premature one. The initial investigation must be to distinguish conjugated from unconjugated causes. Table 13.3 lists investigations for prolonged unconjugated hyperbilirubinaemia.

Management

PREVENTION

Early feeding reduces the incidence of jaundice by preventing dehydration and the elevation of free fatty acids. The maintenance of an adequate fluid intake is an essential part of the care of a jaundiced baby. In addition, feeding will overcome bowel stasis and minimize the effects of the enterohepatic bilirubin circulation. Breastfeeding-associated jaundice is minimized by frequent, early breastfeeding in the first 3 days of life.

PHOTOTHERAPY

This was first used by Cremer in 1958 in the UK, but has only been used widely since 1968, when Lucey (1972) showed its effectiveness in treating unconjugated hyperbilirubinaemia. It is particularly useful in preterm infants with non-haemolytic jaundice, and has resulted in a decline in the number of exchange transfusions being performed.

Phototherapy units, which emit light with a wavelength of about 450 nm, are used. Blue light is most efficient in photodegradation and a combination of blue and white fluorescent tubes is often used. A quartz–halogen light source, with a higher radiant flux in the wavelength 425–475 nm, provides more effective photodegradation than fluorescent lights. Light from this source degrades and photoisomerizes unconjugated bilirubin in the skin to non-toxic bilirubin products. Phototherapy is started after the investigations for the cause of jaundice have been carried out. Once therapy

Table 13.2 Causes of prolonged unconjugated hyperbilirubinaemia

Rhesus and ABO incompatibility
Hereditary spherocytosis
Glucose-6-phosphate dehydrogenase deficiency
Septicaemia and TORCH infection
Extravasated blood and excessive bruising
Twin-to-twin transfusion
Prematurity
Dehydration
Hypothyroidism
Breast milk jaundice
Delayed passage of meconium

Table 13.3 Investigations in an infant with prolonged unconjugated hyperbilirubinaemia

Indirect- and direct-acting bilirubin
Haemoglobin
Blood film for red cell morphology
Maternal and infant blood group
Direct Coombs' test
Maternal haemolysis if ABO mismatch (p. 207)
Infection screen
Urine-reducing substances
Erythrocyte galactose uridyl transferase activity if galactosaemia a possibility
Glucose-6-phosphate dehydrogenase assay
Serum T4 and TSH

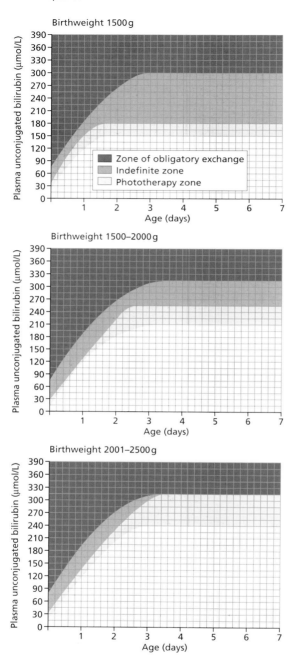

Fig. 13.4 Suggested treatment regimen for unconjugated hyperbilirubinaemia by phototherapy or exchange transfusion for different birthweight groups. (Reproduced from Cockington 1979 with permission.)

has been commenced serum bilirubin estimates will be necessary to assess the severity of jaundice as the skin colour becomes unreliable. Phototherapy may be used in conjunction with other forms of treatment, such as exchange transfusion. The graphs developed by Cockington (1979) provide guidelines for the treatment of hyperbilirubinaemia in low birthweight (LBW) infants (Fig. 13.4). For term infants over 2500 g guidelines modified after Finlay and Tucker (1978) are recommended (Fig. 13.5).

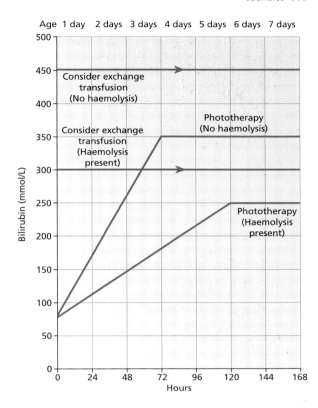

Fig. 13.5 Bilirubin chart modified from Finlay and Tucker (1978).

Complications of phototherapy include:

1 temperature instability;

2 fluid disturbance. The increased insensible water loss may be compensated for by increasing the infant's water intake by 20%;

3 retinal damage. The eyes are thought to be vulnerable to phototherapy but this has never been proved. It is, however, a wise precaution to protect the infant's eyes from the light by a suitable eye shield;

4 diarrhoea. Phototherapy increases bowel transit time and induces lactose intolerance; both are important causes of diarrhoea and consequent fluid loss; and

5 bronze baby. This complication may be seen when an infant with obstructive jaundice receives phototherapy.

EARLY DISCHARGE AND HOME MANAGEMENT OF JAUNDICE

The introduction of early discharge programmes for healthy term infants has resulted in the need for jaundice to be treated at home. Predicting which infants might require treatment using direct and indirect techniques of measuring serum bilirubin at age 24 h has been suggested, but more research is required to identify sensitive methods. Home treatment has been facilitated by the introduction since 1990 of the BiliBlanket® using a fibreoptic phototherapy system. The infant is placed on a mat containing fibreoptic strands, which flood the body with therapeutic light while the infant is clothed normally (Fig. 13.6). More recently (Kappas *et al.* 1995) the use of tin mesoporphyrin (SnMP) as a single intramuscular injection of 6 µmol/kg has been shown to be effective in reducing serum bilirubin levels in candidates for phototherapy.

EXCHANGE TRANSFUSION

This form of therapy was first used in 1951 for the treatment of erythroblastosis fetalis (Diamond *et al.* 1951). Exchange transfusions

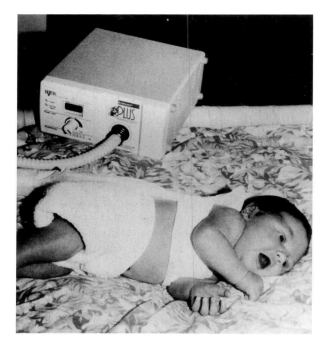

Fig. 13.6 Infant receiving phototherapy using the BiliBlanket®.

may be required in conjunction with phototherapy for infants with severe jaundice, especially when due to rhesus isoimmunization. The exchange transfusion allows:

1 removal of unconjugated bilirubin;
2 removal of immune antibody if present;
3 replacement of sensitized red cells with cells that cannot be haemolysed as easily;
4 restoration of blood volume and correction of anaemia;
5 provision of free albumin for bilirubin binding.

The indications for exchange transfusion depend on the infant's gestational age, postnatal age and state of health. Metabolic compromise with acidosis predisposes to brain damage due to bilirubin toxicity. The level at which bilirubin damages the brain is not known, and the indications for exchange transfusion are therefore arbitrary. Cockington's charts are widely used to decide upon the need for exchange transfusion in LBW infants (see Fig. 13.4). For term infants over 2500 g a chart modified from that used at Hillingdon Hospital is recommended (see Fig. 13.5).

The technique of exchange transfusion is given in Chapter 29.

Complications associated with exchange transfusions include:

1 electrolyte disturbance (hypocalcaemia, hyperkalaemia);
2 blood glucose disturbance—initially hyperglycaemia followed by rebound hypoglycaemia, especially in rhesus immunization;
3 infection—viral (cytomegalovirus (CMV), hepatitis B, human immunodeficiency virus (HIV)) or bacterial (*Staphylococcus aureus* and *Streptococcus* sp.) due to contaminated blood;
4 thromboembolism (air or blood clot);
5 necrotizing enterocolitis (NEC);
6 fluid overload or rarely hypovolaemia;
7 acidosis, hypoxia, bradycardia, cardiac arrest;
8 benign intrahepatic cholestasis in severely growth-restricted infants;
9 haemorrhage.

ALBUMIN

The administration of 1 g/kg of albumin, either intravenously before the exchange transfusion or added to the donor blood, will increase the efficiency of the exchange by binding more free bilirubin.

PHYSIOLOGICAL JAUNDICE

The term 'physiological jaundice' is used by clinicians to describe jaundice which is not severe enough to be treated. It is a diagnosis of exclusion, and if there is any doubt as to the cause, further investigations should be performed. It is presumed to be due to a temporary immaturity of glucuronyl transferase and other factors involved in bilirubin metabolism. Physiological jaundice should not fulfil any of the following criteria:

1 clinical jaundice in the first 24 h of life;
2 total serum bilirubin concentration exceeding 300 µmol/L in a term infant or 255 µmol/L in a preterm infant;
3 a direct-reacting serum bilirubin concentration exceeding 30 µmol/L;
4 clinical jaundice persisting for more than 10 days in a term infant or 2 weeks in a preterm infant;
5 an 'ill' infant.

If any of these features are present, full investigation of the jaundice should be undertaken.

INFECTION

Bacterial infections, particularly septicaemia and urinary tract infections, may cause unconjugated hyperbilirubinaemia. Occasionally severe bacterial infection may cause hepatocellular damage with a conjugated form of jaundice. TORCH (toxoplasmosis, other, rubella, CMV, herpes simplex type II) infections may cause either type of hyperbilirubinaemia, but conjugated is most frequently seen.

BREASTFEEDING AND JAUNDICE

Breastfeeding-associated jaundice is the term used to refer to the increased bilirubin levels seen during the first week of life in almost two-thirds of infants who are breastfed. It is probably due to calorie and fluid deprivation in the first few days of life and delayed passage of stools, as it can be reduced by an increased frequency of breastfeeding during the first few days of life. The importance of recognizing breastfeeding-associated jaundice lies in the fact that it may rarely cause kernicterus if untreated (Maisels & Newman 1995). In itself it is not a contraindication to breastfeeding.

Breast milk jaundice is prolonged jaundice that extends up until the first 3 months of life. It is diagnosed primarily by the exclusion of other aetiologies in a thriving infant and by its time course. It is thought that the high concentrations of non-esterified fatty acids in the breast milk inhibit glucuronyl transferase activity. The milk contains increased lipase activity, which causes free fatty acid elevation and β-glucuronidase enzyme.

DELAYED PASSAGE OF MECONIUM

The jaundice is due to increased enterohepatic absorption of bilirubin.

GILBERT'S SYNDROME

An autosomal dominant condition associated with mild unconjugated hyperbilirubinaemia (< 85 µmol/L). There is no specific test for this and the diagnosis is by exclusion. The prognosis is excellent.

CRIGLER–NAJJAR SYNDROME

An autosomal recessive condition in which hyperbilirubinaemia may become very severe and cause kernicterus. There is no specific investigation and little effective treatment other than prolonged phototherapy. Liver transplantation has been successful in some severe cases; in milder cases phenobarbitone may lower the serum bilirubin.

INSPISSATED BILE SYNDROME

High and prolonged levels of unconjugated bilirubin may cause a condition in which the bilirubin produces cholestasis with progressive conjugated hyperbilirubinaemia. This is usually self-limiting.

Complications of jaundice

KERNICTERUS AND BILIRUBIN ENCEPHALOPATHY

The classic presentation of kernicterus in the newborn is with progressive development of lethargy, rigidity, opisthotonus, a high-pitched cry, fever and convulsions over a period of 24 h. This is followed by death in 50% of the affected infants. At autopsy there is bilirubin staining and necrosis of neurons, especially in the basal ganglia, hippocampus and sub-thalamic nuclei. Survivors of kernicterus often demonstrate choreoathetoid cerebral palsy, high-frequency deafness, mental retardation and paralysis of upward gaze (Parinaud's sign). Preterm infants may manifest more subtle bilirubin brain damage consisting of mild disorders of both motor function and cognitive function (minimal cerebral dysfunction) without demonstrating any of the acute clinical features of bilirubin encephalopathy. High-tone frequency hearing loss is the commonest feature of the bilirubin encephalopathy syndrome and is most commonly seen in premature infants.

The levels at which unconjugated bilirubin causes brain damage are not known, and it is probably only free (non-protein-bound) bilirubin that is dangerous, although bound bilirubin has been reported to cross a leaky blood–brain barrier. Acidosis, asphyxia, prematurity and drugs which compete for bilirubin binding sites predispose infants to kernicterus, possibly by opening the blood–brain barrier to bilirubin molecules.

CONJUGATED HYPERBILIRUBINAEMIA

Causes

This is much less common than unconjugated jaundice in the newborn, but has a much more serious prognosis. Conjugated forms of neonatal jaundice are due to intra- or extrahepatic obstruction (also called cholestasis). It usually presents in the second week of life or later and

Table 13.4 Causes of conjugated hyperbilirubinaemia

Neonatal hepatitis
  TORCH infection
  Metabolic causes
  α_1-Antitrypsin deficiency

Biliary atresia
  Intrahepatic
  Extrahepatic

Inspissated bile

Choledochal cyst

Hepatic necrosis

Cystic fibrosis

Complication of parenteral nutrition

Dubin–Johnson and Rotor syndrome

is associated with greenish skin discolouration, dark bile-stained urine and pale acholuric stools. Hepatosplenomegaly is commonly present and the infant often fails to thrive. Occasionally, conjugated hyperbilirubinaemia is present at birth as a result of TORCH infections or rhesus isoimmunization. The causes of conjugated hyperbilirubinaemia are shown in Table 13.4. Many of these are very rare, but neonatal hepatitis and biliary atresia account for 80% of all cases of conjugated hyperbilirubinaemia.

Investigations

The management of obstructive jaundice in the newborn depends on the diagnosis. The diagnostic dilemma is to distinguish biliary atresia from neonatal hepatitis. Table 13.5 lists the investigations that are of value in distinguishing these conditions. Liver biopsy, radionuclide scanning and further management should be carried out in a specialist children's liver centre.

Management

This depends on the cause of the conjugated hyperbilirubinaemia. Antibiotics are appropriate for the rare cases of bacterial infection.

Table 13.5 Investigations to detect the cause of neonatal conjugated hyperbilirubinaemia

Liver enzymes

Alkaline phosphatase

Serial bilirubin levels

α-Fetoprotein

α₁-Antitrypsin screen and phenotype

¹²³I Rose Bengal excretion test

Abdominal ultrasound

Sweat test

TORCH serology

Amino acid screen

Percutaneous liver biopsy

Radionuclide (HIDA) scan

In general supportive management is all that is available. Steroids are of no real benefit. Cholestyramine (8 g/day) and phenobarbitone (6 mg/kg/day) may have some beneficial effect. An elemental diet (Pregestimil) supplemented with medium-chain triglycerides together with parenteral fat-soluble vitamins (A, D and K) are given to prevent deficiencies. Vitamin D may also be necessary.

Neonatal hepatitis

This is a non-specific condition with a variety of causes which are discussed below, the prognosis depending on the underlying cause. In general, approximately one-third of cases deteriorate and develop hepatic cirrhosis, one-third have evidence of chronic liver disease and one-third recover fully.

CAUSES OF NEONATAL HEPATITIS

1 *Infection.* Most commonly due to TORCH infections contracted in the first trimester, but other viruses may also produce hepatitis (see p. 64). If a mother is positive for hepatitis B, the infant should be protected from infection by immunization (see p. 66).

2 *Metabolic causes.* Fructosaemia and tyrosinaemia may cause severe neonatal hepatitis. Galactosaemia more commonly presents with unconjugated hyperbilirubinaemia, but affected infants later develop cholestasis.

3 *α₁-Antitrypsin deficiency.* This is a relatively common form of conjugated hyperbilirubinaemia. Only infants with the PiZ type are at risk of neonatal hepatitis. This is an autosomal recessive condition.

4 *Cholestatic jaundice of prematurity* relates to lack of enteral feeding and prolonged total parenteral nutrition, especially in the presence of inflammatory bowel disease.

5 *Cystic fibrosis.*

6 *Familial.*

7 *Severe intrauterine growth retardation.* This results in a benign intrahepatic cholestasis.

8 *Idiopathic.*

Biliary atresia

At birth these infants have absent or atretic bile ductules involving the main bile ducts or the main branches of the bile ducts. The deeper in the liver substance that the ducts are abnormal, the more severe is the condition. The commonest variety is extrahepatic biliary atresia. The onset of jaundice may be delayed by up to 4 weeks from birth. It is a surgically operable condition, but because progressive obliteration of the bile ducts occurs rapidly with advancing age, early diagnosis is essential for successful treatment. If surgery is attempted before 60 days of age, there is an 80% chance of achieving biliary drainage by the portoenterostomy operation, known as the Kasai procedure (Kasai *et al.* 1975). Serum bilirubin falls rapidly after successful surgery, but many children develop ascending cholangitis, which is the most serious postoperative complication. Approximately two-thirds of survivors will require liver transplantation by 10 years of age.

Dubin–Johnson syndrome

This is a rare and benign condition in which the neonate may develop low-grade conjugated and unconjugated hyperbilirubinaemia.

REFERENCES

Cockington, R.A. (1979) A guide to the use of phototherapy in the management of neonatal hyperbilirubinaemia. *Journal of Pediatrics* **95**, 281–287.

Diamond, L.K., Allen, F.H. & Thomas, W.O. (1951) Erythroblastosis fetalis VII. Treatment with exchange transfusion. *New England Journal of Medicine* **244**, 39–42.

Finlay, H.V.L. & Tucker, S.M. (1978) Neonatal plasma bilirubin chart. *Archives of Disease in Childhood* **53**, 90–91.

Kappas, A., Drummond, G.S., Henschke, C. & Valaes, T. (1995) Direct comparison of Sn mesoporphyrin, an inhibitor of bilirubin production, and phototherapy in controlling hyperbilirubinemia in term and near-term newborns. *Pediatrics* **95**, 468–474.

Kasai, M., Watanabe, I. & Ohi, R. (1975) Follow-up studies of long-term survivors after hepatic portoenterostomy for 'noncorrectable' biliary atresia. *Journal of Pediatric Surgery* **10**, 173–178.

Kramer, L.I. (1969) Advancement of dermal icterus in the jaundiced newborn. *American Journal of Diseases of Children* **118**, 454–459.

Lucey, J.F. (1972) Neonatal jaundice and phototherapy. *Pediatric Clinics of North America* **19**, 827–839.

Maisels, M.J. (1994) Jaundice. In: *Neonatology. Pathophysiology and Management of the Newborn* (ed. G.B. Avery), 4th edn. Lippincott, Philadelphia.

Maisels, M.J. & Newman, T.B. (1995) Kernicterus in otherwise healthy, breast-fed term newborns. *Pediatrics* **96**, 730–733.

FURTHER READING

American Academy of Paediatrics, Provisional Committee for Quality Improvement and Subcommittee on Hyperbilirubinemia (1994) Practice parameter: Management of hyperbilirubinemia in the healthy term newborn. *Pediatrics* **94**, 558–562.

Milla, P.J. & Muller D.P.R. (1988) (eds) *Harries' Paediatric Gastroenterology*. Churchill Livingstone, Edinburgh.

Mowat, A.P. (ed.) (1994) *Liver Disorders in Childhood*, 3rd edn. Butterworth-Heinemann, Oxford.

14 Congenital abnormalities: malformations and deformations

Estimates of the incidence of congenital abnormalities in all live births vary widely and range from 1% to 7%, depending on the definition of what constitutes an abnormality. Probably about 2% of all babies born have a major congenital anomaly, but the incidence of minor imperfections is about 7% if all skin haemangiomas, preauricular skin tags, etc. are included. The incidence of congenital abnormality is highest in preterm and small for gestational age (SGA) infants.

Congenital abnormalities may be classified into malformations and deformations. *Malformations* result from a disturbance of growth during embryogenesis, e.g. congenital heart disease. *Deformations* result from late changes in previously normal structures by destructive pathological processes or intrauterine (extrinsic) forces, e.g. talipes, hydrocephalus, bowel atresia. Some defects may arise by one or both mechanisms.

DEFORMATIONS

Causes

These may be multiple or single. They have many common aetiological factors, which include:
1 primigravidity;

2 oligohydramnios;
3 abnormal presentation, e.g. breech position;
4 multiple pregnancy;
5 uterine abnormalities, e.g. fibroids, bicornuate or septate uterus;
6 growth restricted.

Extrinsic forces may cause a single localized deformation such as talipes equinovarus or a deformation sequence.

A *deformation sequence* refers to the moulding effects of an intrauterine constraint. Examples are the oligohydramnios sequence, with contractures, facial dysmorphism and pulmonary hypoplasia, or breech deformation sequence.

Intrauterine contractures which give rise to joint fixation are known as arthrogryposis. The types of problems that lead to prenatal joint contractures are demonstrated in Fig. 14.1.

MALFORMATIONS

Incidence

Major congenital abnormalities are either lethal or significantly affect the individual's function or appearance. Minor abnormalities have no functional or major cosmetic importance.

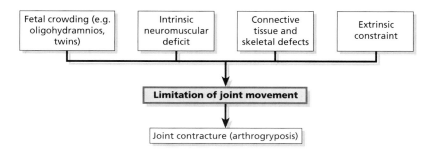

Fig. 14.1 The types of problems that lead to prenatal joint contractures.

National registers of congenital malformations are available for many countries, but it
is difficult to compare overall rates because
of reporting differences. Most registers only
include abnormalities present at birth. Some
do not include data on fetuses aborted after
prenatal diagnosis. There may also be quite
large regional variations within the data from a
single country.

The incidence of congenital malformations
reported for Australia in 1994 was 1.6%. The
figures for the UK are similar. The commonest
major congenital abnormalities involve the
central nervous and the cardiovascular systems. Table 14.1 lists the incidence of some

Table 14.1 Congenital malformations by major
anatomical system, from Day *et al.* 1997

Malformations	Rate per 10 000 births
All malformations	164.4
Nervous system	12.9
Eye	2.9
Heart	35.0
Circulatory system	10.9
Respiratory system	2.2
Cleft palate/lip	14.6
Digestive system	10.3
Genital organs	24.0
Urinary system	19.7
Limbs	14.5
Other musculoskeletal	30.7
Chromosomal	23.1
Other and unspecified	8.3

congenital malformations. Specific congenital
abnormalities are discussed in the appropriate
chapters.

Causes

Causes can be divided into five groups, as
shown in Table 14.2.

TERATOGENESIS

A teratogen is an agent (chemical, drug, virus
or radiation) that causes a malformation or
deformation or affects the wellbeing of the
fetus. A fetotoxin is an agent causing damage
of any kind to the fetus and a mutagen is an
agent which causes a permanent transmissible
change in the genetic material.

The critical periods in embryogenic develop-
ment have been extrapolated from the rubella
experience and are likely to affect different
organs at different times. Some examples of
critical periods are:
Brain   15–25 days.
Eye   25–40 days.
Heart   20–40 days.
Limbs   24–36 days.
Ear   40–60 days.

Drugs

Drugs may act by interfering with embryogenesis or by exerting their pharmacological
actions on developing fetal organs. Adverse

Table 14.2 Causes of congenital malformations

	Estimated incidence (%)
Genetic (Mendelian mode of inheritance)	20
Chromosomal	10
Teratogens	
Infection	2–3
Drugs and chemicals (environmental pollutants & insecticides)	2–3 } 6–9
Radiation	< 1
Maternal metabolic disease	1–2
Unknown	35–40
Polygenic	25–30

Table 14.3 Drugs as teratogens

Definite	
Hormones	Progestogens, diethyl stilboestrol, male sex hormones
Antipsychotics, hypnosedatives	Lithium, haloperidol, thalidomide
Anticonvulsants	Hydantoins, sodium valproate, carbamazepine, primidone, phenobarbitone
Antimicrobials	Tetracycline, chloramphenicol, streptomycin, flucytosine, amphotericin B
Antineoplastics	Alkylating agents, folic acid antagonists
Anticoagulants	Warfarin
Antithyroids	Iodine, carbimazole, propylthiouracil
Antivirals	Ribavarin
Hypoglycaemics	Biguanides, sulphonylureas
Vitamin A analogues	Isotretinoin, etretinate
Others	Toluene, alcohol, marijuana, narcotics

effects are influenced by the timing and dose of agent, the efficiency with which the mother metabolizes the agent, placental transfer and the individual susceptibility of the fetus. Table 14.3 lists some of the commoner teratogenic drugs.

Vitamin A has for many years been known to be a powerful teratogen in animals, but has only recently emerged as a significant clinical problem, with the introduction of oral retinoids for the treatment of severe acne and psoriasis. Teratogenic effects include spontaneous abortion, cleft palate and severe malformations of the ear, heart and brain.

Fetal Alcohol syndrome (alcohol embryopathy)

Excessive alcohol intake in early pregnancy during the period of fetal organogenesis can result in a specific syndrome of facial abnormalities, growth failure, microcephaly, skeletal and visceral abnormalities. This syndrome was identified in 1973 as the fetal alcohol syndrome (Jones & Smith 1973). The facial features that enable the diagnosis to be made include hypoplasia of the mid-face, with beaking of the forehead and a sunken nasal bridge, a small upturned nose, micrognathia, a prominent philtrum and ear deformities (Fig. 14.2).

Growth retardation is usual, with poor postnatal somatic growth. Major abnormalities include cleft lip and palate, and limb, ocular, cardiac and renal malformations. There is usually delayed psychomotor development. Approximately one-third of infants born to chronic alcoholic women develop the fetal alcohol syndrome, whereas others may be growth retarded or demonstrate minor features only. Neonatal withdrawal symptoms, including convulsions, may occur in infants born to alcoholic women. The severity of fetal alcohol syndrome has been described by Majewski (1981) and is shown in Table 14.4.

It is not known whether social drinking of alcohol in pregnancy is associated with intrauterine growth retardation, but in general it is unlikely that the occasional consumption of alcohol during pregnancy will affect the fetus.

Smoking in pregnancy

Although there is overwhelming evidence of harm to the fetus and mother from tobacco smoking in pregnancy, at least one in three pregnant women smoke. Maternal smoking has a dose-dependent effect on decreasing fetal weight owing to impaired uterine perfusion with structural placental changes, an increase in carboxyhaemoglobin and increased fetal

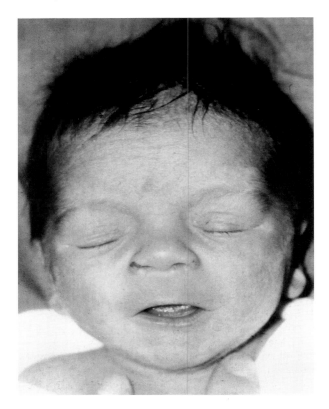

Fig. 14.2 A newborn infant showing the facial features of fetal alcohol syndrome.

Table 14.4 Degrees of fetal alcohol syndrome. (Reproduced from Majewski 1981)

First degree (mild)

Microcephaly, but with normal intelligence (mean IQ 92)

Underweight

No facial features

Second degree (moderate)

Microcephaly with mild intellectual impairment (mean IQ 80)

Mild hyperactivity and minimal cerebral dysfunction

Mild facial abnormalities

No gross developmental organ anomalies

Third degree (severe)—This form is seen in mothers who are chronic alcoholics

Microcephaly with severe intellectual impairment (mean IQ 67)

Severe CNS disturbances

Typical facies (see Fig. 14.2)

Cardiac anomalies

erythropoiesis. Passive exposure to smoking by the father has nearly as great (66%) an effect as maternal smoking in reducing birthweight. Complications in smokers compared to non-smokers include infertility, spontaneous abortion, impaired fetal wellbeing, placenta praevia, abruptio placentae, amniotic fluid infection and premature rupture of the membranes. These are not necessarily causal associations. Follow-up of children born to maternal smokers demonstrates increased rates of hyperactivity at 4 years, deficient stature and mental function, and increased risks of sudden infant death syndrome (SIDS) and malignancy. Excessive smoking is not known to be associated with any specific congenital abnormalities.

The drug-addicted infant

A wide variety of drugs have been abused during pregnancy and neonatal withdrawal symptoms have been reported with alcohol, amphetamines, barbiturates, codeine, ethchlorvynol, heroin, pethidine, methadone, morphine and pentazocine. Heroin and methadone are the narcotic drugs most frequently abused during pregnancy. Their illicit use has been associated with increased fetal and neonatal deaths. The mean birthweight of infants born to heroin addicts is only 2500 g owing to an increased incidence of both prematurity and intrauterine growth retardation. About 70% of the infants exhibit withdrawal symptoms. Symptoms usually occur within 48 h of birth, but can be delayed for up to a week. Signs include extreme jitteriness, tachycardia, vomiting, diarrhoea and fever. Convulsions occur rarely. It has been reported that infants born to drug-addicted mothers may continue to show irritable or restless behaviour for a number of months after birth.

Cocaine Perinatal cocaine intoxication is a major problem in the USA and the use of cocaine or 'crack' in other countries is increasing. This drug is a potent vasoconstrictor affecting the uteroplacental bed as well as the fetal vasculature. It also causes maternal and fetal tachycardia and severe hypertension. The abuse of cocaine in pregnancy results in increased risk of first-trimester abortion, placental abruption and premature birth. Fetal malformations thought to be due to cocaine include hydronephrosis, cryptorchidism, skeletal defects with delayed ossification, exencephaly and eye anomalies. Cerebral artery infarction due to the vasoconstrictive effect of the drug is well described and is most likely to occur in the second and third trimesters.

Management Infants of mothers who abuse drugs in pregnancy should be carefully monitored in the neonatal period for withdrawal symptoms. These are listed in Table 14.5.

About 30% of infants with drug withdrawal can be managed conservatively without the use of drugs. Methods include swaddling, frequent feeds, intravenous fluids and decreased sensory stimulation.

If severe signs of withdrawal are present, drug treatment is necessary, but opinions as to the most effective treatment differ. Opiates such as paregoric (0.2 mL 3-hourly), pethidine

Table 14.5 Withdrawal symptoms seen in neonates born to drug-abusing mothers

Central nervous system

Irritability and high-pitched cry

Hyperactivity with reduced periods of sleep

Tremors

Increased tone

Convulsions (rare)

Gastrointestinal

Poor feeding

Vomiting

Diarrhoea

Other symptoms

Sweating

Fever

Frequent yawning

Snuffles and sneezing

Tachycardia

(1 mg/kg/dose) or morphine (0.1 mg/kg/dose) may be used. Frequently non-specific sedatives such as phenobarbitone (8 mg/kg/day), diazepam (1–2 mg 8-hourly) or chlorpromazine (2–3 mg/kg/day) are used.

Additional assessment of infants of drug-abusing mothers includes screening for hepatitis B and C and human immunodeficiency virus (HIV) infection. When infants are born to mothers with acute hepatitis B in the last trimester of pregnancy or where the mother is surface antigen (HBsAg) positive, hepatitis B immunoglobulin (100 iu) is given as soon as possible after birth. Active immunization with hepatitis B vaccine given with the immunoglobulin injection should be commenced, and repeated at 2 and 6 months.

Prognosis This depends at least in part on the socioeconomic background of the family. Infants of substance-abusing mothers exhibit behavioural and physical features reflecting central and systemic dysfunction. These infants may be at increased risk of SIDS, and they and their families require careful follow-up after discharge by medical and community health and social services.

Infections (see also Chapter 7)

Prenatal maternal infections act by causing inflammatory lesions of the embryo or fetus and interfere with cell division. Maternal infections which may cause congenital abnormalities include:

1 *definite*: rubella, toxoplasmosis, syphilis, cytomegalovirus, herpes simplex, HIV, varicella, parvovirus B19;
2 *probable*: Coxsackie B, herpes zoster; and
3 *possible*: mumps, influenza.

Irradiation

Clinical experience with X-rays and the follow-up studies on pregnant women exposed to atomic bomb irradiation in Hiroshima have confirmed major teratogenic effects, e.g. microcephaly.

Chemicals

Pesticides and waste products have not been subjected to rigorous teratogenic studies in humans. However, recent experience with the dioxin contaminant in the insecticide 2,4,5T and its possible association with spina bifida and Potter's syndrome suggest that a much more rigorous surveillance of chemicals is necessary in the future. The only environmental chemical where there is clear evidence of teratogenicity at present is organic mercury. Long-term prenatal exposure to this chemical has caused neurological damage from disturbed brain development.

Fever

Studies have suggested that it may be the high fever associated with viral infection (e.g. influenza) that causes the malformation. Sauna baths and faulty electric blankets producing very high body temperatures at a critical period of embryogenesis might be teratogenic.

Maternal diseases

Diabetes mellitus Maternal diabetes, especially with coexisting vascular complications, predisposes to many congenital malformations, including the caudal regression syndrome (sacral agenesis), congenital heart disease, idiopathic hypertrophic subaortic stenosis, hypoplastic left colon and renal vein thrombosis.

If the diabetic woman is well controlled on insulin and her blood sugars remain in the normal range before she becomes pregnant, the risk of congenital malformation is reduced.

Maternal hyperthyroidism (graves' disease) This disease results in transient neonatal thyrotoxicosis in approximately 10–20% of pregnancies (see p. 177). The best predictors of neonatal thyrotoxicosis are the outcome of previous siblings and assays of thyroidstimulating immunoglobulin and thyroid receptor-binding inhibitors.

Maternal phenylketonuria The high phenylalanine levels in a pregnant woman with untreated phenylketonuria may have a harmful effect on the fetus, resulting in microcephaly, congenital heart disease and mental retardation.

Polyhydramnios This occurs in 1–2% of all pregnancies. It is usually chronic but may be acute, especially when associated with uniovular multiple pregnancies. Chronic polyhydramnios is often associated with multiple pregnancy, maternal diabetes and a variety of congenital malformations. In a proportion of cases no cause can be found. The commonest associated malformations are oesophageal atresia, duodenal atresia and neural tube defects, but many other conditions have been reported.

Prolonged rupture of membranes Oligohydramnios due to a leak of liquor, as may occur following mid-trimester amniocentesis or prolonged membrane rupture, is associated with lung hypoplasia. An adequate volume of amniotic fluid is necessary for normal lung growth, and any cause of oligohydramnios may be associated with underdeveloped lungs, postural deformities and amnion nodosum of the placenta. Severe renal or bladder outlet obstruction is also associated with oligohydramnios, and a similar clinical appearance which is referred to as Potter's syndrome (see p. 251).

REFERENCES

Day, P., Lancaster, P. & Huang, J. (1997) *Australia's Mothers and Babies 1995.* AIHW National Perinatal Statistics Unit, Sydney.

Jones, K.L. & Smith, D.W. (1973) Recognition of the fetal alcohol syndrome in early infancy. *Lancet* **ii**, 999.

Majewski, F. (1981) Alcohol embryopathy: some facts and speculations about pathogenesis. *Neurobehavioural Toxicology and Teratology* **3**, 129–144.

FURTHER READING

American Academy of Pediatrics, Committee on Drugs (1998) Neonatal drug withdrawal. *Pediatrics* **101**, 1079–1088.

Jones, K.L. (ed.) (1997) *Smith's Recognizable Patterns of Human Malformation*, 5th edn. W.B. Saunders, Philadelphia.

McKusick, V.A. (ed.) (1994) *Mendelian Inheritance in Man. Catalogs of Human Genes and Genetic Disorders*, 11th edn. Johns Hopkins University Press, Baltimore.

Online Mendelian Inheritance in Man, OMIM (TM) (1997) Center for Medical Genetics, Johns Hopkins University, Baltimore and National Center for Biotechnology Information, National Library of Medicine, Bethesda. World Wide Web URL: http://http://www.ncbi.nlm.nih.gov/omim/

15 Genetics and genetic disorders

Genetics is the study of the inheritance of disease or the way in which diseases are transmitted by the parents to their offspring. Terms commonly used in genetics are:

genotype—refers to genetic composition;

phenotype—refers to the physical expression of the genotype;

karyotype—refers to the chromosomal pattern; and

mutation—refers to a random but permanent change in the sequence of genomic DNA.

Many diseases, such as diabetes mellitus, have a genetic background (polygenic), but about 3% of all neonates have an abnormality which is due directly to genetic factors. Genetic problems may be classified as chromosomal, inherited single-gene and multifactorial disorders.

CHROMOSOME DISORDERS

Every cell in the body contains 46 chromosomes (diploid number) in its nucleus: 44 are autosomal and two are sex chromosomes (females XX or males XY). Half (the haploid number) are derived from each parent at the time of fertilization. During meiosis the chromosomes separate and align themselves around the centre of the cell and half migrate into each daughter cell. Occasionally, one of the chromosomes does not separate in time (non-disjunction) and stays with its partner in one daughter cell, leaving the other daughter cell with no chromosomes of this type. Sometimes a process known as translocation occurs, whereby part of one chromosome is added to another during the crossover process of meiosis.

Indications for chromosome analysis

These include the following:

1 recurrent unexplained abortions;

2 fresh stillbirth with physical abnormalities;

3 a neonate with features suggestive of a chromosomal abnormality; and

4 a neonate with two or more dysmorphic features.

Fetal chromosomes may also be tested during pregnancy (prenatal diagnosis). The most common indications are:

1 advanced maternal age;

2 previous chromosome disorder;

3 parent has a balanced translocation;

4 detection of fetal malformation suggestive of a chromosomal disorder.

Chromosome culture techniques

Tissue required:

1 peripheral blood (collected in a heparinized tube), ideally from a patient who has not recently ingested alcohol, antibiotics or drugs of addiction;

2 bone marrow: used for rapid diagnosis;

3 skin (fibroblast culture): useful up to 2 days after death;

4 desquamated cells in amniotic fluid: used for prenatal diagnosis;

5 chorion villus sample: usually 10–12 weeks' gestation.

Culture technique. Phytohaem agglutinin is added to the tissues to stimulate lymphocyte proliferation. Colchicine is then added to arrest cells in the metaphase stage of mitosis.

Staining. A Giemsa stain gives the overall appearance of the karyotype. Banding of the chromosomes gives detailed information about more subtle abnormalities, and this is done by Giemsa and trypsin staining. C banding is performed to detect a heterochromatin body.

Chromosomes are grouped according to banding characteristics, size of chromosomes and centromere position. The larger chromosomes have the lowest numbers. Each chromosome is divided by the centromere into a short arm (p) and a long arm (q).

Fluorescent *in situ* hybridization (FISH): these are special stains used to detect the absence of specific pieces of chromosomes, not visible by microscopic techniques.

Chromosome abnormality classification

With the use of these culture and staining techniques chromosome abnormalities may be classified as numerical abnormalities, structural abnormalities, mosaicism or fragile sites.

NUMERICAL

Aneuploidy

One extra chromosome is called a trisomy. One chromosome deletion is called a monosomy. These abnormalities may occur with autosomes or sex chromosomes.

Trisomy. Autosomal chromosomes: e.g. trisomy 13, trisomy 18, trisomy 21 (Down syndrome) (Table 15.1). Sex chromosomes: e.g. XXY (Klinefelter syndrome), XYY, triple XXX syndrome.

Monosomy. Autosomes: usually incompatible with life and cause spontaneous abortion. Sex chromosomes: e.g. 45,XO (Turner syndrome).

Polyploidy

This is a multiple of the haploid number, e.g. triploidy 69 karyotype usually results in abortion, stillbirth or early neonatal death.

STRUCTURAL

Deletion

Short arm deletion (p–), e.g. *cri du chat* syndrome (5p–). Long arm deletion (q–), e.g. 13q– (rare).

Addition

Rare, compatible with life if the addition is small.

Translocation

Refers to breakage of two non-homologous chromosomes with rejoining of the broken pieces in new ways. When there is significant alteration of genetic material (addition or deletion), the translocation is said to be unbalanced and the individual is phenotypically abnormal. Where there is a normal amount of genetic material, the individual is phenotypically normal and has a balanced translocation. Many individuals with a balanced translocation have only 45 chromosomes and convey a considerable risk to their offspring of spontaneous abortion or unbalanced translocation. The infant may inherit the same balanced translocation.

MOSAICISM

In this condition there is more than one distinct cell line, one line usually being normal and the others abnormal. Thus, only a percentage of the cells will have the abnormal chromosomes. Approximately 2% of Down syndrome babies are mosaics and usually have less obvious stigmata and often higher intellectual ability than in the more common trisomy 21.

FRAGILE X SYNDROME

This is a familial form of mental retardation which has been described in male infants, but one-third of female carriers may be mildly affected. It is the second most common cause of severe mental retardation after Down syndrome. Fragile X syndrome is diagnosed by demonstrating fragile sites on the long arm of a proportion of X chromosomes, although DNA testing is available with the

Table 15.1 Specific chromosomal abnormalities

	Trisomy 21 (Down syndrome, Fig. 15.1)	Trisomy 13 (Patau syndrome)	Trisomy 18 (Edward syndrome, Fig. 15.2)	45,XO syndrome (Turner syndrome, ovarian dysgenesis)	XXY syndrome (Klinefelter syndrome)
Incidence	1 in 600 births	1 in 5000 births	1 in 3500 births (females predominate)	1 in 2500 of live female births (however, majority abort in first few prenatal months)	1 in 500 male births
Karyotype	94% result from non-disjunction, 3.5% translocations, 2.5% mosaicism	75% non-disjunction, 20% translocation, 5% mosaicism	85–95% non-disjunction, 5% mosaicism	60% 45,XO. Remainder—great variety including mosaics, deletions	80% XXY, 10% mosaic, 10% XXYY or XXXY
Maternal age	Important. 1 in 1500 incidence with maternal age 15–29 years, 1 in 50 at 45 years	Older maternal age seems to be important. Mean maternal age approx. 31 years	Mean maternal age 32	No apparent influence	Average maternal age slightly increased
Clinical features	These are too numerous to enumerate here—refer to larger textbooks. Important are: hypotonia, flat faces, slanted palpebral fissures, small ears, etc. Major congenital abnormalities include congenital heart disease (common A-V canal), duodenal atresia	Large 'onion nose', defects of fusion of eyes, nose, lip and forebrain (holoproscencephaly), polydactyly, microcephaly, single umbilical artery; major congenital abnormalities include congenital heart disease, scalp defects	Triangular face, hooked flexion deformity 2nd finger, rocker bottom feet, single umbilical artery, short sternum; major congenital abnormalities: heart disease, kidney malformation	Short stature (length), 'shield-like' chest. Widely spaced nipples, neck webbing, lymphoedema of hands and feet. Major congenital abnormalities: coarctation of aorta, horseshoe kidneys	Appear normal male baby. Usually diagnosed at puberty with failure of appearance of secondary sex characteristics; tall stature. Small testes post puberty
Survival	This will depend on associated malformation. Usually good	Majority die in early infancy	Majority die within first 3 months	Normal except for those with serious cardiac and renal problems	Normal
Recurrence risk	Depends on maternal age. Overall approximately 1 in 100 for non-disjunction type. In translocation depends on karyotype of parents	Low in non-disjunction type. Higher in translocation type depending on karyotype of parents	Less than 1 in 100 recurrence risk	No significant risk	No increased risk

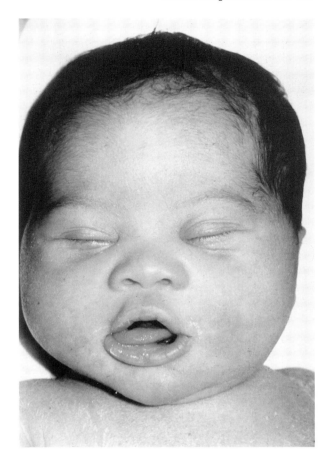

Fig. 15.1 Trisomy 21 (Down syndrome).

more accurate testing methods. It affects 1/1000 newborn males.

CLINICAL FEATURES

Table 15.1 shows the more important features of the commoner chromosomal abnormalities, and these are illustrated in Figs 15.1 and 15.2.

SUMMARY

Chromosome disorders are complex, but in general aneuploidy is better tolerated than polyploidy. Additions are better tolerated than deletions (i.e. trisomy better than monosomy, p+ better than p–); abnormalities of sex chromosomes are better tolerated than abnormalities of autosomes. The higher the chromosome number, the better tolerated the abnormality.

INHERITED SINGLE-GENE DISORDERS

Many diseases may be inherited from parents by Mendelian modes of inheritance. These are single-gene defects or abnormalities, occurring either on autosomes (autosomal disorders) or on sex chromosomes (sex-linked, X-linked disorders). They usually exhibit obvious and characteristic pedigree patterns.

Autosomal disorders

AUTOSOMAL DOMINANT (Fig. 15.3)

The features of this group include:
1 males and females are affected in equal proportion;

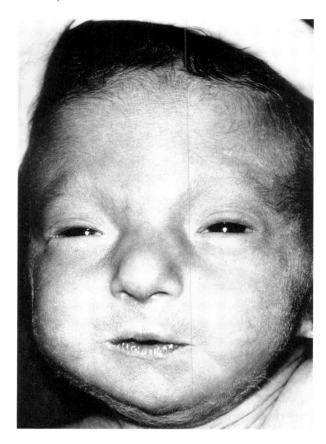

Fig. 15.2 Trisomy 18 (Edward syndrome).

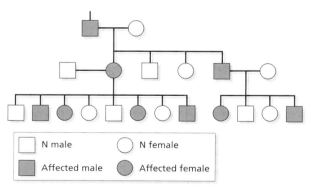

N male		N female
Affected male		Affected female

Fig. 15.3 A family pedigree showing autosomal dominant inheritance.

2 marked variation in expressivity, e.g. osteogenesis imperfecta may range from blue sclerae or deafness to severe bone fragility;
3 inherited from one parent;
4 half the offspring of an affected parent can be expected to have the disorder;

5 new cases commonly arise as spontaneous mutations, more common with advanced paternal age. The mutation may be present in only one chromosome of a pair (matched with a normal allele on the homologous chromosome) or on both. In either case the

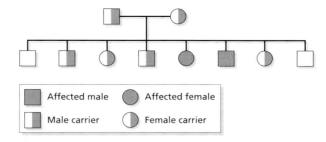

Fig. 15.4 A family pedigree showing autosomal recessive inheritance.

cause is a single critical error in the genetic information.

Autosomal dominant disorders include:
1 major malformation: polycystic kidneys;
2 minor malformations: finger anomalies—shortening, fusion, additions;
3 Central nervous system (CNS) disorders: Huntington's disease, tuberous sclerosis, neurofibromatosis;
4 mesenchymal disorders: osteogenesis imperfecta, achondroplasia, Marfan syndrome;
5 muscular disorders: myotonic dystrophy, other myopathies;
6 tumours: retinoblastoma, colon polyposis;
7 haematological: hereditary (congenital) spherocytosis.

AUTOSOMAL RECESSIVE (Fig. 15.4)

The features of this group include:
1 the disorder is inherited from both parents, who are heterozygotes (carriers);
2 the recurrence risk is 1 in 4;
3 males and females are equally affected;
4 if both parents are heterozygous for the condition, two-thirds of the unaffected offspring can be expected to be heterozygotes and only one in four of the offspring will be genotypically normal;
5 relatively few recessive disorders arise as mutants;
6 consanguinity increases the likelihood of carriers of rare genes mating, thereby increasing the incidence of affected individuals.

The commonest lethal autosomal recessive disease in Europe is cystic fibrosis. The carrier rate in the community of cystic fibrosis is 1 in 25, so that the chance of two carriers mating is 1 in 625. One in four of their offspring will be

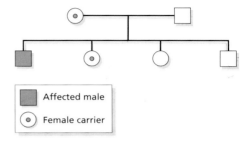

Fig. 15.5 A family pedigree showing X-linked recessive inheritance.

affected, so that the incidence of cystic fibrosis in the community is 1 in 2500.

Other autosomal recessive disorders include:
1 haemoglobinopathies: thalassaemia syndromes, sickle cell disease;
2 storage diseases: glycogen storage, e.g. type I (von Gierke), type II (Pompe); other, e.g. Hurler syndrome;
3 CNS degenerations: white matter, e.g. metachromatic leukodystrophy; grey matter, e.g. Tay–Sachs, hepatolenticular degeneration (Wilson disease);
4 treatable inborn errors of metabolism: phenylketonuria, galactosaemia, adrenogenital syndrome;
5 neuromuscular: spinal muscle atrophy (Werdnig–Hoffman);
6 other: cystic fibrosis, albinism.

Sex chromosome disorders

X-LINKED RECESSIVE (Fig. 15.5)

An X-linked recessive trait is caused by an abnormal gene on the X chromosome. The pattern of X-linked inheritance depends upon the fact that females have two X chromosomes, whereas males have only one. Thus males are said to be 'hemizygous' with respect to X-linked traits, and any gene on the male's single X is expressed. The 'carrier' female is protected from the effects of the recessive gene by the normal gene on her other X chromosome.

The features of this group are:
1 males are predominantly affected;
2 the female carries the trait (rarely the female carrier may be mildly affected);
3 half the male offspring of a female carrier are affected;
4 half the female offspring of a carrier will themselves become carriers;
5 all the female offspring of an affected male will be carriers;
6 often expressed as a new mutation, making genetic counselling difficult (probably 33% of all cases of lethal X-linked recessive diseases);
7 many of the X-linked recessive diseases are lethal (muscular dystrophy, X-linked agammaglobulinaemia, Lesch–Nyhan syndrome), so that the disorder can only be handed on by the carrier female. However, in glucose-6-phosphate dehydrogenase (G6PD) deficiency and colour blindness the disorder may be passed on by the affected males to daughters but not to sons.

X-linked recessive diseases include:
1 haemophilia A, haemophilia B (Christmas disease);
2 Duchenne muscular dystrophy;
3 agammaglobulinaemia;
4 G6PD deficiency;
5 colour blindness.

The Lyon hypothesis

This refers to the random inactivation of one X chromosome in a female (either maternal X or paternal X) at a stage during cell division. This enables heterozygous females to exhibit some features of an X-linked recessive disease, e.g. elevated creatinine phosphokinase in Duchenne muscular dystrophy.

X-LINKED DOMINANT INHERITANCE

These conditions are rare, with the only clinically important disorders being vitamin D-resistant rickets, incontinentia pigmenti and pseudohypoparathyroidism. Some X-linked dominant disorders appear to be lethal to the male, so that only females are affected (e.g. incontinentia pigmenti).

MULTIFACTORIAL OR POLYGENIC DISORDERS

Many congenital abnormalities may be caused by the interaction of multiple factors, both genetic and environmental. These disorders do not exhibit the characteristic patterns of Mendelian inheritance, although their recurrence within families is greater than that predicted for the general population.

Such diseases include:
1 anencephaly;
2 spina bifida;
3 cleft lip;
4 cleft palate;
5 cleft palate without cleft lip;
6 clubfoot (talipes equinovarus);
7 congenital dislocation of the hip;
8 congenital heart diseases;
9 Hirschsprung's disease;
10 pyloric stenosis.

Some diseases which present later in life, such as diabetes mellitus, schizophrenia and hypertension, are probably examples of multifactorial inheritance.

In general, the incidence of conditions associated with multifactorial inheritance is approximately 1/1000 live births. However, once the entity has occurred there is said to be an increased recurrence risk in first-degree relatives of about 1/20–40.

Environmental factors known to cause birth defects include maternal disease, such as insulin-dependent diabetes mellitus, medications taken during pregnancy and pregnancy infections such as rubella. It is also presumed that vascular accidents during organogenesis can be associated with defects.

Birth defects are a major cause of perinatal and postnatal mortality and morbidity, which have a significant impact on family life and the community as a whole. It is therefore important to have an approach to preventing such defects and identifying causes when they occur.

PREVENTION OF BIRTH DEFECTS

Strategies used to prevent birth defects include:
1 preconceptual counselling in mothers with insulin-dependent diabetes mellitus;
2 prenatal diagnosis using ultrasound, chorionic villus sampling, amniocentesis, maternal serum, fetal blood sampling and fetal biopsy. Early prenatal diagnosis will provide an opportunity for counselling and possibly termination of pregnancy;
3 the administration of folic acid (0.4 mg daily) for at least 1 month before conception in planned pregnancies and in the early months of pregnancy to reduce the incidence of neural tube defects (see p. 218);
4 rubella immunization of adolescent girls;
5 avoidance of drugs known to be teratogens (see Table 14.3);
6 avoidance of maternal exposure to known chemical teratogens and irradiation (see p. 148). There is currently no sound evidence that paternal exposure to environmental chemicals is teratogenic. Theoretically, it is possible that environmentally induced mutations could contribute to the known paternal age-related risk of new dominant mutations, such as for achondroplasia;
7 community education in the avoidance of harmful practices and the use of potential teratogens, including smoking, alcohol and cocaine during pregnancy;
8 neonatal screening for the early detection and treatment of diseases or conditions before permanent damage is incurred, for example phenylketonuria, galactosaemia, hypothyroidism, cystic fibrosis and congenital dislocation of the hip;
9 genetic counselling where there has been an affected child can prevent recurrence.

GENETIC COUNSELLING

Genetic counselling aims to provide parents

or prospective parents with sufficient knowledge to make an informed decision about their reproduction options and provide information about issues they may have to face.

Indications for genetic counselling include:
1 previous stillbirth or multiple miscarriages;
2 previous child with a birth defect, mental retardation or chromosomal abnormality;
3 family history of known genetic disorder;
4 advanced maternal age;
5 exposure to teratogenic drugs, teratogenic chemicals or irradiation during pregnancy;
6 history of neoplastic conditions with genetic implications, e.g. retinoblastoma, colon polyposis.

MOLECULAR GENETICS

Recent advances in molecular genetics using DNA-based and other techniques have given an added dimension to the diagnosis of genetic disease and counselling. The list of genetic loci and mutations which may cause genetic disease, many of paediatric importance, is ever expanding (see Online Mendelian Inheritance in Man, OMIM).

A detailed discussion of the causes and types of mutations that may occur is beyond the scope of this book. For further information the reader should refer to specific texts on the molecular basis of genetic disease.

Mutations of developmental genes have been identified as a cause of birth defects. Examples include homeotic (HOX) and paired box (PAX) gene families. HOX genes are involved in the formation of structures developing from specific segments of the embryo. For example, mutation of the HOXD13 gene is associated with dominant polysyndactyly; PAX genes are important in eye development, for example mutant PAX6 is associated with aniridia.

The types of mutations occurring during DNA replication are complex. Although this is an oversimplification, they may be classified into groups according to the scale of the mutation (a portion of DNA sequence vs. entire chromosomes) and the type of mutation (affecting primarily the structure or regulation of the genetic information). Examples of gene structural errors include Duchenne muscular dystrophy, Charcot–Marie–Tooth disease, Hurler syndrome and Crouzon syndrome. Examples of gene function errors include thalassaemia, Beckwith–Wiedemann syndrome and fragile X syndrome. Structural errors of chromosomes involve monosomy (deletion), e.g. Turner syndrome, trisomy (duplications), e.g. Down syndrome, or triploidy, e.g. miscarriages. Function errors of chromosomes occur with uniparent disomy, e.g. Prader–Willi syndrome.

Direct methods involve testing the DNA from an individual, usually using polymerase chain reaction (PCR), to see whether or not it carries a known mutation associated with the suspected disease. For prenatal diagnosis the DNA can be obtained in the first trimester of pregnancy by chorionic villus sampling, or in the culturing of cells obtained at amniocentesis. Examples of diseases that may be detected in this way include β-thalassaemia, cystic fibrosis and Duchenne muscular dystrophy. In some situations *in utero* treatment may be possible, e.g. with congenital adrenal hyperplasia due to 21-hydroxylase deficiency, prenatal diagnosis and treatment of an affected female fetus with dexamethasone may prevent virilization.

Indirect testing (gene tracing) uses closely linked molecular markers in family studies to discover whether or not an individual inherited the disease-carrying chromosome from a parent. An example of this is seen in the preclinical diagnosis of retinoblastoma, 20–40% of which is hereditary where the risk for the child is 50%. If the child has inherited the parent's retinoblastoma gene, regular ophthalmological review is mandatory. The same principles apply for adolescent- or adult-onset disease, such as polycystic kidney or polyposis coli.

DIAGNOSTIC APPROACH TO THE DYSMORPHIC NEONATE

In some instances the suspected cause of dysmorphism in a neonate may be obvious from classic clinical features, such as with Down syndrome. In others the cause may be more subtle, with unusual facies or single

and multiple birth defects, some of which may appear unrelated. In all cases a systematic approach to diagnosis which may aid treatment is mandatory.

The diagnostic procedure involves:

1 a detailed medical history to obtain information about the pregnancy and the possibility of exposure to teratogens. A family pedigree should be obtained when a genetic disorder is suspected;

2 a detailed clinical examination should be carried out and all abnormalities documented;

3 investigations, which include:

(a) chromosomal analysis where two or more dysmorphic features are present;

(b) metabolic studies on blood and urine in suspected inborn errors of metabolism; and

(c) radiology, including head, renal ultrasound and X-rays to distinguish bone dysplasia. Autopsy if the infant dies;

4 database consultation may aid in the diagnosis with multiple birth defects, e.g. OMIM, London Dysmorphology Database;

5 consultation with specialists: radiologist, geneticist, biochemist, ophthalmologist, neurologist.

FURTHER READING

Buyse, M.L. (ed.) (1990) *Birth Defects Encyclopedia: The Comprehensive, Systematic, Illustrated Reference Source for the Diagnosis, Delineation, Aetiology, Biodynamics, Occurrence, Prevention, and Treatment of Human Anomalies of Clinical Relevance.* Blackwell Scientific Publications, Cambridge, Mass.

Connor, J.M. & Ferguson-Smith, M.A. (1993) *Essential Medical Genetics*, 4th edn. Blackwell Scientific Publications, Oxford.

Davies, K.E. (1992) *Molecular Basis of Genetic Disease*, 2nd edn. IRL Press at Oxford University Press, Oxford.

Emery, A.E.H. & Mueller, R.F. (1992) *Elements of Medical Genetics*, 8th edn. Churchill Livingstone, Edinburgh.

Friedman, J.M., Dill, F.J., Hayden, M.R. & McGillivray, M.D. (eds) (1996) *Genetics*, 2nd edn. Williams & Wilkins, Baltimore.

Jones, K.L. (ed.) (1997) *Smith's Recognizable Patterns of Human Malformation*, 5th edn. W.B. Saunders, Philadelphia.

McKusick, V.A. (ed.) (1994) *Mendelian Inheritance in Man. Catalogs of Human Genes and Genetic Disorders*, 11th edn. Johns Hopkins University Press, Baltimore.

Online Mendelian Inheritance in Man, OMIM (TM) (1997) Center for Medical Genetics, Johns Hopkins University, Baltimore and National Center for Biotechnology Information, National Library of Medicine, Bethesda. World Wide Web URL: http://www.ncbi.nlm.nih.gov/omim/

Winter, R.M. & Baraitser, M. (eds) (1996) *London Dysmorphology Database and London Neurogenetics Database* [computer file]. Oxford University Press, Oxford.

GLUCOSE HOMEOSTASIS AND ITS ABNORMALITIES

The fetus has a continuous supply of glucose from the mother via the placenta, and consequently fetal blood glucose levels are the same as the mother's. At birth the infant has to rapidly switch to endogenous gluconeogenesis until feeding is established. At birth the newborn's blood glucose falls to approximately 75% of the maternal blood glucose level.

Glucose and oxygen are the main metabolic substrates of the mature brain, but in the neonate the brain can use alternative metabolic fuels such as lactate and ketones. This is why the brain may be able to function normally, or near normally, despite very low levels of blood glucose. Profound neurological compromise and irreversible damage occur if the brain is deprived of glucose and alternative metabolic substrates.

Glucose Metabolism

Figure 16.1 summarizes the main metabolic pathways involved in gluconeogenesis.

1 *Glycogen production and glycogenolysis.* These occur largely in the liver and muscles, but only liver glycogen is available for rapid breakdown to glucose.

2 *Gluconeogenesis.* The most important substrates are amino acids (particularly alanine), lactate, pyruvate and glycerol. The points at which these are metabolized are shown in Fig. 16.1.

3 *Lipolysis.* Glycerol is metabolized from adipose tissue and can be directly utilized in gluconeogenesis metabolism. Other products of lipolysis (fatty acid and triglycerides) are metabolized to ketone bodies, which may be used directly in energy production, particularly by the brain.

These mechanisms are under the control of the endocrine system and are affected by insulin, glucagon, cortisol and growth hormone. Therefore, so that the neonate can regulate his blood sugar within the physiological range, he must be endowed with adequate liver glycogen, lipid stores and effective metabolic pathways including glycogenolysis and gluconeogenesis, as well as overall endocrine control. Hypoglycaemia will rapidly develop if any of these processes are disturbed.

Measurement of Blood Glucose

It is essential to measure blood glucose rapidly and accurately in high-risk infants and a variety of techniques have been developed to give cotside values. Glucose concentrations in plasma or serum are 10–15% higher than in whole blood, and many bedside techniques rely on whole-blood methods, whereas the laboratory techniques are more likely to measure serum glucose levels. In the neonatal unit strip reagents are most widely used, but these are generally unreliable in the presence of low blood glucose, which is the range of most importance in the newborn. Strip tests use glucose oxidase-sensitive blocks, which change colour depending on the blood glucose concentration and are specific for glucose alone. Blood glucose estimation by Dextrostix is critically affected by the time the block is in contact with the blood, whereas this is less critical with BM stix. Recent developments in reagent strip tests (e.g. Accutrend and Advantage) promise more accurate estimates of true blood sugar. More recently a number of portable devices for measuring glucose at or near the cotside have been introduced. These devices (Yellow Springs Instruments Reflolux II, Kodak Ektachem) are also prone to over-read low levels, but are probably more consistently

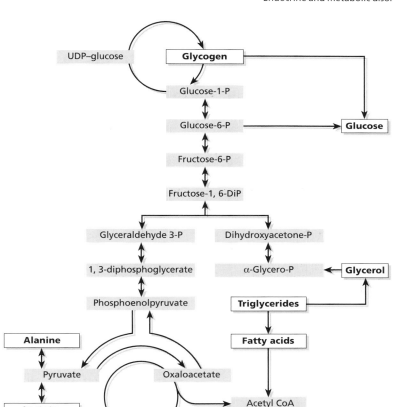

Fig. 16.1 Metabolic pathways involved in gluconeogenesis. (Reproduced from Aynsley-Green *et al.* 1981, with permission.)

reliable than strip tests. Low levels recorded in the nursery should be confirmed by sending a specimen to the laboratory.

Hypoglycaemia

Historically, hypoglycaemia has been defined as a whole-blood glucose concentration of < 1.7 mmol/L in term infants and < 1.1 mmol/L in preterm neonates (Cornblath & Schwartz 1976). More recently hypoglycaemia has been defined in term infants as 2.2–2.5 mmol/L after the first 24 h of life. There is little evidence to suggest that preterm infants are more resistant to hypoglycaemia than premature infants.

In a retrospective study, Lucus *et al.* (1988) found that premature infants (birthweight < 1850 g) with blood sugar levels < 2.6 mmol/L were at increased risk of lower neurodevelopmental scores, particularly when blood sugar values were below this figure on repeated occasions. Others have shown that a deterioration in neurological function (measured by evoked potentials) occurred with a blood sugar level < 2.6 mmol/L (Koh *et al.* 1988). These studies can be used to define normoglycaemia in the newborn as blood sugar levels of 2.6 mmol/L and above, but levels below this do not necessarily indicate potentially damaging hypoglycaemia.

We recommend maintaining the blood sugar of preterm infants and term infants who are at risk of hypoglycaemia (see below) above 2.5 mmol/L.

SYMPTOMS

The symptoms of hypoglycaemia in the newborn can be divided into major and minor.
1 *Major*. Apnoea, convulsions and coma. Rarely prolonged hypoglycaemia may cause congestive heart failure or persistent pulmonary hypertension.
2 *Minor*. Jitteriness, irritability, tremors, apathy, cyanotic spells and temperature instability.

It is not possible to confidently diagnose neonatal hypoglycaemia clinically as the symptoms are non-specific and similar to those of infection. Hypoglycaemia may remain entirely without clinical signs or symptoms, and this is referred to as asymptomatic hypoglycaemia. It is unusual for a newborn with hypoglycaemia to have a classic autonomic nervous system response, with sweating, pallor and tachycardia, as occurs in adults. A low blood sugar detected by a stick test should be checked by a laboratory blood assay for glucose.

CAUSES

These can be considered under five major headings, which are summarized in Table 16.1.

MANAGEMENT

The major aim is to prevent hypoglycaemia developing, and this is done by recognizing babies who are at higher risk of this condition and giving early and appropriate feeding. However, if hypoglycaemia does occur it should be detected early, before symptoms are apparent.

Prevention

Frequent heel-stick test estimations of blood sugar are recommended for 'at-risk' infants, e.g. infants of diabetic mothers, small for gestational age (SGA) and preterm infants. A useful regimen is a blood glucose estimate done before the second feed (assuming that the baby receives its first feed within 2 h of birth),

Table 16.1 Causes of neonatal hypoglycaemia

Decreased substrate availability

SGA infants (see p. 83)

Premature infants. Second twin, especially if growth retarded

Increased glucose utilization

Hyperinsulinaemia
  Infant of a diabetic mother
  Rhesus isoimmunization
  Nesidioblastosis
  Islet cell tumour
  Beckwith–Wiedemann syndrome

Polycythaemia

Inability to utilize glucose

Glycogen storage disease type I

Galactosaemia

Fructose intolerance

Inborn errors of amino acid metabolism

Iatrogenic

Inappropriate infusion of glucose

Miscellaneous

Birth asphyxia

Endocrine deficiencies (e.g. rare types of congenital adrenal hyperplasia)

Hypopituitarism

and then 2–3-hourly before further feeds. When blood sugar levels are satisfactory, the frequency of heel-prick estimations may be reduced to 4-hourly and then 8-hourly before ceasing.

Early feeding. 'At-risk' infants should be fed within 2 h of birth with high glucose-containing solutions. A suitable regimen would be: glucose 10% or full-strength formula given 2-hourly. SGA infants often tolerate up to 100 mL/kg on day 1 of life.

Treatment of established hypoglycaemia

If asymptomatic hypoglycaemia fails to be corrected by early, frequent feeds, an infusion with 10% dextrose will be necessary.

A baby with symptomatic hypoglycaemia will require a dextrose infusion. An initial bolus dose of dextrose 0.1 g/kg is given over 10 min as 1 mL/kg of 10% dextrose or 0.4 mL/kg of 25% dextrose. This is usually followed by a steady-state infusion of 10% dextrose at a rate of 80–100 mL/kg/24 h. If the blood glucose estimate is less than 2.6 mmol/L (40 mg/100 mL), the dextrose concentration may need to be increased to 15% dextrose. Up to 15% dextrose may be infused via a peripheral intravenous line, but if more than 15% dextrose is required a central intravenous line will be necessary. Where possible oral feeding should be continued, but if hypoglycaemia persists with solutions of more than 10% dextrose, feeds should probably be discontinued.

Resistant hypoglycaemia

Rarely, the above regimen fails to control hypoglycaemia and hyperinsulinaemia should be suspected (see p. 170). Under these circumstances other forms of treatment are necessary to control the hypoglycaemia, used in the following sequence:
1 hydrocortisone—25 mg/kg/day intravenously (i.v.);
2 glucagon (100 µg/kg/dose) may be useful when the infant has adequate glycogen stores, e.g. infant of diabetic mother (IDM);
3 diazoxide—5 mg/kg/dose, given i.v. every 6 h;
4 laparotomy and subtotal pancreatectomy when an insulinoma or nesidioblastosis is strongly suspected (see p. 170);
5 somatostatin analogue SMS 201–995 is useful in the short-term management of neonatal hyperinsulinism due to nesidioblastosis.

INVESTIGATIONS

Hypoglycaemia in most infants resolves spontaneously within a few days, but is sometimes more severe or fails to resolve rapidly. Hyperinsulinaemia is suspected clinically when a baby with severe non-ketotic hypoglycaemia requires a glucose infusion rate exceeding 10 mg/kg/min to maintain normoglycaemia.

These babies have a very brisk response to glucagon injections, with the blood glucose increasing to > 1.7 mmol/L above baseline. The definitive diagnosis of hyperinsulinism is made by measurement of serum insulin (> 10 mU/mL) during an episode of hypoglycaemia (< 2.2 mmol/L). The plasma should be separated and frozen immediately after taking the sample if reliable results are to be obtained. A screen for inborn errors of metabolism may be necessary in some cases. An exploratory laparotomy may be necessary in infants suspected of having islet cell tumours or nesidioblastosis (see p. 170).

PROGNOSIS

Severe symptomatic hypoglycaemia carries a very poor prognosis. Approximately half of these babies will die and half of the survivors will have severe neurodevelopmental abnormalities, including mental retardation, convulsions, spasticity and microcephaly. The prevention of symptomatic hypoglycaemia is one of the most important factors in preventing brain damage in the whole of neonatal medicine.

It has been widely understood that infants with asymptomatic hypoglycaemia are not at risk of adverse neurodevelopmental outcome, but recent interest in redefining the level of normoglycaemia is based on a reassessment of the importance of asymptomatic hypoglycaemia. At present the data are not clear, and until a randomized controlled trial is carried out of various levels of blood glucose control the question will not be answered. There is currently evidence of neural dysfunction with blood sugar levels < 2.6 mmol/L, and repeated levels below this may have a cumulative adverse effect on neural function, although the baby may not show clinical symptoms.

Specific causes of hypoglycaemia

INFANTS OF DIABETIC MOTHERS

Maternal diabetes is classified as follows:
1 pregestational;
2 type I: the basic cause is β cell destruction;

Table 16.2 Frequency of complications (percentages) in infants of diabetic mothers (IDM) and infants of gestational diabetic mothers (IGDM). Complications are related to the quality of glucose control in pregnancy

Complications	IDM (%)	IGDM (%)
Uneventful course	50	80
RDS	30	10
Hypoglycaemia (asymptomatic and symptomatic)	60	16
Symptomatic hypoglycaemia	20	10
Hypocalcaemia	25	15
Polycythaemia	40	30
Hyperbilirubinaemia	50	25
Congestive heart failure	10	Unknown
Congenital abnormalities	10	3

3 type II: this is due to insulin resistance with an insulin secretory defect;
4 gestational diabetes.

IDM have unique problems and require specialized neonatal care. The prognosis for the diabetic pregnancy depends on the severity of the diabetes and the quality of diabetic control during pregnancy.

The two main factors determining whether maternal diabetes will have an effect on the fetus and baby are the vascular complications that the diabetes causes the mother, and the blood glucose control during pregnancy.
1 *Vascular disease.* Mothers with vascular complications as a result of diabetes are much more likely to develop hypertension in pregnancy, which may affect fetal growth and wellbeing.
2 *Glucose control.* The outcome of pregnancy in diabetic women also depends on glucose control both before conception and during gestation. Diabetic women should have their diabetes very carefully managed prior to conception, and combined care through pregnancy by a physician and obstetrician is essential. The blood sugar should be maintained below 8 mmol/L, with soluble insulin if necessary, and hypoglycaemia avoided. On this regimen the complications for the fetus are reduced and may be avoided completely.

Clinical features of an IDM

Complications to the fetus are likely to occur in diabetic women in whom glucose control has been less than adequate. The frequency of complications in IDM and in gestational diabetic mothers is given in Table 16.2. Complications include:
1 congenital malformations. The most frequent congenital abnormalities in IDM are:
(a) congenital heart disease, especially ventricular septal defect, transposition of the great vessels, coarctation of the aorta;
(b) renal vein thrombosis;
(c) sacral and coccygeal agenesis (caudal regression syndrome);
(d) left microcolon;
(e) hypertrophic cardiomyopathy. This mainly affects the intraventricular septum and may cause ventricular outflow obstruction. It is a transient condition which resolves in the first few months of life. Inotropic drugs such as digoxin should be avoided;
2 stillbirth. There is an increased risk of intrauterine fetal death during pregnancy;
3 infants born to mothers with diabetic vascular disease are more likely to be SGA;
4 macrosomia. Insulin is a major trophic hormone influencing fetal growth, and

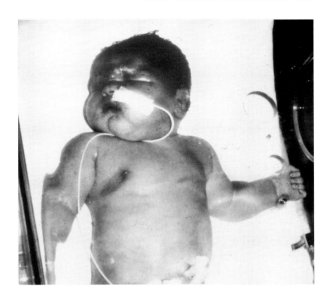

Fig. 16.2 Characteristic appearance of the macrosomic infant of a poorly controlled diabetic mother.

hyperinsulinaemic fetuses become macrosomic. These infants are plethoric, obese and 'Cushingoid' in appearance, and have an enlarged heart, liver and spleen (Fig. 16.2). There is an increased body length and birthweight, but the head circumference and brain weight are appropriate for gestational age. They have excessive fat stores and inhibition of lipolysis and β-oxidation resulting from hyperinsulinaemia. The large size predisposes to birth-related problems, including:

(a) birth trauma from cephalopelvic disproportion, difficult instrumental delivery and shoulder dystocia. Injuries include intracranial haemorrhage, fractured bones and nerve palsies;

(b) birth asphyxia may occur in a poorly controlled diabetic pregnancy and may be related to cephalopelvic disproportion;

5 neonatal hypoglycaemia. Chronically elevated maternal glucose levels cause hyperplasia of the islet β cells in the fetal pancreas with fetal hyperinsulinism. Once the baby is born the high circulating insulin causes neonatal hypoglycaemia lasting for several days. There are three common patterns:

(a) transient hypoglycaemia which lasts 1–4 h, followed by a spontaneous rise in the blood sugar;

(b) prolonged initial hypoglycaemia lasting 24–48 h;

(c) rarely there may be a mild initial hypoglycaemia, followed in 12–24 h by more severe hypoglycaemia which may be symptomatic;

6 insulin has an antagonistic effect on surfactant development and hyperinsulinaemic babies are at much greater risk of developing respiratory distress due to surfactant deficiency, retained lung fluid or polycythaemia, even at full term.

Management

Careful control of diabetes during pregnancy decreases many of the complications. Management of the pregnancy involves obsessional diabetic control, planned delivery in a suitably equipped hospital, examination for congenital abnormalities and screening for expected complications, especially hypoglycaemia.

Prognosis for IDM

Published studies give perinatal mortality rates of about 30/1000 for diabetic pregnancies. There is a 1% incidence of overt diabetes mellitus in childhood, although 10% will have abnormal glucose tolerance when tested in childhood.

NESIDIOBLASTOSIS

This term has been used to describe excessive numbers of isolated β cells and islets within the pancreas. This causes hyperinsulinaemia with profound hypoglycaemia. Nesidioblastosis is now thought to be a disorder in the regulatory function of β cells. This condition should be considered in infants who require glucose infusion to prevent hypoglycaemia exceeding 15 mg/kg/min (Aynsley-Green *et al*. 1981), and confirmed by showing high levels of insulin during hypoglycaemia (see p. 167). Few ketone bodies are produced during the hypoglycaemic episodes.

Severe hypoglycaemia can be temporarily reversed by glucagon, but cure requires total or subtotal pancreatectomy with removal of up to 95% of the pancreas.

BECKWITH–WIEDEMANN SYNDROME

This refers to the association of macroglossia, umbilical hernia (or exomphalos) and macrosomia. The infants almost invariably show a crease or fissure in their earlobes. There is often hyperinsulinaemia due to β-cell hyperplasia. Hypoglycaemia occurs in the neonatal period in about a third of cases. Later malignant disease occurs in about 6% of cases.

IATROGENIC HYPOGLYCAEMIA

This occurs most commonly in infants at risk of hypoglycaemia in whom low blood sugar is detected and aggressive treatment started. Treatment with rapid intravenous injection of concentrated (25% or 50%) dextrose will cause a rapid increase in blood glucose, and in the presence of hyperinsulinism there may be a rebound hypoglycaemia. When the blood glucose is next measured, hypoglycaemia is found as a result of this rebound effect, and another rapid infusion of concentrated dextrose is given with similar effect.

The management of hypoglycaemia is discussed on p. 166. Rapid or concentrated injections of dextrose are rarely necessary and should be avoided if possible. When absolutely necessary, they should be followed by a continuous infusion to avoid rebound hypoglycaemia.

When insulin is used to treat hyperglycaemia or hyperkalaemia, hypoglycaemia may be induced. Regular blood glucose measurements must be performed on all infants receiving insulin.

Hyperglycaemia

Hyperglycaemia is usually defined as a blood sugar greater than 9 mmol/L, at which level glycosuria may occur. Hyperglycaemia frequently occurs in the preterm infant who is receiving 10% dextrose intravenously, or in any infant receiving parenteral nutrition.

Usually hyperglycaemia responds to a reduction in the glucose concentration or the infusion rate. Hyperglycaemia must be considered to be a sign of septicaemia. A full infection screen should always be performed on neonates with high glucose levels or glycosuria. Glycosuria induces an osmotic diuresis and may cause electrolyte imbalance.

Rarely insulin is required to treat hyperglycaemia. Soluble insulin 0.1 U/kg should be given intravenously and repeated as necessary to keep the blood sugar below 9 mmol/L (165 mg/dL).

TRANSIENT NEONATAL DIABETES MELLITUS

This is very rare and occurs in severely growth-retarded infants. Non-ketotic hyperglycaemia develops as a result of inadequate insulin production by the pancreatic β cells. Treatment is by correction of electrolyte disturbances and the administration of insulin (0.1 U/kg) intravenously. Later, chlorpropamide can be substituted for insulin until normal pancreatic function develops (Kuna & Addy 1979).

DISORDERS OF CALCIUM, PHOSPHATE AND MAGNESIUM METABOLISM

The metabolism of these three electrolytes is interrelated and not completely understood.

Calcium. Half the total serum calcium is in ionized form and half is protein bound. Ionized calcium is most physiologically active. Fetal calcium levels are higher than maternal levels but drop rapidly, reaching a low point 18–24 h after birth, largely as a result of calcitonin. This fall in serum calcium stimulates parathormone, with resultant bone resorption and an increase in serum calcium to approximately adult levels.

Phosphate. Most inorganic phosphate is in ionic form (PO_4) or complexed as either HPO_4 or H_2PO_4 ions.

Magnesium. Half the total body magnesium is in bone and most of the rest is intracellular. Neonatal levels are higher than maternal levels. Low levels of magnesium inhibit parathyroid hormone secretion, and hypomagnesaemia is commonly found together with hypocalcaemia.

Parathormone (PTH). This is secreted from the parathyroids in response to low ionized calcium levels. PTH increases serum calcium and lowers serum phosphate levels by the following actions:
1 increases the reabsorption of calcium and phosphate from bone;
2 increases tubular reabsorption of calcium and reduces the reabsorption of phosphate;
3 stimulates the production of renal 1,25-dihydroxyvitamin D.

Vitamin D. This compound requires skin, liver and renal metabolism. Oral cholecalciferol is converted in the liver to 25-hydroxyvitamin D and then further metabolized in the kidney to 1,25-dihydroxyvitamin D. 1,25-Dihydroxyvitamin D increases the intestinal absorption of calcium and phosphate. Low maternal vitamin D levels cause the fetus to be born with relatively low levels.

Calcitonin. This hormone is produced in the thyroid and is secreted in response to a high ionized calcium level. Calcitonin reduces serum calcium and phosphate levels.

Hypocalcaemia

Hypocalcaemia is usually defined as a serum calcium concentration less than 1.8 mmol/L (7.5 mg/dL). It is the ionized fraction that determines whether symptoms occur, but few laboratories can routinely measure ionized calcium. Furthermore, acidosis causes more calcium to be ionized and alkalosis decreases ionized calcium. For these reasons, infants may exhibit few or no symptoms of hypocalcaemia despite low serum calcium levels, provided ionized calcium is normal. This is particularly common in hypoproteinaemic states.

Hypocalcaemia may present early or late.

Early hypocalcaemia. This occurs within the first 72 h of life, although the reasons for this are not fully understood. It is most liable to occur in the following cases:
1 prematurity;
2 associated with respiratory distress syndrome (RDS);
3 birth asphyxia;
4 IDM;
5 neonatal sepsis.

Persistent hypocalcaemia is due to hypoparathyroidism. This is a rare condition and may be inherited in either an X-linked or an autosomal recessive manner. It also occurs in the DiGeorge syndrome. Hypocalcaemia is associated with hyperphosphataemia and requires lifelong vitamin D treatment.

Late hypocalcaemia. This is often referred to as neonatal tetany and occurs after the first week of life. In the past it was commonly due to feeding with an unmodified cows' milk preparation containing a high phosphate/

calcium ratio. Dietary-induced hyperphos-phataemia caused hypocalcaemia and tetany. As the practice of feeding infants unmodified cows' milk has declined, this form of hypocalcaemia is now rarely seen.

Rarely, late hypocalcaemia is due to maternal hyperparathyroidism. Maternal hypercalcaemia causes fetal hypercalcaemia with suppression of the fetal parathyroid. This predisposes the infant to hypocalcaemia in the second or third week of life. It is a transient condition.

Iatrogenic Hypocalcaemia This may occur following exchange transfusion with citrated blood or as a result of inadequate vitamin D supplementation.

CLINICAL FEATURES

Low ionized calcium levels produce neuromuscular irritability. Tremors, tetany, jitteriness and convulsions may occur. Seizures may be identical to those due to hypoglycaemia or other cerebral causes. Occasionally, bradycardia and apnoea may be due to hypocalcaemia.

DIAGNOSIS

Serum calcium and magnesium levels should be measured in 'at-risk' or symptomatic infants.

An electrocardiogram (ECG) will show a prolonged Q–T interval (this needs to be corrected for heart rate).

MANAGEMENT

1 *Asymptomatic hypocalcaemia.* The low serum calcium should be corrected with oral calcium gluconate supplements, or if there is an intravenous line *in situ* by i.v. calcium gluconate (dose is 300 mg/kg/day).
2 *Abnormal movements or apnoea* due to hypocalcaemia should be corrected by a slow infusion of 10% calcium gluconate (100 mg/kg) over 20 min, with ECG monitoring.

Severe and resistant hypocalcaemia, as occurs in congenital hypoparathyroidism, may

require vitamin D supplementation in the form of 1-α-vitamin D.

Some cases of hypocalcaemia will not respond to calcium gluconate infusion and require magnesium sulphate (see below).

PROGNOSIS

Most children with neonatal hypocalcaemia recover completely with no adverse neurodevelopmental sequelae (compare hypoglycaemia). Severe dental caries is seen in the primary dentition of some infants with tetany due to hypocalcaemia.

Metabolic Bone Disease (Rickets of Prematurity)

This condition, also referred to as osteopenia of prematurity, was formally known as rickets of prematurity. Rickets implies a deficiency or abnormality of vitamin D metabolism, which is now known not to be an important factor in metabolic bone disease and is a term that is no longer appropriate.

Metabolic bone disease was reported in the late 1980s to occur in over 40% of very immature babies, but is now considerably less common than this. Metabolic bone disease is due to a nutritional deficiency (mainly phosphate) and is most likely to occur in infants who have been fed diets with too little phosphorus or an inappropriate phosphorus/calcium ratio. With the widespread use of modern low birthweight formula feeds and supplementation of breast milk, severe metabolic bone disease is less of a problem than formerly.

RISK FACTORS

1 Very premature infants fed on unmodified milks and during parenteral nutrition.
2 Placental insufficiency.
3 Steroid administration.
4 Long-term diuretic therapy.
5 Copper and zinc deficiency causes a condition indistinguishable from the osteopenia due to phosphate deficiency.

CLINICAL FEATURES

Most babies are asymptomatic and the condition is only diagnosed on radiography of a long bone. The main feature of this condition is bone undermineralization (osteopenia), which is seen on X-ray. Skeletal deformities involving the rib cage or alteration in head shape may occur and, in its most severe form, fractures and frank rickets may be present, but these latter abnormalities are now uncommonly seen radiographically. Biochemical abnormalities include elevation of alkaline phosphatase and hypophosphataemia.

DIAGNOSIS

The condition may be diagnosed on radiography of a wrist or knee. Rarely frank rickets is seen (Fig. 16.3), with cupping and splaying of the metaphysis.

The biochemical features include:

1 hypophosphataemia (plasma phosphate < 1.0 mmol/L);

2 hypophosphaturia due to very high renal tubular reabsorption of phosphorus (> 90%), so that there is virtually no measurable phosphate in the urine. Excessive urinary calcium loss may occur;

3 elevated serum alkaline phosphatase due to osteoblast activity. The serum alkaline phosphatase activity is normally elevated in newborn babies and remains high for several months. Alkaline phosphatase activity five times the normal adult upper limit suggests metabolic bone disease, and an X-ray should be performed.

MANAGEMENT

The key to this condition is its prevention. Metabolic bone disease can be avoided by appropriate dietary intake of phosphorus. All enterally fed preterm infants should receive 2 mmol/kg/day of phosphate. A baby on full milk feeds of an adapted low birthweight formula will receive this intake. Premature babies exclusively fed breast milk will become phos-

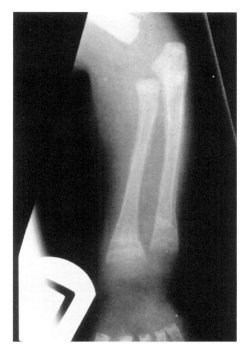

Fig. 16.3 Radiograph of an infant's wrist showing the metaphyseal flaring of neonatal rickets.

phorus deficient and, in these, supplementation with phosphorus is necessary. This is most easily done with a powdered breast milk fortifier (p. 53). Additional phosphate supplementation is recommended for the first 6 months of life if the baby remains on breast milk alone.

Babies on total parenteral nutrition also need phosphate supplementation. Enhancement to 1.9 mmol/kg/day of calcium and 2.4 mmol/kg/day of phosphorus is associated with a reduction in the incidence of hypophosphataemia (Ryan 1996).

The treatment of established metabolic bone disease is to increase phosphate intake so that serum phosphate levels are normal and phosphorus is excreted in the urine. In some cases additional calcium will also be required. There is no need to give more than 1000 iu/day of vitamin D (cholecalciferol) unless there is evidence of liver disease.

LONG-TERM CONSEQUENCES

In most babies with osteopenia of prematurity the bones subsequently appear to mineralize normally. There is no increased risk of fractures in the first few years of life, but babies with undermineralized bones grow less well over the first few years.

Hypercalcaemia

Hypercalcaemia is defined as a serum calcium greater than 2.75 mmol/L (11 mg/dL). This is often iatrogenic due to the excessive use of calcium gluconate in intravenous fluid therapy. Other rare causes include renal failure, inappropriate antidiuretic hormone secretion, hyperparathyroidism, vitamin D intoxication and Williams syndrome (idiopathic hypercalcaemia with elfin facies and often supravalvar aortic stenosis or peripheral pulmonary stenosis).

Disorders of magnesium metabolism

HYPOMAGNESAEMIA

Hypomagnesaemia is defined as a serum magnesium less than 0.6 mmol/L (1.5 mg/dL). It is always associated with hypocalcaemia. Sometimes hypocalcaemia will not respond to calcium gluconate infusion, but rapidly increases following magnesium sulphate injections. The dose is 50–100 mg/kg of a 50% magnesium sulphate solution by deep intramuscular injection or intravenous infusion over 1 h with ECG monitoring.

HYPERMAGNESAEMIA

Hypermagnesaemia is defined as a serum magnesium greater than 1.5 mmol/L and may be associated with hypotonia, bradycardia and apnoea. It may occur as the result of magnesium sulphate administration to the mother for severe maternal pre-eclampsia or given to the baby for pulmonary hypertension (p. 199).

DISORDERS OF SODIUM AND POTASSIUM METABOLISM

Sodium metabolism

The full-term newborn infant requires 2–3 mmol/L of sodium per day. Preterm infants have greater requirements because of the immaturity of renal tubular reabsorption. Requirements in these infants are in the order of 5–6 mmol/kg/day.

HYPONATRAEMIA

This is defined as a serum sodium less than 125 mmol/L and may cause apnoea and convulsions. The causes of hyponatraemia are listed in Table 16.3, and are discussed in detail elsewhere in this book. Care must be taken in the interpretation of serum sodium, as red cell haemolysis may lower the apparent serum level.

In the assessment of infants with hyponatraemia, serum potassium, creatinine and osmolality should be measured as well as urinary sodium and osmolality (or specific

Table 16.3 Causes of neonatal hyponatraemia

Inadequate sodium intake

Vomiting and diarrhoea

Inappropriate intravenous fluids

Inappropriate antidiuretic hormone secretion (see p. 44).

Maternal hyponatraemia following excessive administration of 5% dextrose or oxytocin in labour

Congestive cardiac failure (e.g. patent ductus arteriosus)

Diuretic treatment

Indomethacin (due to increased intravascular volume)

Renal failure

Sepsis

Cystic fibrosis

Bowel obstruction

Congenital adrenal hyperplasia (salt-losing variety)

gravity). A careful fluid input and output chart should be kept for these infants.

Treatment

Treatment depends on the cause. If due to haemodilution (inappropriate antidiuretic hormone secretion or excessive intravenous water) then water restriction is necessary. If due to sodium loss then carefully replace with hypertonic saline according to the equation:

Na required (mmol) = 135 − actual Na × weight (kg) × 0.3

0.3 represents the 'Na space', which may vary between 0.3 and 0.7 depending on birth-weight, gestation and postnatal age.

HYPERNATRAEMIA

Hypernatraemia is defined as a serum sodium greater than 150 mmol/L. Newborn infants, particularly preterm ones, rapidly become dehydrated and hypernatraemic if fluid intake is reduced or abnormal losses occur where water loss exceeds sodium loss. There are two main causes of hypernatraemia:
1 reduced renal excretion. The newborn kidney is less efficient at excreting excess salt than water, and so hypernatraemia is more likely in very immature infants than in older children;
2 excessive water loss. The lack of keratin in the skin of very tiny babies causes excessive transepidermal water loss. Phototherapy and radiant warmers aggravate this loss.

With hypernatraemia the serum osmolality is high and this may be associated with intra-cerebral haemorrhage. The causes of hyper-natraemia are:
1 mismanaged intravenous fluids;
2 dehydration;
3 vomiting and diarrhoea;
4 bowel obstruction: necrotizing enterocolitis (NEC);
5 osmotic diuresis: hyperglycaemia;
6 excessive use of sodium bicarbonate;
7 congenital hyperaldosteronism;

8 faulty technique in making up formula feeds.

Treatment

The serum sodium is reduced by slow infusion of dextrose solution. Too rapid reduction in hypernatraemia may be deleterious, resulting in cerebral fluid shifts and convulsions.

Potassium metabolism

HYPERKALAEMIA

This is defined as a serum potassium greater than 6.5 mmol/L and may cause life-threatening ventricular dysrhythmias if levels exceed 7.5 mmol/L. Spurious hyperkalaemia occurring with haemolysis during blood sampling should not be confused with true hyperkalaemia.

Pathological causes include renal failure, acidosis, shock, hypoxia and blood transfu-sion. It is particularly likely to occur sponta-neously in very ill, premature infants within 72 h of birth.

Treatment

The underlying cause should be corrected wherever possible.
1 Calcium resonium enemas when the potas-sium exceeds 7.5 mmol/L.
2 Insulin infusion started when the potassium is over 8.0 mmol/L, or in the presence of dys-rhythmias. Give 0.1 U soluble insulin per kg body weight at the same time as starting an infusion of 1 g/kg of glucose intravenously.
3 Salbutamol infusion (4 µg/kg over 20 min) has been shown to reduce serum potassium by 1 mmol/L in the first hour after starting the infusion.

The prognosis for severe hyperkalaemia is very poor in terms of both mortality and mor-bidity. This reflects the fact that hyperkalaemia is most likely to occur in the sickest and small-est of babies, as well as the fact that high levels of potassium may provoke spontaneous car-diac dysrhythmias.

HYPOKALAEMIA

This is defined as a serum potassium less than 2.5 mmol/L (depends on laboratory standards). The causes are:
1 diuretic treatment;
2 alkalosis;
3 inadequate intake of potassium;
4 vomiting and diarrhoea;
5 congenital adrenal hyperplasia.

Treatment

If the hypokalaemia is due to dietary potassium deficiency, it can be replaced orally by adding it to the milk. The normal requirements are 2–3 mmol/kg/day.

Intravenous potassium replacement must only be given in the presence of known and adequate renal function, according to the formula:

K required (mmol) = (3.5 − actual K) × weight (kg) × 0.3

This is given by slow intravenous infusion up to a maximum of 0.5 mmol/kg/h under ECG control.

ENDOCRINE GLAND DISORDERS

Disorders of thyroid function

HYPOTHYROIDISM

Untreated hypothyroidism is associated with severe intellectual impairment and as such is an important cause of subsequent disability. Because early recognition and effective treatment offer an excellent outcome in the majority of cases, the early detection of congenital hypothyroidism is essential.

The incidence of congenital hypothyroidism in the UK and Australia is approximately 1/4000 liveborn infants. Causes (Table 16.4) can be divided into:

Screening tests

The aim of screening is to detect all infants

Table 16.4 Causes of hypothyroidism in the neonate

Primary, affecting the thyroid gland (90%)	
Dysgenesis (75%)	Ectopic thyroid (30%)
	Absent thyroid (30%)
	Hypoplastic thyroid (15%)
Dyshormonogenesis (20%)	Multiple causes involving biochemical defects in thyroid gland function. These are usually associated with a goitre at birth and are autosomal recessive in inheritance
Isoimmune (5%)	Occurs as the result of transplacental antibodies and may cause permanent or transient hypothyroidism
Secondary, affecting the pituitary or hypothalamus (10%)	
Transient neonatal hypothyroidism	This is the cause of 10–20% of all positive screening tests (see below)

with clinically significant congenital hypothyroidism at an early stage in order to effect appropriate treatment to avoid brain damage. Screening is performed on heel-prick blood obtained at the same time as the Guthrie test. In the UK and Australia, thyroid-stimulating hormone (TSH) is assayed. Deficiency of circulating thyroid hormone causes the pituitary to release more TSH to stimulate the thyroid. It is more sensitive in screening for hypothyroidism than thyroxine, but fails to detect the rare cases due to pituitary/hypothalamic failure. It does not detect deficiency of thyroid-binding globulin. If TSH levels are high (> 40 mU/L), the infant is urgently referred for definitive investigations of thyroid function. A borderline assay (15–40 mU/L) requires a repeat Guthrie card screen. The median age of notification for congenital hypothyroidism in Scotland following a screening programme is 10 days (Donaldson 1998).

Clinical features

Most infants detected by a screening programme will be clinically normal. The classic signs of severe or untreated hypothyroidism include poor feeding, constipation, abdominal distension, umbilical hernia, mottled skin, coarse puffy facies with a large protruding tongue, hypotonia, hypothermia, failure to thrive, persistent jaundice and both growth and developmental retardation.

Transient hypothyroidism

This refers to babies who have a positive screening test but whose thyroid function subsequently normalizes without treatment. Prenatally acquired causes include maternal thyroid deficiency, antithyroid drugs and thyroid antibodies acquired transplacentally. In the neonatal period the most common transient abnormality is due to topically applied iodine-containing antiseptics. Elevated TSH levels are related to the surface area swabbed and the frequency of skin swabbing.

Investigations

Once a positive screening test has been notified, the following investigations are required:
1 serum thyroxine and TSH;
2 thyroid autoantibodies in mother and baby;
3 radioactive isotope scan to localize the position of an ectopic or hypoplastic thyroid;
4 ultrasound scan of the thyroid gland;
5 bone age X-ray. This is delayed in hypothyroidism;
6 enzyme assays may be required in the investigation of inborn errors of thyroid metabolism.

Treatment

Treatment consists of L-thyroxine 7–10 µg/kg/day initially. Monitoring of the dose will be by growth assessment, bone age, physical appearance and thyroid function tests. Treatment is lifelong in all but transient cases.

Prognosis

The outcome for congenital hypothyroidism depends on the severity of intrauterine hypothyroidism and the delay in establishing effective treatment after birth. The pretreatment venous thyroxine level is the best predictor of eventual IQ (Donaldson 1998) and, in those with high levels, even with effective treatment after birth, mild educational, motor and behavioural problems are likely at 10 years.

If diagnosis and treatment are delayed until 3–6 months of age, only 50% of treated children achieve an IQ greater than 90. If diagnosis and treatment are commenced by 3 months, 75% will achieve an IQ greater than 90.

NEONATAL HYPERTHYROIDISM

This is a rare condition that occurs in about 1–10% of infants born to women with Graves' disease. Women suffering from thyrotoxicosis (or who have been treated with subtotal thyroidectomy) may have circulating immunoglobulin G (IgG) thyroid-stimulating antibodies which may cross the placenta. Long-acting thyroid stimulator (LATS) and LATS-protector are two such agents. If the maternal level of LATS-protector at delivery exceeds 20 U/mL, then neonatal thyrotoxicosis is likely to occur (Munro et al. 1978). If serum TSH receptor antibody is detected, approximately 75% of the offspring will develop neonatal thyrotoxicosis.

Clinical features

The infant usually has a small goitre at birth and develops irritability and diarrhoea, with failure to gain weight despite feeding well. The most important feature is tachycardia, which may not be present at birth but develops rapidly within 48 h. This may be severe enough to precipitate cardiac failure.

Management

All infants born to thyrotoxic women should be carefully monitored for tachycardia for the first 48 h of life. If symptoms develop, propranolol (2 mg/kg/day) is the treatment of choice. The condition is self-limiting and it should be possible to stop treatment by 2–3 months.

Abnormalities of the adrenal gland

Neonatal adrenal disorders fall into the categories of hyperplasia and hypoplasia.

CONGENITAL ADRENAL HYPERPLASIA

Congenital adrenal hyperplasia (CAH) is a rare but important autosomal recessive disorder of adrenal function with an incidence of 1/20 000; 95% of cases are due to 21-hydroxylase deficiency. Figure 16.4 shows the metabolic pathway for adrenal hormones. An enzyme block causes failure of cortisol production, which results in central overstimulation of the adrenal by adrenocorticotropic hormone (ACTH). This leads to the overproduction of adrenal hormones produced downstream to the enzyme block, and it is the effect of this overproduction that produces the clinical features of CAH.

Clinical presentation

21-Hydroxylase deficiency presents in one of two ways:
1 *Virilization.* This is usually most obvious in

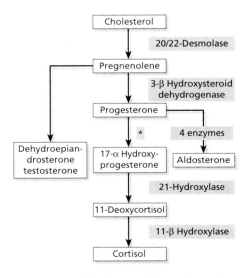

Fig. 16.4 A simplified diagram to illustrate the synthesis of adrenal hormones. The asterisk represents the enzyme 17-α-hydroxydehydrogenase.

male infants, who may be born with hypertrophic, pigmented genitalia. Female virilization may be missed, as on cursory examination the virilized clitoris may be mistaken for a penis;
2 *Salt-losing.* This is due to an excessive aldosterone effect on the renal tubules and occurs in 75% of cases. Hyponatraemia does not usually become obvious until the second week of life, and is associated with a high serum potassium. Symptoms of vomiting and poor feeding precede shock in these babies.

The other forms of CAH are excessively rare but may present with poor virilization and hypertension (Table 16.5).

Investigations

Plasma 17-α-hydroxy-progesterone is markedly raised in the common 21-hydroxylase deficiency type of CAH. Biochemical abnormalities for the other enzyme defects are shown in Table 16.5. Countries with a high incidence of this condition may screen the entire population of newborn babies.

Treatment

Emergency. Intravenous fluid replacement, electrolyte correction and mineralocorticoids such as DOCA (if available) and hydrocortisone.

Long term. Medical management consists of replacement therapy with fludrocortisone and other corticosteroids, usually under the supervision of a paediatric endocrinologist.

Surgical treatment may be required for the enlarged clitoris in virilized females.

Prenatal therapy

It is now possible to determine whether a fetus is affected by 21-hydroxylase deficiency where there is a family history of this condition. Diagnosis may be made by identifying the gene mutation on tissue obtained at chorionic villus biopsy, or by assay of hormones in amniotic fluid. Dexamethasone given to the mother from 10 weeks of gestation inhibits

Table 16.5 Clinical and biochemical features of enzymatic defects in congenital adrenal hyperplasia.

Enzyme defect	Virilization	Poor virilization	Salt loss	Hypertension	Urinary 17-ketosteroids	Plasma 17-OH progesterone
20/22-Desmolase	−	+	++	−	↓	↓
3-β OH steroid dehydrogenase	+	+	+	−	↑	Normal or ↑
17-α OH steroid dehydrogenase	−	+	−	+	↓	↓
21-Hydroxylase	+	−	+−	−	↑	↑++
11-β-Hydroxylase	+	−	−	+	↑	↑

ACTH overstimulation and reduces the extent of fetal virilization.

ADRENAL HYPOPLASIA

This is a rare condition and may arise as primary adrenal failure or secondary to pituitary hypoplasia (as occurs in anencephaly), but may occur in infants with an otherwise normal brain. Adrenal hypoplasia is most often suspected by absent oestriol estimation performed during pregnancy. The infant of any such pregnancy should have adrenal function carefully assessed postnatally. There are also X-linked and autosomal recessive forms of adrenal hypoplasia.

At birth the infant may show hyperpigmentation and hypoglycaemia. Alternatively, symptoms may be delayed until later in infancy. Severe metabolic collapse with profound hypotension may be the first feature of this condition. Adrenal hypoplasia may be confused with CAH, but virilization is not seen and salt loss rarely occurs.

Infants with a family history or low oestriols during pregnancy should have short and long Synacthen tests to investigate the cortisol response to stimulation. Treatment involves lifelong replacement with cortisol and possibly aldosterone.

INBORN ERRORS OF METABOLISM

The term inborn error of metabolism was introduced by Garrod in 1896 to describe a group of genetically determined biochemical disorders caused by specific defects in the structure or function of protein molecules. Some of these have no clinical manifestation, such as histidinaemia, whereas others have major clinical sequelae, e.g. phenylketonuria. The majority are inherited as autosomal recessive disorders but some are sex linked, e.g. Hunter syndrome, Lesch–Nyhan disease, Menkes syndrome and ornithine transcarbamylase deficiency.

Metabolic disorders may be understood if the hypothetical biochemical reaction shown in Fig. 16.5 is considered.

This reaction may be interfered with at the following sites:

1 failure of substance A to cross into cells, e.g. Hartnup disease (failure of tryptophan to enter cell);

2 deficiency of enzyme a. This may cause disease by the accumulation of precursor A, as happens in galactosaemia with the build-up of galactose-1-phosphate (see p. 183);

3 alternatively, a deficiency of enzyme a may be associated with the build-up of alternative metabolic products derived from the metabolites of high levels of precursors of A. An example of this is phenylketonuria, with

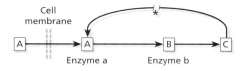

Fig. 16.5 Representation of metabolic pathways with a negative feedback loop.

the production of high levels of phenylketones (see p. 182);

4 deficiency of end-metabolic products as occurs in albinism, where there is failure to produce melanin C in Fig. 16.5;

5 failure of positive feedback control. This occurs when the end product of metabolism is required to switch off a hormone-controlled loop system. CAH is an example of this condition (see p. 178). Failure of cortisol production by an enzyme block results in failure to inhibit ACTH, with consequent adrenal hyperplasia. This is represented by the asterisk in Fig. 16.5.

The inborn errors of metabolism may be diagnosed clinically, in either an asymptomatic phase or an acute early symptomatic phase. Preferably they are diagnosed by newborn screening programmes.

NEWBORN SCREENING

There are many important principles inherent in newborn screening. The following criteria should be satisfied:

1 the disease is a significant health problem;

2 the disease has a latent or asymptomatic phase;

3 there is a commonly accepted and successful therapy;

4 the natural history of the disease is understood;

5 the test is suitably sensitive (few false negatives) and specific (few false positives);

6 the screening programme is cost effective;

7 the test sample is acceptable to the patient and easily obtained;

8 adequate facilities for diagnosis and therapy exist;

9 there is a commitment to careful follow-up.

The incidence of diseases which have been considered for newborn screening is shown in Table 16.6.

Screening programmes that have been adopted in parts of Europe, Australia and the USA include:

1 phenylketonuria (p. 182);

2 hypothyroidism (p. 176);

3 galactosaemia (p. 182);

Table 16.6 Incidence of diseases considered for newborn screening

Specific metabolic disease	Approximate incidence
Cystic fibrosis	1/2500
Hypothyroidism	1/4000
Phenylketonuria	1/15 000
MCAD deficiency	1/15 000
Hartnup disease	1/18 000
Histidinaemia	1/18 000
Galactosaemia	1/30 000
Homocystinuria	1/150 000
Maple syrup urine disease	1/250 000

4 CAH (p. 178);

5 cystic fibrosis. Neonatal screening by elevated immunoreactive trypsin on a dried blood spot detects 90% of cases with severe disease. Positive cases can then be screened by analysis for the $\delta F508$ mutation, which accounts for 80% of cases of cystic fibrosis. Although screening for this condition is available in some countries, it is not yet widespread in the UK because of doubts over the benefits of early treatment. In fact, the evidence does support better lung function in children who had been screened as neonates;

6 medium-chain acyl-CoA dehydrogenase (MCAD) deficiency. This condition is as common as phenylketonuria and presents with collapse (implicated in some cases of sudden infant death syndrome (SIDS)) and severe hypoglycaemia. If the condition is recognized, hypoglycaemia can be avoided by careful attention to carbohydrate intake, and the prognosis is excellent. Screening on a newborn dried blood spot is possible using a tandem mass spectrometer, and screening may be adopted in the near future once this new technique is more widely available.

PRESENTATION IN THE ACUTELY ILL CHILD

Inborn errors of metabolism as a group are

very rare and may present in a number of different ways. In the newborn, presentation is usually dramatic and the infant is very ill. Inborn errors of metabolism must always be considered in the differential diagnosis of an acutely ill infant when there is no obvious alternative diagnosis.

In infants in whom inborn errors of metabolism are considered, particular attention should be paid to the following:

1 *family history.* Most are inherited as an autosomal recessive disorder and consanguinity should be asked about. A family history of unexplained stillbirth or neonatal deaths is important;

2 *onset of illness related to feeds.* Some of the disorders only become manifest when the infant ingests milk (e.g. galactosaemia);

3 *is there a characteristic smell?* Infants with isovaleric acidaemia smell of sweaty feet, and in maple syrup urine disease the baby smells of curry;

4 *dysmorphic features.* Peroxisomal disorders (e.g. Zellweger syndrome) show characteristic facial features. Cataracts are features of galactosaemia.

DIAGNOSIS

Affected infants present in a variety of ways, but the most frequent are:

1 *encephalopathy.* Symptoms include convulsions, apathy, coma and profound hypotonia. Early onset of severe seizures suggests pyridoxine deficiency and non-ketotic hyperglycinaemia;

2 *hypoglycaemia.* This is seen particularly in the organic acidaemias and type I glycogen storage disease. Ketonuria in the absence of hypoglycaemia suggests an organic acidaemia;

3 *acid–base disturbance.* This is seen frequently in any sick baby and is usually not related to inborn errors of metabolism. Calculation of the anion gap may be helpful:

Anion gap = serum $(Na^+ + K^+)$ mmol/L – serum $(Cl^- + HCO_3^-)$ mmol/L

If the anion gap is > 25 mmol/L then the patient is likely to have a specific organic acidaemia;

4 *hepatic failure.* Rapidly progressive liver disease with rising levels of conjugated bilirubin suggests galactosaemia, α_1-antitrypsin deficiency or tyrosinaemia.

If an inborn error of metabolism is suspected, the following investigations should be undertaken as a matter of urgency:

1 amino acid concentrations in blood and urine. Freeze all additional urine specimens for more detailed subsequent examination;

2 organic acid analysis;

3 plasma ammonia;

4 serum lactic acid level;

5 urine for ketone estimate.

MANAGEMENT

Definitive treatment depends on the precise underlying condition. While awaiting a diagnosis the following management points are important:

1 stop all milk feeds;

2 treat metabolic acidosis with infusions of sodium bicarbonate;

3 prevent catabolism by giving 10–15% dextrose infusions, together with insulin if necessary;

4 removal of toxic waste products by peritoneal dialysis (see p. 324);

5 if there is hyperammonaemia (> 600 µmol/L), give sodium benzoate 250 mg/kg as a loading dose followed by an infusion of 250 mg/kg/day;

6 megavitamin cocktail. Some of the inborn errors of metabolism are responsive to large doses of vitamins. The megavitamin doses are shown in Table 16.7.

Table 16.7 Megavitamin dosages for infants with suspected inborn errors of metabolism

Vitamin	Dose (mg/day)
Vitamin B_{12}	1.0
Biotin	100
Thiamine	50
Riboflavine	50
Nicotinamide	600
Pyridoxine	100

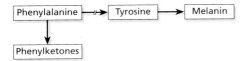

Fig. 16.6 Metabolism of phenylalanine. The broken arrow represents the enzyme defect in phenylketonuria.

Phenylketonuria

Phenylketonuria (PKU) is an autosomal recessive condition and, in its classic form, is caused by a deficiency of the enzyme phenylalanine-hydroxylase, which converts phenylalanine to tyrosine. Absence of the enzyme results in the accumulation of phenylalanine and its metabolites (see Fig. 16.6). In untreated patients the accumulation of phenylalanine and phenyl-ketones produces a clinical picture of neonatal convulsions, later mental impairment, epilepsy and eczema. Affected children usually have fair hair and skin with blue eyes, owing to a relative lack of melanin, which is metabolized downstream from tyrosine.

Malignant hyperphenylalaninaemia has recently been described and is due to a deficiency of biopterin in the liver. This is required as a cofactor for the enzyme phenylalanine-hydroxylase.

DIAGNOSIS

This may be suspected from screening tests and confirmed by definitive investigations.

Screening

This is done by the Guthrie test, which is a bacterial inhibition assay on blood absorbed on to blotting paper from a heel-prick sample. The infant needs to be on an adequate milk diet for 48 h prior to testing. This is particularly important in preterm and ill infants. Antibiotic treatment of the infant may inhibit the bacteria that produce the Guthrie reaction. Alternative methods for mass screening are used in some centres.

Definitive diagnosis

This involves recalling the infant for definitive biochemical investigations of blood phenylalanine and tyrosine levels, together with urinary phenylketones.

TREATMENT

This consists of a diet low in phenylalanine and tryptophan instituted within 20 days of age.

With early treatment the prognosis is good, provided careful control is maintained. Diet should probably be lifelong, but at least into the early adolescent years. In the rare malignant hyperphenylalaninaemia treatment with biopterin will be necessary.

Such conditions are best managed in specialized metabolic clinics.

MATERNAL PKU

Undiagnosed maternal PKU may cause the infant to be brain damaged owing to the passage of toxic phenylpyruvate products across the placenta. All women with seizures or low IQ should be tested at booking in the antenatal clinic for urinary phenylketones by means of a simple stick test (Phenistix, Ames Ltd). Women known to have PKU should be well controlled on their diet before conception in order to prevent neurological compromise of the fetus.

Galactosaemia

This rare autosomal recessive condition has many variants, but only classic galactosaemia presents early in the neonatal period. Classic galactosaemia is due to a deficiency of the enzyme galactose-1-phosphate uridyl transferase. It presents with severe illness in the first week of life, with vomiting, encephalopathy, jaundice, failure to thrive, cataracts, hepatomegaly and a coagulation disorder. If treatment is not started the infant will die.

DIAGNOSIS

If galactosaemia is suspected clinically, the urine should be tested for reducing substances. If the urine is positive on Clinitest tablet testing, but negative to glucose on a glucose oxidase stick test, then assay of galactose-1-phosphate uridyl transferase should be performed. A proportion of children with galactosaemia do not show reducing substances in their urine, and enzyme assay should be performed if the condition is suspected.

TREATMENT

This consists of careful dietary control using galactose-free milk (see p. 60).

PROGNOSIS

Unlike other inborn errors of metabolism early diagnosis does not appear to significantly improve outcome, as the fetus has been damaged prior to birth. Most have significant developmental delay despite adequate dietary management.

SCREENING

Outcome is not markedly improved by early diagnosis, which weakens the argument for screening all newborns.

AMBIGUOUS GENITALIA

This is a complex subject and one where the neonatologist, the paediatric endocrinologist and the paediatric surgeon must work together to achieve the optimal physical and psychological result for the child and family.

The neonate with ambiguous genitalia may represent a medical emergency. Assessment and subsequent gender assignment must consider the future physical and sexual development of the child.

Parents are informed of the medical concern and the baby is examined in their presence.

Terms such as 'underdeveloped' or 'overdeveloped' should be used, and 'intersex' and 'pseudohermaphrodite' avoided. The naming of the baby should be delayed until the definitive sex of rearing has been determined.

CLINICAL ASSESSMENT

The following are useful guidelines that should be followed.
1 Is the baby a female who has been virilized?
2 Is the baby a male who is undervirilized?
3 Are gonads palpable in the inguinogenital region? If gonads are present it is almost certain that they are testes.

A diagnostic flow chart can be based on these observations (Fig. 16.7).

Discussion of the various conditions and their individual treatment is beyond the scope of this text. CAH has been discussed above.

REFERENCES

Aynsley-Green, A., Polak, J.M., Bloom, S.R. *et al.* (1981) Nesidioblastosis of the pancreas: definition of the syndrome and the management of the severe neonatal hyperinsulinaemic hypoglycaemia. *Archives of Disease in Childhood* **56**, 496–508.

Cornblath, M. & Schwartz, R. (1976) *Disorders of Carbohydrate Metabolism in Infancy.* W.B. Saunders, Philadelphia.

Donaldson, M.D.C. (1998) Neonatal screening for congenital hypothyroidism. *Seminars in Neonatology* **3**, 35–47.

Koh, T.H., Aynsley-Green, A., Tarbit, M. & Eyre, J.A. (1988) Neural dysfunction during hypoglycemia. *Archives of Disease in Childhood* **63**, 1353–1358.

Kuna, P. & Addy, D.P. (1979) Transient neonatal diabetes mellitus. *American Journal of Diseases of Childhood* **133**, 65–66.

Lucus, A., Morley, R. & Cole, T.J. (1988) Adverse neurodevelopmental outcome of moderate neonatal hypoglycaemia. *British Medical Journal* **297**, 1304–1308.

Munro, D.S., Dirmikis, S.M., Humphries, H., Smith, T. & Broadhead, G.D. (1978) The role of thyroid stimulating immunoglobulins of Graves' disease in neonatal thyrotoxicosis. *British Journal of Obstetrics and Gynaecology* **85**, 837–843.

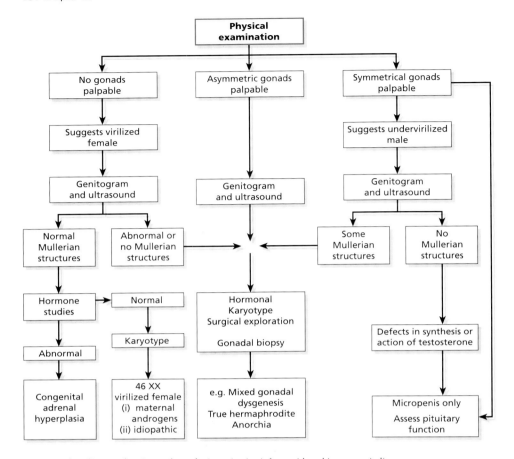

Fig. 16.7 Flow diagram showing a scheme for investigating infants with ambiguous genitalia.

Ryan, S. (1996) Nutritional aspects of metabolic bone disease in the newborn. *Archives of Disease in Childhood* 74, F145–F148.

FURTHER READING

Brook, C.G.D. (ed.) (1981) *Clinical Paediatric*

Endocrinology. Blackwell Scientific Publications, Oxford.

Lippe, B.M. (1979) Ambiguous genitalia and pseudohermaphroditism. *Paediatric Clinics of North America*, **26**, 91–106.

Visser, H.K. (1981) Sexual differentiation in the fetus and newborn. In: *Scientific Foundations of Paediatrics* (eds J.A. Davis & J. Dobbing), 2nd edn. Butterworth-Heinemann, Oxford.

17 Disorders of the cardiovascular system

PHYSIOLOGY

The cardiovascular system undergoes major changes in the hours and days after birth. The transition of the circulation from fetal to neonatal is described in Chapter 2. Failure of organ perfusion is a major part of many neonatal disorders and an understanding of cardiovascular physiology is important in analysing what are the most appropriate management strategies.

Cardiac Output

Cardiac output is the total amount of blood ejected from both ventricles, but in the neonatal period reciprocal changes occur in the two ventricles. Pulmonary vascular resistance falls rapidly after birth, with a consequent reduction of right ventricular afterload, whereas systemic vascular resistance gradually increases, resulting in an increasing left ventricular afterload; this leads to a doubling of left ventricular stroke volume with no significant change in right ventricular stroke volume. This means that neonatal cardiac output increases after birth with cardiac performance near the upper limit of its range.

Cardiac output (CO) is dependent on stroke volume (SV) and heart rate (HR):

$$CO = SV \times HR$$

Stroke Volume

This is a complicated function which is dependent on the stretch undergone by individual heart myofibrils.

$$SV \sim preload + afterload + contractility$$

PRELOAD

This represents the passive stretching of the resting heart prior to ventricular filling, and is largely influenced by vascular volume. The myocardium contracts most efficiently at a certain preload volume. Underfilling (reduced preload) or overfilling (increased preload) causes the contraction to be less efficient.

AFTERLOAD

This is the resistance to ventricular contraction distal to the ventricles and a variety of factors are involved, including peripheral vascular resistance and the viscosity of the blood.

CONTRACTILITY

This refers to the metabolic state of the heart muscle itself and is largely independent of both pre- and afterload.

Cardiac output can be increased by increasing myocardial contractility (inotropy) or increasing the heart rate (chronotropy). These changes are mediated through adrenergic receptors, either α, β or dopaminergic. These effects include the following:

1 β_1 *stimulation* increases myocardial contractility and heart rate;

2 β_2 *stimulation* increases pulmonary and systemic vasodilatation;

3 α_1 *stimulation* causes arteriolar constriction;

4 *dopaminergic stimulation* causes vasodilatation in vascular beds such as the kidney, brain and gut.

HYPOTENSION

Blood pressure is the product of flow and resistance according to the formula:

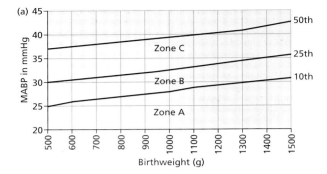

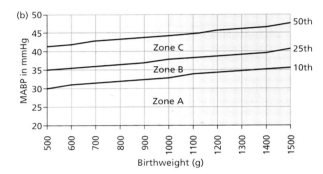

Fig. 17.1 (a) Range of mean arterial blood pressure (MABP) measurements in very low birthweight infants less than 36 h of age and (b) more than 36 h old. Zone A: Hypotension requiring treatment (see Fig. 17.2). Zone B: Possible hypotension requiring clinical assessment. Zone C: Blood pressure unlikely to require treatment but clinical signs should be assessed.

Blood pressure = blood flow × peripheral resistance

Hypotension is a common and important complication of the sick newborn infant, but blood pressure in itself is not the critical physiological function in which the clinician is interested. It is the maintenance of organ perfusion that is essential, because once this falls below a critical limit, organ function will fail. The clinical measurement of blood flow and vascular resistance is not possible, and so blood pressure is the physiological measurement that is used to monitor physiological integrity. Failure to perfuse an organ normally will cause that organ system to fail, and clinical features of this failure may be evident. Such features include:

1 increasing metabolic acidosis, which may indicate tissue hypoxaemia;

2 reducing urine output. Failure to adequately perfuse the kidneys will cause a reduction in urine production and this may indicate a low output state;

3 poor skin perfusion. This can be assessed by blanching the skin over the chest to see how long it takes to recover its colour. Reperfusion within 3 s is normal.

Normal range

Blood pressure varies normally with gestational age and postnatal age, and both may need to be considered when deciding whether a baby needs treatment for low blood pressure. The normal range for blood pressure is shown in Fig. 17.1.

Zone A represents the mandatory need for treatment because the blood pressure is critically low.

Zone B represents possible hypotension and is a level of uncertainty, as the baby may either cope without support or show signs of failing organ perfusion. If clinical signs are present, such as metabolic acidosis, decreasing peripheral perfusion, poor capillary return, poor colour and low peripheral temperature, then treatment should be given.

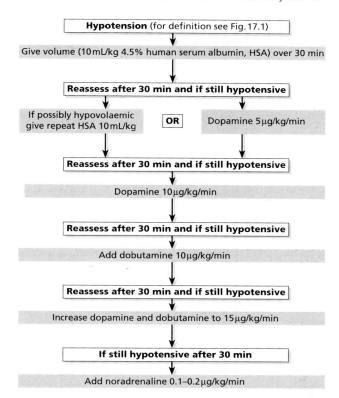

Fig. 17.2 Flow diagram showing a suggested graded management response to neonatal hypotension.

Zone C represents satisfactory blood pressure and treatment is only required if there are obvious and overriding clinical signs of poor perfusion.

A widely used rule of thumb is to maintain the minimum mean arterial blood pressure (MABP) above the infant's gestational age in weeks. Therefore, a 27-week infant should have a MABP no lower than 27 mmHg.

Management

There are two important factors to consider.
1 What is the cause of the hypotension? This must be identified and the underlying cause treated.
2 What is the best therapeutic option in restoring adequate blood pressure? In considering the first-line management of hypotension it is important to think through the possible physiological mechanisms:

(a) preload. Is the vascular compartment adequately filled?
(b) afterload. Should vascular resistance be increased?
(c) contractility. Is the myocardium working to maximum advantage?
(d) heart rate. Is the heart rate fast enough to maintain adequate cardiac output?
Figure 17.2 illustrates the incremental management of neonatal hypotension.

VOLUME REPLACEMENT

Many ill premature infants are hypovolaemic. It is difficult to measure circulating blood volume, but serum electrolytes, urinary concentration and weight changes may be helpful in determining this factor (p. 43). If the baby is thought to be hypotensive due to volume depletion, an infusion of either a colloid or a crystalloid fluid should be given (10 mL/kg, repeated once if necessary). There is considerable controversy as to what fluid should be used. Traditionally, human serum albumin is given, but if the vasculature is 'leaky' the colloid can be rapidly lost into the tissues, which will cause a further loss of fluid from the vascular compartment owing to osmotic effect. Gelufusin and normal saline can also be used to expand intravascular volume.

Giving fluid to a baby who already has increased preload may precipitate further cardiac output decompensation, and positioning a central venous pressure line by advancing an umbilical venous catheter into the right atrium may be useful in the further assessment of some babies in cardiac failure where uncertainty exists about whether they remain fluid depleted.

INOTROPIC AGENTS

Dopamine acts in a complicated way depending on its dosage. In low dose (1–5 μg/kg/min) it has primary dopaminergic actions and vasodilates the renal, coronary and possibly the cerebral circulation. In higher dose (5–10 μg/kg/min) it stimulates β_1 receptors, enhances myocardial contractility and increases heart rate. At yet higher dosage (10–20 μg/kg/min) the main effects are α-adrenergic, with an increase in peripheral vascular resistance and a reduction in renal blood flow.

Dobutamine (5–20 μg/kg/min by continuous infusion) has mainly β_2 effects, and increases blood pressure by increasing myocardial contractility with some reduction in systemic resistance, thereby reducing afterload, which may be valuable in the failing heart. There is little effect on heart rate.

Noradrenaline (0.1–0.2 μg/kg/min by continuous infusion) is sometimes used once dopamine and dobutamine have been given in maximum dosage. It has both α and β effects, causing an increase in contractility, tachycardia and vascular resistance.

HYPERTENSION

Neonatal hypertension is not a rare phe-

Table 17.1 Causes of neonatal hypertension. (Adapted from Adelman 1988)

Vascular
Renal artery thrombosis
Coarctation of the aorta
Renal
Renal dysplasia
Obstructive uropathy
Polycystic/multicystic disease
Drugs
Steroids
Theophylline
Endocrine
Congenital adrenal hyperplasia (rare forms)
Phaeochromocytoma
Miscellaneous
BPD
Intracranial hypertension
Essential

nomenon in sick newborn infants. It is rarely due to essential hypertension and is most commonly related to an underlying anatomical or endocrine abnormality, or arises as the result of a complication of drug treatment. Table 17.1 lists the commoner causes of neonatal hypertension.

Management is directed at the underlying cause of the condition, and includes renal or aortic surgery where appropriate. At present there is no evidence that thrombolysis is useful in the treatment of renal artery thrombosis.

The medical management of hypertension is largely empirical. Drugs include frusemide (1–2 mg/kg), chlorothiazide (20–40 mg/kg), propranolol (0.5–5.0 mg/kg), hydralazine (0.5 mg/kg 8-hourly) and captopril (0.1–1.6 mg/kg/day).

CONGENITAL HEART DISEASE

Congenital heart disease (CHD) refers to an abnormality in the structure or function of the heart that is present at birth. Many congenital cardiac abnormalities remain asymptomatic and undetected in the neonatal period, only to be diagnosed weeks or years later. The incidence of CHD based on the definition given above is

Table 17.2 Frequency of the commoner congenital heart malformations

Ventricular septal defect	25%
Patent ductus arteriosus	15%
Atrial septal defect	15%
Pulmonary stenosis	10%
Aortic stenosis	5%
Coarctation of the aorta	5%
Transposition of the great arteries	5%
Tetralogy of Fallot	5%
Tricuspid atresia	1%
Other individually rare conditions	14%

therefore higher than previously reported, when only lesions diagnosed at birth were included. The generally accepted incidence is 4–10/1000 births, and represents the commonest form of major congenital abnormality in developed countries. Table 17.2 lists the frequency of different congenital cardiac anomalies.

Aetiology

The aetiology of CHD is multifactorial and depends on the type of abnormality, but overall 75% have no identifiable cause. There is an increased incidence with the following factors:
1 chromosomal disorders. These account for approximately 5% of all children with CHD;
   (a) Down syndrome—30% have CHD, most commonly atrioventricular defects, ventricular septal defect (VSD) and atrial septal defect (ASD);
   (b) trisomy 18—90% have major cardiac defects;
   (c) trisomy 13—80% have major cardiac defects;
   (d) Turner syndrome—10% have coarctation of the aorta;
2 single-gene defects. These account for approximately 3% of children with CHD. The following are the most common:
   (a) Noonan syndrome (pulmonary valve abnormalities are particularly common);

   (b) Marfan syndrome (aortic valve and aortic dissections);
   (c) Holt–Oram syndrome (VSD and ASD);
3 polygenic factors. These are poorly understood but are probably the most important factors in the development of CHD, which may recur in successive generations;
4 infection—rubella infection in the first trimester may cause a patent ductus arteriosus (PDA) or pulmonary artery stenosis. Coxsackie B and influenza A may cause myocarditis;
5 drugs—maternal lithium is associated with tricuspid valve anomalies. Thalidomide, amphetamines, antimetabolites and phenytoin have been associated with CHD;
6 alcohol—30% of infants with fetal alcohol syndrome have CHD;
7 maternal diabetes—transposition of the great vessels, VSD, coarctation and idiopathic hypertrophic subaortic stenosis.

Familial incidence

In a family with one child who has CHD there is a 2–5% risk of recurrence in siblings. There is a 5–10% risk of an affected individual transmitting the condition to the next generation, reflecting the polygenic nature of the condition.

Mode of presentation

Cardiac disease in the newborn presents in the following ways:
1 cyanosis. This may be due to either cardiac or respiratory causes, which can usually be easily distinguished;
2 congestive cardiac failure;
3 murmur heard on routine examination;
4 circulatory maladaptations at birth;
5 dysrhythmias.

Investigations

Investigations are triggered by symptoms or abnormal signs such as a cardiac murmur. In many centres where there is no direct access to paediatric cardiologists, it is necessary to undertake basic investigations in order to determine which babies require referral to a paediatric cardiologist for further evaluation. These basic investigations include chest X-ray, electrocardiography and nitrogen washout test. Modern echocardiography has supplanted the need for many of the investigations that were formerly performed, but this technique requires considerable expertise which is not readily available in many centres.

CHEST X-RAY

This is used to assess:
1 heart size. This is assessed by measuring the cardiothoracic ratio. The widest cardiac diameter is measured and compared to the maximal internal thoracic diameter of the chest, usually at the costophrenic angles. In the newborn a ratio of up to 0.6 is normal. CHD may exist in the presence of a normal heart size;
2 abnormal heart shape;
3 lung field vascularity. This may be difficult in the newborn, especially if the film is not cor-rectly exposed. If there is increased vascularity (pulmonary plethora) then there is a left-to-right shunt, and if reduced (oligaemia) there is obstruction of right-sided flow to the lungs;
4 situs inversus (stomach gas bubble on the right) may indicate serious underlying heart disease. Vertebral anomalies may also suggest cardiac anomalies.

ELECTROCARDIOGRAPH (ECG)

This may be helpful in elucidating the nature of a cardiac abnormality prior to transfer to a cardiac centre for full assessment. In infants it is necessary to record from the V4R position (over the right nipple) as well as the traditional chest leads V1–V6. Normal values for various ECG variables are shown in Table 17.3.

Heart rate. The heart rate normally varies with gestational and postnatal age. Normal heart rates for premature and full-term infants are shown in Table 17.4.

Table 17.3 Normal range for P–R interval, R and S waves for various postnatal ages (Scott 1981)

Age	P–R interval (s)	R wave		S wave	
		V1	V6	V1	V6
0–24 h	0.07–0.13	7–20	2–7	3–27	2–10
1–7 days	0.07–0.13	9–27	2–13	5–19	0.8–10
8–30 days	0.07–0.17	4–20	2–21	3–13	0.6–9
1–3 months	0.07–0.17	4–18	4–13	2–17	0.8–6
3–6 months	0.07–0.13	6–17	5–16	2–12	0.6–5

Table 17.4 Range of normal heart rates for premature and full-term infants at different postnatal ages

Age	Premature infants (Moss & Adams 1968)	Full-term infants (Scott 1981)
0–24 h	109–173	94–145
1–7 days	134–200	100–175
8–30 days	133–200	115–190
1–3 months	128–203	124–190
3–6 months	—	111–179

Axis. The mean QRS axis in neonates is further to the right than in older children, but moves to the left within the first month of life. The QRS vector is markedly abnormal in tricuspid atresia (left axis −45°, i.e. maximal positive QRS deflection in the direction of aVL). The axis is also vertical (−90°) in endocardial cushion defects.

P wave. The P wave precedes atrial contraction. A tall P wave exceeding 3 min in lead II indicates right atrial hypertrophy, and a broad P wave suggests left atrial hypertrophy but is rarely seen in the newborn.

P–R interval. This measures the time from the onset of atrial contraction to the onset of ventricular contraction. A prolonged P–R interval indicates a degree of heart block (Table 17.3).

Right ventricular hypertrophy (RVH). This is estimated from the right chest leads. The criteria for diagnosis of RVH are:
1 upright T wave in V4R or V1 with dominant R after the first 5 days of life;
2 the voltage of R or S in V1 or V6 exceeds the normal range (see Table 17.3);
3 Q wave in V1;
4 right axis deviation.

Left ventricular hypertrophy (LVH). This is diagnosed according to the following criteria, but left axis deviation on its own does not necessarily indicate LVH:
1 tall R waves in V6 and deep S waves in V1 above the normal range (see Table 17.3);
2 a combined voltage of R in V5 or V6 and S in V1 exceeding 30 mm;
3 inverted T waves in the left chest leads. This suggests ischaemia, but digoxin may also cause this appearance.

NITROGEN WASHOUT TEST

This may be helpful in distinguishing congenital cyanotic heart lesions from respiratory pathology. Blood-gas estimations are performed before and after the infant has been breathing 100% oxygen for 10 min. In normal babies the Pa_{O_2} should rise to 80 kPa (600 mmHg). With intrinsic lung disease the Pa_{O_2} increases to 20–53 kPa (150–400 mmHg), depending on the severity of disease. In the presence of cardiac abnormalities with a right-to-left intracardiac shunt there is little increase in Pa_{O_2}.

There is a potential danger in this technique if the patient is dependent on maintaining right-to-left mixing through a PDA. Hyperoxia may cause the ductus to close, thereby seriously compromising the infant. Prostaglandin E_1 (PGE_1) (see p. 194) should be available during this procedure.

More specialized investigations

In specialist centres a definitive diagnosis can be made in most cases using echocardiography. More rarely cardiac catheterization is required for diagnosis or therapy in transposition of the great vessels (p. 192).

ECHOCARDIOGRAPHY

The investigation of CHD has been revolutionized by the introduction of high-resolution, real-time, two-dimensional (2D) echocardiography. This allows the heart to be scanned in a number of standard planes, giving fine detail of anatomical structure. Most lesions can be diagnosed using this technique alone, and increasingly cardiac abnormalities are recognized on prenatal ultrasound assessment.

The heart can be studied in a number of planes which highlight anatomical structures:
1 parasternal long-axis view shows the left-sided structures, including left atrium, mitral valve, ventricle, septum, aortic valve and ascending aorta (Fig. 17.3a);
2 parasternal short-axis view shows the structure of the aortic and pulmonary valves and the main pulmonary artery (Fig. 17.3b); and
3 the apical four-chamber view shows all four chambers simultaneously: the atrio-ventricular (a-v) valves are particularly well seen (Fig. 17.3c).

Most abnormalities can be readily recognized by an experienced cardiologist using ultrasound. Cardiac Doppler with colour flow

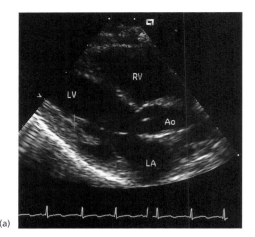

(a)

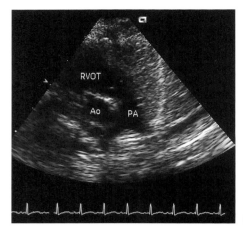

(b)

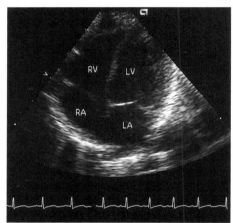

(c)

Fig. 17.3 Real-time, two-dimensional echocardiograms of the normal neonatal heart. (a) Parasternal long-axis view. RV, right ventricle; LV, left ventricle; Ao, aorta; LA, left atrium. (b) Parasternal short-axis view. RVOT, right ventricular outlet tract; PA, pulmonary artery. (c) Apical four-chamber view, RA, right atrium.

imaging is also very helpful in highlighting cardiac function and blood turbulence through small lesions.

CARDIAC CATHETERIZATION

This is only undertaken in a specialist children's cardiac unit. Cardiac catheterization in the newborn has an approximately 1–2% mortality rate and a significant morbidity rate, including infection and necrotizing enterocolitis (NEC).

Cyanotic heart disease

Persistent central cyanosis in the newborn infant is usually due to respiratory or cardiac disease, but rarely may be due to methaemoglobinaemia or shock. Central cyanosis occurs when there is more than 5 g/dL of deoxygenated haemoglobin in the blood. This must be distinguished from peripheral cyanosis with a poor circulation due to cold, shock or polycythaemia with hyperviscosity.

Most neonates presenting with cyanotic heart disease do not pose a diagnostic problem as they show central cyanosis with little or no respiratory distress. However, if there is difficulty distinguishing pulmonary disease from cyanotic CHD, a hyperoxia test or nitrogen washout test (see above) should be performed. The causes of cyanotic CHD are shown in Table 17.5. An approach to the diagnosis of cyanotic CHD is shown in Fig. 17.4.

Table 17.5 Causes of cyanotic CHD

TGA

Tricuspid atresia

Pulmonary atresia or pulmonary stenosis

Hypoplastic right heart syndrome

Tetralogy of Fallot with severe pulmonary stenosis

Ebstein's anomaly

Total anomalous pulmonary venous drainage

Truncus arteriosus

Some causes of cyanotic heart disease rarely present in the neonatal period as cyanosis does not develop for several months (see Fallot's tetralogy).

TRANSPOSITION OF THE GREAT ARTERIES

Transposition of the great arteries (TGA) is the commonest congenital heart defect presenting in the newborn period. The aorta arises from the right ventricle and the pulmonary artery from the left, with the aorta lying in front of the pulmonary artery. The degree of cyanosis depends on the mixing of pulmonary and systemic blood. If a VSD is present a murmur may be heard, but in TGA murmurs are usually absent.

Investigations

There is a characteristic chest X-ray appear-ance with a narrow pedicle (an egg on its side). The lung markings may be normal but are often increased. The ECG shows right axis deviation and RVH.

Treatment

Metabolic acidosis may be severe due to tissue hypoxaemia and should be corrected with bicarbonate. Maintaining the ductus arterio-sus open with PGE_1 infusion may be life-saving prior to elective surgery. The treatment of choice for simple transposition is the arterial switch operation. In experienced hands this has a mortality of $< 5\%$ and involves a full anatomical correction by switching the two major arteries and reconstructing the insertion of the coronary arteries. This procedure must be performed within 10–14 days of birth. Previously the condition was treated by atrial septostomy (Rashkind procedure), with defini-tive surgery (Mustard's repair or Senning's procedure) carried out at 9–12 months, but this produces a less satisfactory anatomical correction than the switch procedure.

TRICUSPID ATRESIA

In tricuspid atresia (TA) there is obstruction at the level of the right atrium to ventricle, often with hypoplasia of the right ventricle. Pulmonary stenosis commonly accompanies TA, together with a VSD. Pulmonary blood flow is often poor and the pulmonary arteries

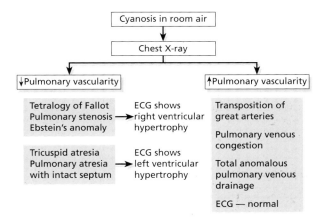

Fig. 17.4 A diagnostic approach to cyanotic CHD.

small. A systolic murmur is usually heard and the infant is severely cyanosed. Pulmonary blood flow is from the left ventricle via an open ductus arteriosus.

Investigations

There is pulmonary oligaemia but no cardiomegaly. ECG shows left-axis deviation and LVH. There are usually tall P waves in lead II. Echocardiography should confirm the diagnosis.

Treatment

Maintaining the ductus open with PGE_1 may keep the infant relatively pink in the hope that growth will occur until a palliative shunt operation can be performed. When the child is older a further procedure will be necessary, but the long-term results of surgery are reasonably good and up to 90% will survive over 10 years, and many into adult life.

PULMONARY ATRESIA OR STENOSIS

A number of abnormalities of the pulmonary valve occur and the symptoms depend on associated cardiac abnormalities. Pulmonary atresia or stenosis (PA or PS) with VSD is very similar to Fallot's tetralogy but usually presents with cyanosis earlier. Rarely the ventricular septum is intact: the right ventricle is then hypoplastic and the prognosis is very poor.

Investigations

The heart is not enlarged on X-ray but the lung fields are oligaemic. There is right-axis deviation with right atrial and right ventricular hypertrophy if there is a coexistent VSD. Left ventricular hypertrophy is seen in PA without VSD.

Treatment

PGE_1 infusion may be of value in the acute stages to maintain the ductus arteriosus open and allow pulmonary perfusion. Later a shunt operation may be of value in relieving cyanosis.

TETRALOGY OF FALLOT

This does not classically present with cyanosis in the newborn period, but a murmur may be detected early and on investigation some infants are found to be cyanosed. After the age of 1 month it is the commonest cause of cyanotic heart disease. Treatment is initially with a Blalock–Taussig shunt and later total repair. The long-term prognosis following successful surgery is excellent.

EBSTEIN'S ANOMALY

In this condition there is an abnormal tricuspid valve with obstruction to right ventricular ejection, and diminished pulmonary blood flow. In some children presentation occurs in the first days of life with intense cyanosis and cardiac failure.

Investigations

The chest X-ray shows a very large heart with oligaemic lung fields. The ECG is often pathognomonic, with complete bundle branch block and right atrial hypertrophy (very tall P waves).

TOTAL ANOMALOUS PULMONARY VENOUS DRAINAGE (TAPVD)

The pulmonary veins drain either directly or indirectly into the right rather than the left atrium. If the drainage is obstructed, little oxygenated blood enters the right atrium and the infant is cyanosed. There is also pulmonary congestion, and the infant often shows features of cardiac failure with respiratory distress. This condition may be very difficult to distinguish from primary lung disease and may require extensive investigation.

Investigations

Chest X-ray shows a normal-sized heart with

Table 17.6 Causes of congestive heart failure presenting in the newborn period (the commoner ones are discussed in the text)

Structural lesions (the most common in order of frequency)

PDA

Hypoplastic left heart syndrome (e.g. aortic valve stenosis)

Coarctation of the aorta (includes interrupted aortic arch)

VSD

Endocardial cushion defects

Persistent truncus arteriosus

Total anomalous pulmonary venous drainage (non-obstructive)

Aortic stenosis

Non-structural lesions

Transient myocardial ischaemia (association with prenatal asphyxia or severe respiratory distress)

Viral myocarditis (especially Coxsackie, echo, rubella, CMV)

Endocardial fibroelastosis

Polycythaemia

Hydrops fetalis

Fluid overload

Hypertrophic subaortic stenosis (especially in infant of diabetic mother)

Hypoglycaemia, hypocalcaemia

Arrhythmias

---

pulmonary oedema, which may be so severe as to be confused with respiratory distress syndrome (RDS). The ECG usually shows RVH. Echocardiography may be diagnostic, but the diagnosis may require cardiac catheterization.

Treatment

Urgent surgery is necessary but carries a high mortality.

PROSTAGLANDIN TREATMENT

PGE_1 causes the ductus arteriosus to open and can be given as an emergency to any severely cyanosed infant in an attempt to improve pulmonary blood flow. If successful and the ductus opens, the infant rapidly 'pinks up' as soon as the infusion is started. Dosage is 0.01–0.05 µg/kg/min by intravenous infusion,

and this can later be given orally (62.5–250 µg) 2–3-hourly. PGE_1 may also be life-saving in left-sided obstructive lesions, such as hypoplastic left heart and critical coarctation of the aorta, when systemic blood flow is achieved from the right ventricle through the ductus.

Prostaglandins may cause pyrexia, jitteriness and apnoea requiring ventilation. Great care should be taken to avoid flushing the intravenous infusion, thereby giving a bolus of prostaglandin. Prolonged use may result in periostitis.

Congestive heart failure

Acute left ventricular failure rapidly progresses to congestive heart failure and occasionally to cardiovascular collapse. Table 17.6 lists causes of congestive cardiac failure in the neonatal period, according to whether they are structural or non-structural.

CLINICAL FEATURES

Congestive heart failure may present with feeding or respiratory difficulties, excessive sweating or failure to thrive. The cardinal signs of congestive heart failure in the newborn are tachypnoea (respiratory rate greater than 60/min) with mild chest retractions, tachycardia (heart rate greater than 180/min), hepatomegaly (liver more than 3 cm below costal margin), a vigorous precordium and cardiomegaly (often only detected on chest X-ray).

Other signs, such as oedema or excessive weight gain, triple or gallop rhythm, crepitations on chest auscultation, sweating, peripheral cyanosis and cardiovascular collapse, are variable. The position, quality and radiation of any murmurs may be useful in identifying the cardiac lesion.

HYPOPLASTIC LEFT HEART

In this condition there is failure of development of the left atrium and ventricle and the aortic and mitral valves are usually atretic. The ascending aorta is hypoplastic and blood reaches the systemic circulation retrogradely through the ductus arteriosus. The infant usually develops severe cardiac failure in the first week of life when the ductus closes. The pulses are weak and there is often cyanosis with pallor. There is marked hepatomegaly.

Investigations

Chest X-ray shows a large heart with plethoric lung fields. The ECG shows little left ventricular activity and RVH. The diagnosis can be made by echocardiography.

Treatment

Many centres offer palliative surgery to establish a viable haemodynamicly stable heart, and this may require a series of operations in the first 2 years of life. In some centres cardiac transplantation is offered following palliative management if the brain and other organs are intact.

COARCTATION OF THE AORTA (COA)

If outflow obstruction is severe, then cardiac failure occurs in infancy. Blood enters the aorta retrogradely through the ductus arteriosus, but if this closes then the infant rapidly deteriorates, presenting breathless and in cardiac failure. The femoral pulses are weak and the blood pressure considerably higher in the arms than in the legs. About half of patients with COA have a VSD or aortic stenosis, and a murmur is usually audible.

Investigations

Radiographs show a large heart with pulmonary plethora. ECG reveals severe RVH with little evidence of left ventricular activity. Echocardiography may confirm the diagnosis, but requires special training. Cardiac catheterization is necessary to show the extent of the coarctation, as well as the presence of hypoplasia of the ascending aorta.

Treatment

PGE_1 may be life-saving in maintaining ductal flow. Dopamine infusion (5 µg/kg/min) will improve compromised renal blood flow. Surgery is urgent and angioplasty of the aorta may be remarkably successful. Inotropic support with digoxin and frusemide is best started early and continued postoperatively.

VENTRICULAR SEPTAL DEFECT

VSD accounts for 30% of all cardiac abnormalities. Lesions may vary in size, but only large defects cause symptoms in infancy. Cardiac failure due to VSD occurs very rarely in the neonate because of a relatively high pulmonary vascular resistance. Usually the only sign is a cardiac murmur in the first weeks of life.

Table 17.7 Dosage regimen for digoxin in the neonate. (From Hastreiter *et al.* 1988)

	Loading dose (μg/kg)	Maintenance dose (μg/kg)
Preterm infants (< 1500 g)	20*	2.5
Preterm (1500–2500 g)	20*	5.0
Full-term infants	30	7.5

* Avoid if possible, see text.

Investigations

If there is a significant left-to-right shunt, the heart is enlarged on X-ray and pulmonary plethora may be seen. The ECG shows RVH and LVH. A large VSD will be seen on echocardiography and an assessment of flow through the defect may be made at that time.

Treatment

Digoxin (see below) and diuretics are useful in cardiac failure. Banding of the pulmonary artery will protect the pulmonary circulation in the presence of a large left-to-right shunt. In some cases primary closure may be performed rather than banding. Later surgery to patch the defect will always be necessary after banding of the pulmonary artery, and also in large septal defects.

AORTIC STENOSIS

This rarely presents in the neonatal period unless it is very severe, and it is then likely to be associated with a hypoplastic left ventricle. The prognosis is poor, although valvular surgery may be of some benefit.

MANAGEMENT OF CONGESTIVE HEART FAILURE

General management

Supportive treatment consists of oxygen therapy, elevation of the head of the cot, the provision of a thermoneutral environment, correction of metabolic acidosis with sodium bicarbonate, administration of glucose or calcium when indicated, and tube feeding.

Blood transfusion

An increase in oxygen to the tissues can best be obtained by ensuring an adequate haemoglobin. Anaemia should be treated with blood transfusion of packed cells and the haemoglobin should be maintained at 12–14 g/dL.

Digitalization

This is a time-honoured method of treating cardiac failure by improving myocardial contraction. Often the newborn myocardium has little inotropic reserve and digoxin is not as effective as in older children. Its main value is the treatment of cardiac failure due to a large VSD and for supraventricular tachycardia (see p. 201). Digitalis toxicity frequently occurs in the preterm infant, especially with ischaemic and viral myocarditis. The signs are vomiting, lack of interest in feeding and cardiac dysrhythmias.

Digitalizing dose. In order to avoid the risk of digoxin toxicity, it is preferable to start the baby on maintenance therapy rather than giving a loading dose. Maintenance doses (Table 17.7) take a week to reach steady state. Avoid giving digoxin intramuscularly.

Diuretics

Frusemide in a dose of 1 mg/kg is the usual diuretic used in acute heart failure. Maintenance diuretic therapy consists of frusemide 2 mg/kg/day and spironolactone 2 mg/kg/day, with electrolyte monitoring. Spironolactone may interact with digoxin, leading to toxicity.

Fluid restriction to 100–120 mL/kg/day will act as an adjunct to other therapies.

Captopril, an angiotensin-converting enzyme inhibitor, may be of value in patients who continue to show signs of cardiac failure after maximum diuretic therapy. Captopril causes the blood pressure to fall (p. 185), and this must be carefully monitored.

MURMUR HEARD ON ROUTINE EXAMINATION

Heart disease may present with a cardiac murmur heard on routine examination in an apparently healthy infant. In such cases evidence of other cardiac disease should be excluded, including a check on the blood pressure in the arms and legs. A chest X-ray and ECG (or echocardiography if available) should be done in all cases but the softest murmurs. It is necessary to give a full explanation and adequate reassurance to the parents. Most murmurs detected in the neonatal period will disappear in infancy, but arrangements for follow-up must be made.

Circulatory maladaptation at birth

PATENT DUCTUS ARTERIOSUS

Normally the ductus arteriosus is functionally closed by 10–15 h after birth and is anatomically closed by 5–7 days of age. In preterm infants who sustained birth asphyxia or hypoxia after birth, patency of the ductus arteriosus is common. It is rare in term infants unless they are born at high altitude or have rubella embryopathy. A relatively high proportion of very low birthweight (VLBW) infants requiring intermittent positive-pressure ventilation (IPPV) develop delayed closure of the ductus. High fluid volumes are a major factor in its development, and congestive cardiac failure is seen in about half of these cases.

Clinical features

Preterm infants with respiratory distress develop clinical features of a PDA within the first week or two of life, unlike term infants, who present at 4–6 weeks when the pulmonary vascular resistance has decreased to adult levels.

The classic signs are bounding (collapsing) pulses, a hyperdynamic precordium, a loud second heart sound, and initially a systolic murmur at the upper left sternal edge, with the diastolic component developing later. The absence of a murmur in a clinically significant ductus arteriosus is well recognized (the silent duct), but the peripheral pulses are always abnormal.

Once cardiac decompensation occurs congestive heart failure develops, with tachycardia, tachypnoea, cardiomegaly, hepatomegaly, gallop rhythm and crepitations. Preterm infants with a PDA often develop increasing apnoea, and ventilator and oxygen dependence, sometimes predisposing to NEC.

Investigations

Chest X-ray may show an enlarged heart, and pulmonary oedema is present in large shunts. ECG is usually unhelpful. The diagnosis is confirmed with echocardiography, which shows ductal size. Doppler assessment of flow through the ductus may also be helpful in quantifying the shunt.

Treatment

Careful fluid management with avoidance of fluid overload is essential in preventing this condition. Once the infant shows evidence of a haemodynamically significant shunt (collapsing pulses, abnormal echocardiographic findings), fluid restriction should be instituted. Frusemide and top-up blood transfusion if anaemic may be beneficial.

Medical treatment with indomethacin is often successful, and is most likely to close the ductus if administered in the first 2 weeks of life and if the gestational age is between 30 and 34 weeks.

Indomethacin. PGE_1 relaxes the ductus arteriosus and prostaglandin synthetase inhibitors such as indomethacin reverse this effect. Unfortunately, indomethacin has an effect on all vascular beds, reducing renal blood flow and gut perfusion. The standard dose is 0.2 mg/kg intravenously given every 24 h for three doses. An alternative regimen of six doses of 0.1 mg/kg 8-hourly has been suggested to have a reduced effect on other vascular beds. A closure rate of up to 80% has been claimed with early intravenous indomethacin (Gersony *et al.* 1983).

Indomethacin reduces renal blood flow and glomerular filtration rate, thereby increasing the circulating blood volume. For this reason, it is recommended that the fluid volume given to the infant be reduced by 20% when indomethacin 0.2 mg/kg is given, and this is continued for 6 h following the dose. Contraindications to indomethacin include NEC, thrombocytopenia (< 100 000 mm^{-3}), creatinine > 200 μmol/L, and severe unconjugated hyperbilirubinaemia (> 200 μmol/L).

If medical closure fails and the infant remains ventilator dependent owing to the large left-to-right shunt, then surgical ligation is necessary.

PERSISTENT PULMONARY HYPERTENSION OF THE NEWBORN

The normal changes in the circulation with birth are described in Chapter 2. Conditions that interfere with normal oxygenation or lung expansion after birth may delay the physiological drop in pulmonary vascular resistance which results in persistent pulmonary hypertension of the newborn (PPHN). Failure of the pulmonary vascular resistance to fall, with persistence of the intracardiac shunts, leads to severe hypoxia and cyanosis. This condition is sometimes referred to as persistent fetal circulation (PFC), but this terminology is incorrect as the placental component of the fetal circulation has been removed.

The tone of pulmonary arterioles is in balance, depending on the opposing influence of vasoconstrictors (e.g. leukotrienes, endothelin-1) and vasodilators (nitric oxide (NO), prostacyclin). It is now recognized that NO has the major influence on pulmonary vasodilatation after birth.

Aetiology

1 Primary (or idiopathic) accounts for 20% of all cases of PPHN and is due to a primary abnormality of the pulmonary arterioles, which have thick walls with a narrowed lumen.
2 Secondary:
  (a) hypoxia with metabolic acidosis (e.g. birth asphyxia, RDS, pneumothorax) is a major cause;
  (b) underlying CHD;
  (c) hypothermia;
  (d) metabolic: hypoglycaemia, hypocalcaemia;
  (e) polycythaemia with hyperviscosity;
  (f) fetal exposure to prostaglandin synthetase inhibitors, e.g. aspirin, indomethacin. Under these circumstances the ductus arteriosus may close *in utero*, leading to persistent pulmonary hypertension, but in practice this is very rare;
  (g) many lung diseases, such as diaphragmatic hernia, pneumonia and meconium aspiration, may be associated with PPHN.

Clinical features

The clinical features depend to some extent on the underlying cause, but affected babies usually present shortly after birth with cyanosis and respiratory distress (tachypnoea, grunting and sternal and intercostal recession). In some cases cyanosis may be delayed by several hours, and may initially be intermittent, with wide fluctuations in Pao_2 from normal to severe hypoxia because of arteriolar lability.

Arterial blood gases show hypoxaemia, acidaemia and variable hypercarbia. These infants resemble those with cyanotic CHD. Untreated their hypoxaemia may become extreme, despite assisted ventilation with high inspiratory pressures. In the survivors the respiratory distress decreases after some days.

It has been suggested that the following conditions should be satisfied before a diagnosis of PPHN can be made:
1 sustained systemic or suprasystemic pulmonary artery pressure;

2 profound hypoxaemia with or without acidosis, while breathing 100% oxygen;
3 normal cardiac anatomy on echocardiographic examination;
4 evidence of right-to-left shunting of blood through either the ductus arteriosus or the foramen ovale.

Management

Management should be directed towards the underlying cause of the PPHN if this can be recognized, as well as methods directed towards pulmonary vasodilatation.

General principles

1 Correct hypothermia, hypocalcaemia, hypomagnesaemia and hypoglycaemia.
2 Correct metabolic acidosis with sodium bicarbonate or trishydroxyaminomethane (THAM).
3 Treat polycythaemia (packed cell volume (PCV) > 65%) with a partial exchange transfusion.
4 Correct systemic hypotension with volume expanders, isoprenaline or dopamine.

Specific management

1 Ventilatory support should be used to treat hypoxia if the Pao_2 is < 7 kPa (50 mmHg) in 100% oxygen. Hyperventilation and alkalinization to maintain the pH at 7.45–7.50 is recommended, as this reduces pulmonary vascular resistance. Muscle paralysis is useful. Curare has a histamine-releasing effect and may be used initially, followed later by pancuronium. High peak inspiratory pressures may be necessary.
2 Ensure adequate systemic blood pressure. Shunting will be reduced by increasing the differential pressure between the systemic and pulmonary circulations. Inotrope infusion (dopamine and/or dobutamine) is given to increase the systemic blood pressure by at least 20%.
3 Pulmonary vasodilators. There is now a range of vasodilating agents available, which are discussed below.

4 Extracorporeal membrane oxygenation (ECMO). This therapy is aimed at supporting the cardiorespiratory system until pulmonary hypertension settles. It is therefore only indicated for potentially recoverable conditions and is not recommended in diaphragmatic hernia with severe pulmonary hypertension due to lung hypoplasia. A recent British randomized study has shown clearly that the outcome in term babies with severe respiratory failure is twice as good with ECMO than with conventional ventilatory techniques.

Pulmonary vasodilators

The pulmonary artery pressure in PPHN is always higher than systemic, and right-to-left shunting occurs through the ductus arteriosus and/or foramen ovale. For therapy to be successful, this shunt must be reduced by selectively reducing the pulmonary vascular resistance while maintaining systemic vascular resistance.

Tolazoline. This acts as a vasodilator by α_1 antagonism and histamine-like effects, but almost always causes a reduction in systemic blood pressure, often with no consequent reduction in the right–left shunt. Close blood pressure monitoring at the time of tolazoline infusion is essential, and preloading the circulation with volume expanders or simultaneous dopamine infusion may be necessary. The initial dose of tolazoline is 1–2 mg/kg intravenously (i.v.), followed by a continuous infusion of 1–2 mg/kg/h. Gastric erosions with gastrointestinal bleeding are a common complication, and an H_2 antagonist (ranitidine) is usually given with tolazoline.

Prostacyclin. This acts as a vasodilator, but has a very short half-life. There is some evidence that it stimulates endothelial NO release. It is given by continuous intravenous infusion (5–20 mg/kg/min). Like tolazoline it is not a selective pulmonary vasodilator, and systemic hypotension should be anticipated.

Magnesium sulphate. This also acts as a non-specific vasodilator. The recommended dose of $MgSO_4 \cdot 7H_2O$ is 250 mg/kg as a loading dose over 20 min, followed by 20–50 mg/kg/h.

Nitric oxide (NO). As mentioned above, NO has a major effect as an arteriolar vasodilator and has been shown to be effective in the management of PPHN when given in low concentration through the ventilator circuit. The therapeutic dose is 5–40 p.p.m. (parts per million) and careful monitoring of inhaled concentration is necessary, as methaemoglobinaemia may occur with higher concentrations. Exhaled gases should be scavenged so that they do not contaminate the air within the nursery.

Dysrhythmias

The newborn infant is subject to disorders of cardiac rate and rhythm, some of which may be detectable before birth with antepartum monitoring. Many are transient, especially following birth asphyxia and birth trauma.

The most important dysrhythmias in the newborn are:
1 supraventricular tachycardia;
2 congenital atrioventricular block; and
3 ventricular tachycardia and fibrillation.

SUPRAVENTRICULAR TACHYCARDIA

This is the commonest form of tachycardia and is becoming increasingly more frequently recognized *in utero* as a result of cardiotocography monitoring and real-time ultrasound examinations. It is often sensitive to intravenous digoxin, and the fetus can be treated by digoxin administered to the mother. Prolonged fetal supraventricular tachycardia leads to congestive cardiac failure and hydrops fetalis.

In the newborn it may be idiopathic or due to irritation of the sinoatrial node by inadvertent catheterization of the right atrium during umbilical catheterization. Heart failure may develop after a few hours, and treatment includes one of the following:

1 vagal stimulation by eyeball pressure or an ice pack applied to the face may occasionally be enough to cause reversion to sinus rhythm;
2 digoxin (see p. 197);
3 verapamil (0.1–0.3 mg/kg);
4 amiodarone: 500 mg/m^2 for 5–10 days, then 250 mg/m^2. This drug has not been widely used in the neonatal period and is probably best avoided;
5 D.c. cardioversion (10 J).

An interval ECG may demonstrate the Wolff–Parkinson–White syndrome (short P–R interval and a wide QRS complex).

CONGENITAL HEART BLOCK

In 50% of cases this is due to a major congenital cardiac anomaly, such as transposition of the great vessels or Ebstein's anomaly. Some cases are associated with maternal systemic lupus erythematosus, which may be subclinical. Heart block is only likely to cause clinical problems in the newborn period if it is complete (third degree) and associated with profound bradycardia.

Treatment is initially with an infusion of isoprenaline to increase the heart rate. A number of cases are transient and recover fully, but in some infants an electronic pacemaker may be necessary.

VENTRICULAR TACHYCARDIA AND FIBRILLATION

If these occur they must be rapidly recognized and efficiently treated to avoid cerebral ischaemia. The commonest cause of ventricular tachycardia is hyperkalaemia (p. 175). This occurs spontaneously in some critically ill VLBW infants and may develop if the potassium exceeds 7.5 mmol/L. Treatment of the tachycardia includes:

1 calcium gluconate (10%): 1–2 mL i.v. under ECG control;
2 correct acidosis with sodium bicarbonate infusion;
3 lignocaine 2 mg/kg by bolus i.v. injection followed by 4 mg/kg by slow i.v. infusion for 1 h;
4 cardioversion (5–10 J).

Usually calcium gluconate is successful in reverting the ventricular tachycardia to sinus rhythm. The treatment of the hyperkalaemia is discussed on p. 176.

Ventricular fibrillation should be treated with external cardiac massage and electrical cardioversion.

REFERENCES

Adelman, R.D. (1988) The hypertensive neonate. *Clinics in Perinatology* **15**, 567–585.

Gersony, W.M., Peckham, G.J., Ellison, R.C., Miettinen, O.S. & Nadas, A.S. (1983) Effects of indomethacin in premature infants with patent ductus arteriosus: results of a national collaborative study. *Journal of Pediatrics* **102**, 895–906.

Hastreiter, A.R., John, E.G. & van der Horst, R.L. (1988) Digitalis, digitalis antibodies, digitalis-like immunoreactive substances, and sodium homeostasis: a review. *Clinics in Perinatology* **15**, 491–522.

Moss, A.J. & Adams, F.H. (eds) (1968) *Heart Disease in Infants, Children and Adolescents.* Williams and Wilkins, Baltimore.

Scott, O. (1981) Advances in paediatric cardiology. In: *Recent Advances in Paediatrics* (ed. D. Hull), **6**, 71–95. Churchill Livingstone, Edinburgh.

FURTHER READING

Field, D.J. (1997) Persistent Pulmonary Hypertension of the Newborn. *Seminars in Neonatology* **2**, 1–79.

Gillette, P.C (ed.) (1990) *Congenital Heart Disease.* Paediatric Clinics of North America. W.B. Saunders, Philadelphia.

Jordan, S.C. & Scott, O. (1989) *Heart Disease in Paediatrics*, 3rd edn. Butterworth-Heinemann, Oxford.

Lone, W.A. (1990) *Fetal and Neonatal Cardiology.* W.B. Saunders, Philadelphia.

18 Haematological disorders

The blood volume and red cell mass at birth and in the neonatal period depend on the volume of the placental transfusion and subsequent readjustments of blood volume.

PLACENTAL TRANSFUSION

This occurs within 3 min of delivery and contributes 25% of the total neonatal blood volume. This amount will be increased in the following situations:
1 elevated maternal blood pressure;
2 use of oxytocic drugs;
3 late clamping or milking of the cord;
4 infant held in a low, dependent position.

It will be reduced by early cord clamping, or holding the infant above the level of the attached placenta.

The average blood volume of a newborn infant is 85–90 mL/kg, but ranges from 75 to 100 mL/kg. The practice of delay in clamping the umbilical cord or milking the cord from the placenta to the baby may rarely result in symptomatic pulmonary plethora as well as hyperbilirubinaemia.

READJUSTMENT OF BLOOD VOLUME

Within the first 3–4 h after birth there is haemoconcentration to compensate for rapid expansion of intravascular volume.

ANAEMIA

The causes of neonatal anaemia are shown in Table 18.1 and will be discussed under the following headings:
1 physiological anaemia;
2 haemorrhage;
3 haemolysis; and
4 aplasia.

Physiological anaemia

The full-term infant is born with a haemoglobin in the range 15–23.5 g/dL, whereas in the premature infant the haemoglobin level is slightly lower. Initially there is a slight increase due to haemoconcentration, but over the first week the haemoglobin drops and remains low for most of the first year of life (Fig. 18.1). This is known as physiological anaemia.

In term infants the lowest haemoglobin level occurs between 6 and 10 weeks, when it falls to 10–11 g/dL. In premature infants the anaemia occurs earlier and lasts longer, with a nadir of 7–8 g/dL (Fig. 18.1).

Table 18.1 Causes of neonatal anaemia

Physiological anaemia
Anaemia of prematurity
Haemorrhage
Antepartum haemorrhage
Fetomaternal transfusion
Twin-to-twin transfusion
Neonatal internal haemorrhage
Haemolysis (see Table 18.2)
Aplasia: Blackfan–Diamond syndrome

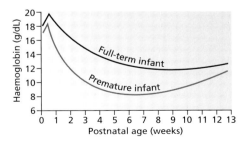

Fig. 18.1 Physiological anaemia. The two graphs show the normal fall in haemoglobin with postnatal age in mature and premature infants.

Anaemia of prematurity

In the preterm infant physiological anaemia occurs earlier, is more severe and prolonged than in the term infant, and is termed anaemia of prematurity. It is caused by a number of factors.

Lack of erythropoietin. At birth the infant moves from a relatively hypoxic fetal state to become relatively hyperoxic. This suppresses erythropoietin secretion for the first 7–8 weeks of life. In addition the bone marrow is probably more resistant to the stimulatory effect of erythropoietin. This phase is terminated when reticulocytes are seen in the peripheral blood film.

Venesection. The preterm infant is subjected daily to repeated blood sampling for laboratory investigation.

Haemodilution. There is an increase in plasma volume over the first months of life and, together with poor red cell production, the haemoglobin falls. This is referred to as 'early anaemia'.

Iron deficiency. The full-term infant is born with sufficient iron stores for the first 4 months of life, but in preterm infants these stores are exhausted more quickly because of their rapid growth rate. An infant of 1.5 kg at birth has half the iron stores of a 3.0-kg neonate. Iron deficiency causes the 'late anaemia' which accounts for low haemoglobin levels after 4 months of age, when hypochromic red cells are seen on a blood film.

Haemolysis. Haemolysis may occur in preterm infants as a result of vitamin E deficiency. Administration of vitamin E (25 mg/day) may reduce the extent of late anaemia of prematurity.

TREATMENT

Iron should be given to preterm infants from about 3 weeks of age. A daily dose of 1–2 mg/kg/day of elemental iron (equivalent to 30–60 mg of ferrous salt) is recommended until the baby is 12 months of age.

Transfusion (10 mL/kg) may be necessary in premature infants if the haemoglobin falls below 7–8 g/dL and the infant is symptomatic. Symptoms include breathlessness with feeds, tachycardia, apnoea and bradycardia or failure to gain weight. Blood transfusion will suppress erythropoietin activity, and if the infant shows a reticulocyte count of more than 5% then transfusion may be delayed, depending on the infant's condition.

The following formula may be used to calculate the volume of blood to be transfused for an anaemic infant (Hct, haematocrit):

$$\text{Donor blood required (mL)} = \frac{\text{desired Hct} - \text{actual Hct}}{\text{donor Hct}} \times \text{body weight (kg)} \times 90$$

The administration of subcutaneous recombinant human erythropoietin to preterm infants has been shown to stimulate red blood cell production and avoid the need for frequent blood transfusions, but this form of treatment has not been shown to be cost-effective and is not widely used.

Haemorrhage

This may be due to:
1 haemorrhage before and during delivery from:
   (a) placenta: placenta praevia, placental abruption, incision into the placenta during caesarean section;
   (b) cord: rupture or torn vessels on insertion into the placenta;
   (c) fetal: fetomaternal, twin-to-twin transfusion;
2 neonatal haemorrhage:
   (a) trauma: bleeding may occur into brain, lung, peritoneum or bowel;
   (b) haemorrhagic disease of the newborn (see p. 213).

INVESTIGATIONS

These will depend on the likely diagnosis, but include:

1 haemoglobin and haematocrit;
2 blood group (mother and baby);
3 cross-matched blood (against mother's and baby's blood);
4 Kleihauer's test (to assess the presence of fetal cells in maternal blood, indicating feto-maternal transfusion);
5 coagulation studies (indicated if a bleeding diathesis is suspected);
6 investigations to determine site of bleeding, e.g. lumbar puncture, ultrasound of head or abdomen, testing stools for blood.

TREATMENT

The clinical examination for hypovolaemia and shock includes assessment of colour, blood pressure, heart rate, tissue perfusion and urine output.

Severe haemorrhage may be a neonatal emergency and may require an immediate blood transfusion to prevent irreversible shock. If blood is not immediately available, plasma or plasma substitute (purified protein fraction 20 mL/kg) may be given via a peripheral vessel. Umbilical transfusion via the umbilical vein may be life-saving in the shocked patient. In an emergency, group O rhesus-negative blood may be used, but formal cross-matching should be done whenever possible.

Haemolysis

The causes of neonatal haemolysis are shown in Table 18.2. Unconjugated hyperbilirubinaemia and reticulocytosis are usually associated with haemolysis, the causes of which can be divided into immune and non-immune.

RHESUS HAEMOLYTIC DISEASE

This occurs because the mother's immune system has been sensitized by rhesus-positive cells from her fetus. Sensitization may be due to:
1 fetomaternal transfusion;
2 rhesus-incompatible transfusions.

The rhesus factor is complex, comprising CDE/cde antigens. The commonest antigen is D, and this accounts for 95% of cases. Approximately 83% of the population are D positive, i.e. rhesus positive (Rh +ve). If sensitization occurs, maternal immunoglobulin G (IgG) crosses the placenta to cause haemolysis of 'foreign' fetal erythrocytes. IgG remains present in the neonatal circulation for up to 3 months and neonatal haemolysis may occur for some weeks after birth.

Prevention

Anti-D gammaglobulin in a dose of 100–200 μg is administered within 72 h of delivery to all rhesus-negative women who give birth to rhesus-positive infants. If antibodies are already present anti-D is not given. The dose is sufficient for a 5–10 mL fetomaternal transfusion. Women should have a Kleihauer test after anti-D gammaglobulin to test whether the dose was adequate to neutralize all rhesus-positive red blood cells.

Anti-D gammaglobulin should also be given to at-risk rhesus-negative women after abortions and after amniocentesis if the Kleihauer test shows a fetomaternal transfusion.

Table 18.2 Causes of immune and non-immune neonatal haemolysis

---

Immune haemolysis (positive Coombs' test)

Rhesus incompatibility

ABO incompatibility

Minor blood group incompatibility (e.g. Kell, Duffy, Kidd)

Maternal autoimmune diseases (e.g. SLE)

Non-immune haemolysis (negative Coombs' test)

Congenital infection

DIC

G6PD deficiency

Pyruvate kinase deficiency

Hereditary spherocytosis

α-Thalassaemia

Infantile pyknocytosis

Vitamin E deficiency

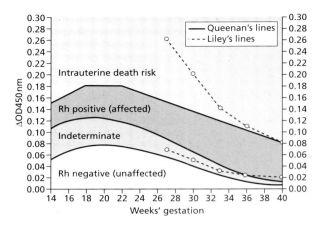

Fig. 18.2 Superimposed 'Queenan' and 'Liley' charts of the deviation of optical density at a wavelength of 450 nm in amniotic fluid (OD450) vs. gestation. Note that 'Liley's' lines only started at 27 weeks. These lines are not linear on this graph because the scale for OD450 is not logarithmic on 'Queenan's' chart. Also note that the division lines for 'Queenan's' chart are lower at all gestations compared to 'Liley's'. (From Scott and Chan 1998, copyright of John Wiley & Sons Limited. Reproduced with permission.)

Anti-D gammaglobulin is ineffective against non-D rhesus antigen (usually C, E). If a large transfusion of fetal blood occurs, the standard dose of 200 µg/kg may be insufficient.

Management during pregnancy

Routine testing. Rhesus-negative women should be screened for rhesus antibodies at their first antenatal visit, and at 28, 32 and 36 weeks' gestation. If antibodies are detected at any of these times, more frequent testing will be necessary.

Antibodies present. If antibodies are present, then depending on the level and/or whether the titre is rising, an amniocentesis should be performed. This should also be done if there is a history of a previously affected infant who required exchange transfusion, or if there has been a previous stillbirth because of rhesus disease. Amniocentesis is commonly done at 30–32 weeks but may be performed earlier, depending on the level of antibodies, and particularly on the history of previous pregnancies. Amniocentesis is carried out under ultrasound control so that the placenta can be localized and avoided. A Kleihauer test is done before and after amniocentesis, and a lecithin/sphingomyelin (L/S) ratio will be done on the amniotic fluid obtained. The timing of delivery will depend on the antibody levels, amniocen-

tesis result and previous history of affected infants.

Assessment of bilirubin in liquor amnii. Traditionally the amount of bilirubin in the amniotic fluid was assessed by a spectrophotometric technique at a wavelength of 450 nm, which is the region of maximal absorption of bilirubin. The optical density difference between the patient's amniotic fluid and normal amniotic fluid at a specific gestational age is plotted on either the Liley (Liley 1961) or the Queenan (Queenan *et al.* 1993) chart. Figure 18.2 superimposes Queenan and Liley charts (Scott & Chan 1998).

The Liley chart provides guidelines for the severity of rhesus isoimmunization, treatment and expected cord blood haemoglobin. It allows the obstetrician to plan when to deliver the infant. This chart, which starts at 27 weeks' gestation, has been largely superseded by the Queenan chart, which commences at 14 weeks' gestation. Maternal fetal medicine specialists often also use liver length and assessment of fluid in visceral cavities to estimate the timing of fetal blood transfusion. If the fetus is severely affected and is too immature to deliver, then *in utero* blood transfusion into the fetal peritoneal cavity may be life-saving and may be required on a number of occasions until the fetus is mature enough to be delivered. An alternative technique is to inject blood directly into the fetal umbilical vein under ultrasound control.

Management of the rhesus-immunized infant

The baby should be assessed for maturity, pallor, jaundice, hepatosplenomegaly, oedema, ascites, ecchymoses, heart failure and respiratory distress. The placenta is examined for the presence of oedema, weighed and sent to the pathology department for confirmation of the diagnosis.

Investigations at birth. Cord blood is taken for grouping, direct Coombs' test, haemoglobin and platelet count and total bilirubin estimation. The Coombs' test is always positive in rhesus incompatibility, unless an intrauterine transfusion with rhesus-negative blood has been performed. The more positive the Coombs' test, the more severely affected the infant is likely to be.

Indications for immediate exchange transfusion

1 Cord haemoglobin < 8 g/dL.
2 Hydrops fetalis.

Early exchange transfusion

1 Cord bilirubin > 8.5 μmol/L (5 mg/100 mL).
2 Cord haemoglobin 8–12 g/dL.
3 Rapidly rising serum bilirubin which crosses the level for exchange transfusion on the charts shown on p. 140.
4 A very strongly positive Coombs' test.

Interval exchange transfusion. This is done to prevent the serum unconjugated bilirubin reaching a potentially dangerous level (250 μmol/L in preterm, 340 μmol/L in term infants). This is usually carried out as an adjunct to phototherapy, and guideline graphs are useful (see p. 140).

Exchange transfusion. This is performed with less than 5-day-old warmed (37°C) whole blood. The infant is given a double-volume exchange (180 mL/kg). The blood should be rhesus negative and ABO compatible with the mother's blood. The method for exchange transfusion is described on p. 140.

Complications of rhesus incompatibility

These include:
1 kernicterus and bilirubin encephalopathy (see p. 137);
2 hyaline membrane disease;
3 β cell hyperplasia of the pancreas, resulting in hypoglycaemia;
4 hypoalbuminaemia and lung oedema;
5 thrombocytopenia and disseminated intravascular coagulopathy;
6 inspissated bile syndrome;
7 complications of exchange transfusion (see p. 141);
8 anaemia. This results from ongoing haemolysis and possibly folic acid deficiency. The anaemia, which reaches its lowest level by the age of 6–8 weeks, will require careful assessment with haemoglobin levels and reticulocyte counts. Treatment includes folic acid and 'top-up' transfusions. Iron therapy is not necessary unless the infant is born prematurely.

ABO INCOMPATIBILITY

Haemolytic disease caused by ABO incompatibility is now the commonest cause of isoimmune haemolytic anaemia, but is generally less severe than that caused by rhesus incompatibility.

The naturally occurring anti-A or anti-B antibody is of the IgM type, which does not cross the placenta. Approximately 10% of women carry 'immune' anti-A or anti-B antibodies of the IgG class. It is in the pregnancies of these women that ABO incompatibility occurs, as the IgG crosses the placenta to haemolyse fetal red cells. Women with blood group O are most likely to have anti-A and anti-B IgG agglutinins, and it is this maternal blood group that accounts for the vast majority of ABO incompatibility. The mechanisms of development of this antibody are disputed. ABO incompatibility may occur in the first

Table 18.3 Blood group combinations causing ABO incompatibility

Mother	Infant	Frequency
O	A or B	Common
A	B or AB	Rare
B	A or AB	Rare

pregnancy, and subsequent pregnancies may be relatively unaffected.

ABO incompatibility generally occurs with the blood group combinations listed in Table 18.3.

Clinical features

The usual presentation is with jaundice on the first day or two of life but without hepatosplenomegaly. Kernicterus is an unusual complication and hydrops fetalis has only occasionally been reported. Unlike rhesus disease, late anaemia is seldom a problem but folic acid is recommended because of ongoing haemolysis.

Investigations

ABO incompatibility is usually suspected in the presence of maternal blood group O and the infant is either blood group A or, less commonly, group B.
1 The direct Coombs' test on the infant's blood is usually negative or only weakly positive, but the indirect Coombs' test may be positive.
2 A blood smear from the infant may show features of haemolysis, often with microspherocytes. Spherocytes are rarely seen in rhesus disease.
3 If the mother's serum causes haemolysis of adult A or B cells, this strongly suggests that she carries α or β haemolysins. Maternal blood should be examined for haemolysins.
4 Immune anti-A or anti-B may be eluted from fetal red blood cells or cord blood.

Treatment

This is as for rhesus haemolytic disease but intrauterine fetal transfusion is much less likely to be required (see p. 206).

MINOR BLOOD GROUP INCOMPATIBILITIES

Rarely blood group incompatibilities are caused by Duffy, Kell, Kidd and C and E antibodies. They usually present with mild jaundice, but hydrops fetalis has been reported.

GLUCOSE-6-PHOSPHATE DEHYDROGENASE (G6PD) DEFICIENCY

This disease is inherited in an X-linked recessive manner and is due to a deficiency of the enzyme within the red blood cells which renders the cells more susceptible to haemolysis. More than 100 million people throughout the world, mainly Chinese, southern Mediterranean, black American or black African, have this abnormality. It usually occurs in males, although the heterozygote female may manifest mild features of the disease (an example of the Lyon hypothesis—see p. 159). There are many variants of this condition, some requiring an oxidizing agent to trigger haemolysis and others that cause haemolysis spontaneously. Some infants with the enzyme deficiency develop jaundice in the newborn period without exposure to oxidant drugs, but in other variants of the condition oxidant drugs are required to trigger haemolysis. In later years otherwise healthy children may become acutely ill with anaemia when exposed to drugs.

Table 18.4 lists the more commonly used drugs which may cause haemolysis in susceptible neonates. Some drugs excreted in breast milk are liable to haemolyse red cells in G6PD-deficient infants, including nitrofurantoin, sulphonamides and sulphasalazine. In addition, respiratory viruses, viral hepatitis and fava beans cause haemolysis in susceptible infants. Naphthalene in mothballs is a potent inducer of haemolysis in susceptible infants. Routine administration of 1 mg vitamin K_1 to G6PD-deficient infants is safe.

Clinical features

Haemolysis may occur spontaneously or after exposure to infection or drugs. Jaundice and

Table 18.4 Drugs that may cause haemolysis in infants with G6PD deficiency

Antimalarials (primaquine, quinine)

Nitrofurantoin

Sulphonamides

Phenacetin

Acetylsalicylic acid

Nalidixic acid

Methylene blue

Naphthalene

Vitamin K (large doses)

Chloramphenicol

pallor may be the only clinical signs. It may be severe and require exchange transfusion. Hepatosplenomegaly is uncommon.

Investigations

Anaemia with spherocytosis, reticulocytes and crenated red cells is seen. Heinz bodies are another feature of the haemolytic anaemia. A screening test for G6PD deficiency is available and is reliable in infants of Chinese and Mediterranean extraction. In black infants, once haemolysis has occurred a population of young red cells may remain with normal enzyme activity, and this makes the screening test unreliable. Black infants and those positive on the screening test should have the enzyme level directly assayed.

Treatment

Infants born into families known to have G6PD deficiency should not be exposed to agents likely to cause haemolysis. Spontaneous haemolysis may occur, and the treatment is as for any cause of unconjugated hyperbilirubinaemia. Anaemia may require transfusion.

PYRUVATE KINASE DEFICIENCY

This is an autosomal recessive condition affecting glucose metabolism within the red cell

membrane. Spontaneous haemolysis occurs in the neonatal period with anaemia and jaundice. Splenomegaly is always present. Diagnosis is made by enzyme assay.

HEREDITARY SPHEROCYTOSIS (HS)

This is an autosomal dominant condition which may cause early neonatal haemolysis. The blood film shows spherocytes with little splenomegaly initially. ABO incompatibility may present in a similar way, and a family history of HS is an important diagnostic point. The spherocytes show an increased osmotic fragility, although this may not be apparent in the first few months of life. Severe haemolysis with very high levels of hyperbilirubinaemia may occur suddenly.

α-THALASSAEMIA

Classic β-thalassaemia major does not affect neonates because the majority of the haemoglobin is in the fetal (HbF) form, which comprises α and γ chains only. α-Thalassaemia is a rare and severe condition that causes hydrops and severe anaemia. The α chain is manifested by a double allele, so that four different types of α-thalassaemia may be recognized:
Hb Barts = hydrops fetalis is homozygous for both alleles and is denoted -/-
HbH disease is both homozygous and heterozygous for alleles α-/--
α-thalassaemia minor may be α-/α-; or −/αα- and α-thalassaemia trait αα/α-.

INFANTILE PYKNOCYTOSIS

This is a rare cause of neonatal haemolysis and is diagnosed by finding large numbers of small distorted 'pyknocytes' in the peripheral blood film. The greater the numbers of pyknocytes, the greater the tendency to haemolysis. This condition may be due to vitamin E deficiency and is self-limiting.

HYDROPS FETALIS

This term is used to describe an infant who shows severe and generalized oedema and fluid in at least two visceral cavities (pleural effusions, ascites, pericardial effusions).

Causes

1 Immune: severe haemolytic disease of the newborn (rhesus, ABO, minor blood groups).
2 Non-immune:
  Severe chronic anaemia *in utero*
    fetomaternal haemorrhage
    homozygous α-thalassaemia
    chronic fetomaternal transfusion or twin-to-twin transfusion;
  Cardiac failure
    severe congenital heart disease
    premature closure of foramen ovale
    large atrioventricular (A-V) malformation (haemangioma)
    fetal supraventricular tachycardia;
  Hypoproteinaemia
    renal disease
      congenital nephrosis
      renal vein thrombosis
    congenital hepatitis;
  Infections (intrauterine)
    syphilis
    toxoplasmosis
    cytomegalovirus
    parvovirus B19;
  Miscellaneous
    maternal diabetes mellitus
    parabiotic syndrome (multiple pregnancy)
    sublethal umbilical or chorionic vein thrombosis
    fetal neuroblastomatosis
    Chagas' disease
    choriocarcinoma *in situ;*
  Congenital malformations
    cystic adenomatoid malformation of the lung
    obstructive uropathy
    achondroplasia
    pulmonary lymphangiectasia
    Gaucher's disease.

Idiopathic

This may account for up to 50% of cases where after extensive investigations no obvious cause is found.

Management

Investigations are done to determine the cause of the hydrops fetalis and include:
1 Coombs' test and full blood count;
2 haemoglobin electrophoresis;
3 Kleihauer test;
4 TORCH (toxoplasmosis, other, rubella, cytomegalovirus, herpes simplex type II)/ syphilis investigations;
5 placental examination;
6 chest X-ray;
7 echocardiography;
8 total serum proteins and serum albumin.

Treatment

This will include paracentesis of the abdomen and chest, transfusion, intubation and positive-pressure ventilation, and diuretic and intravenous albumin therapy.

Aplasia

Impaired erythrocyte production is an unusual cause for anaemia in the newborn. The most common cause is the Diamond–Blackfan syndrome, also known as congenital hypoplastic anaemia.

POLYCYTHAEMIA

Polycythaemia in the newborn is common and is defined as a venous haematocrit of 65% or more (approximating to a haemoglobin of 22 g/dL), during the first week of life. Polycythaemia does not mean the blood is hyperviscous. Blood viscosity depends largely on packed cell volume (haematocrit), but the deformability of red blood cells and the plasma viscosity may also be significant factors. The relationship between viscosity and haematocrit is linear below a haematocrit of 60–65%, but increases exponentially above this (Oski & Naiman 1982). Viscosity is much greater in small vessels than in large ones.

Polycythaemia should only be diagnosed on a free-flowing venous specimen and not from a heel-prick sample.

Table 18.5 Causes of neonatal polycythaemia

Chronic intrauterine hypoxia:
  SGA infants
  Post-maturity

Excessive transfusion of blood
  Placental transfusion due to delayed clamping
  Twin-to-twin transfusion
  Maternofetal transfusion

Infants of diabetic mothers

Down syndrome

Neonatal thyrotoxicosis

Congenital adrenal hyperplasia

Beckwith–Wiedemann syndrome

The causes of polycythaemia are listed in Table 18.5.

Clinical features

The infant looks plethoric and polycythaemia may cause problems in a number of organ systems owing to diminished blood flow through small vessels.

The clinical signs associated with polycythaemia/hyperviscosity are illustrated in Fig. 18.3.

Management

Infants at risk of polycythaemia should have a haematocrit measured on free-flowing venous blood. Babies without symptoms of polycythaemia but a venous haematocrit greater than 70% should have a dilutional exchange transfusion. Those with a venous packed cell volume (PCV) of 65–70% may require dilutional exchange if symptoms are present (4–5% salt-poor albumin).

A dilutional exchange is performed with plasma and is aimed at reducing the haematocrit (Hct) to about 50% by the following formula:

$$\text{Volume to be exchanged} = \frac{\text{actual Hct} - \text{desired Hct}}{\text{actual Hct}} \times \text{body weight (kg)} \times 90$$

where 90 refers to the blood volume per kg.

BLEEDING AND COAGULATION DISORDERS

These may be due to thrombocytopenia, clotting factor deficiency, abnormal capillaries or a combination of these. Coagulation is a complicated process and is relatively less efficient in the newborn (particularly prematures) than in older children.

When the vascular endothelium is damaged specific factors are released which cause platelet aggregation, upon which thrombus is deposited. This induces fibrin formation,

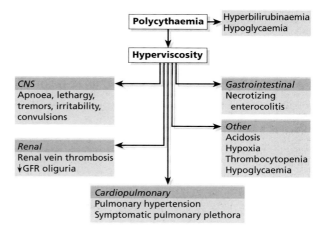

Fig. 18.3 The interrelationship between polycythaemia and hyperviscosity and their contribution towards clinical signs. CNS, central nervous system; GFR, glomerular filtration rate.

which further induces platelets to be deposited, ending in a platelet–fibrin syncytium which prevents further bleeding. Thrombin is formed from prothrombin by the action of factor X. Factor X may be activated by either the intrinsic or the extrinsic pathway to precipitate a cascade of clotting factors, culminating in the production of fibrin. Plasminogens act to remove fibrin (fibrinolysis), and in the healthy state this system is balanced with the clotting mechanism by a series of inhibitors.

CLINICAL FEATURES

Bleeding may be overt, from venepuncture sites or the umbilical stump. Bruising (ecchymoses), purpura or petechial haemorrhages may be present at birth or develop in the neonatal period.

A careful maternal history should be taken, including a family history of bleeding, drugs (warfarin, aspirin), idiopathic thrombocytopenic purpura (ITP) and recent viral illness.

Neonatal examination includes:
1 site of bleeding: examination will determine the origin of bleeding, such as the gastrointestinal tract, umbilicus or circumcision;
2 purpura suggesting thrombocytopenia;
3 hepatosplenomegaly: infection (TORCH, bacterial);
4 congenital anomaly, e.g. giant haemangioma, thrombocytopenia with absent radii (TAR) syndrome.

INVESTIGATIONS

Platelet count. A platelet count less than 100 000/mm³ is usually classified as thrombocytopenia. A useful guide to severity is:
50–100 000: mild thrombocytopenia (bleeding with surgery);
20–50 000: moderate thrombocytopenia (bleeding with minor trauma);
< 20 000: severe thrombocytopenia (spontaneous bleeding is likely). Infants with longstanding thrombocytopenia may have no spontaneous bruising even with platelets as low as 10 000.

Coagulation profile

Bleeding time. This measures the time to stop bleeding after a standard small wound, as from an Autolet device. The upper limit of normal for this test in the neonate is 3.5 min (Rennie *et al.* 1985). Prolonged bleeding time is seen in thrombocytopenia, Von Willebrand's disease and disseminated intravascular coagulation (DIC).

Prothrombin time (PT). This assesses the extrinsic clotting pathway (factors II, V, VII and X). This is not markedly affected by heparin.

Partial thromboplastin time (PTT). This assesses the intrinsic clotting pathway (most factors except VII and XII) but is prolonged by heparin contamination. It is the most sensitive test for coagulation disturbances.

Thrombin clotting time. This assesses fibrinogen activity and requires calcium for activation.

Fibrinogen degradation products (FDPs). Fibrin is deposited during coagulation and is simultaneously degraded by plasminogens to FDPs. The presence of increased levels of FDPs indicates that fibrinolysis is occurring, usually following thrombosis.

Clotting factor analysis. Specific factors can be assayed individually, but interpretation may be difficult because of uncertainty as to the normal range in very immature infants.

The normal ranges for some of these tests are shown in Table 18.6.

Thrombocytopenia

Petechiae and ecchymoses which may be present at birth or appear after birth are the characteristic lesions produced by platelet deficiencies. Whereas bleeding may occur from any site, intracranial haemorrhage is the most devastating complication. Table 18.7 lists the causes of neonatal thrombocytopenia.

Table 18.6 Normal results for some of the more commonly used tests of coagulation

Test	Preterm (30–36 weeks)	Term
PT (s) (I, II, V, VII, X)	13–23	13–17
Thrombotest (TT;%) (II, VII, IX, X)	15–50	15–60
PTT (s) (I, II, V, VII, IX, X, XI, XII)	35–100	35–70
Thrombin time (s)	12–24	12–18
Reptilase time (s)	18–30	18–24
Fibrinogen concentration (g/L)	1.2–3.8	1.5–3.5

Table 18.7 Causes of neonatal thrombocytopenia

Infection:
  Any bacterial infection
  TORCH infections

Isoimmune

Maternal disease:
  Severe toxaemia of pregnancy
  ITP
  Systemic lupus erythematosus
  Drug induced (hydralazine, thiazides)

Neonatal drug exposure:
  Thiazide diuretics
  Quinine
  Sulphonamides

DIC

Thrombocytopenia with absent radii (TAR syndrome)

Giant haemangioma (Kasabach–Merritt syndrome)

Fanconi's anaemia

Leukaemia

Pancytopenias

ALLOIMMUNE THROMBOCYTOPENIA

This is analogous to rhesus isoimmunization but is a much rarer condition. A transfusion of fetal A1 antigen-positive platelets into the maternal circulation may produce maternal IgG antibodies if the mother is platelet A1 antigen negative. The mother has normal numbers of platelets. Thrombocytopenia in the neonate may be severe, but is transient. The disease presents with intracranial haemorrhage (often fetal) in 20%. *In utero* treatment consists of fetal platelet transfusion and regular gammaglobulin therapy. Neonatal treatment is valuable with platelet transfusions, gammaglobulin and steroids.

MATERNAL IDIOPATHIC THROMBOCYTOPENIA

Transplacental maternal antibodies cause thrombocytopenia in the neonate and the mother will usually have thrombocytopenia. The lower the maternal platelets, the more severely affected the infant may be. Prenatal administration of corticosteroids or high-dose intravenous IgG has been advocated to reduce the incidence and severity of neonatal thrombocytopenia, but the response to these treatments is uncertain and unpredictable. The use of IgG infusion in the thrombocytopenic neonate may rapidly cause the platelet count to increase.

It has been suggested that delivery by caesarean section should be undertaken in severely thrombocytopenic fetuses to avoid trauma, but recent evidence suggests that intracerebral bleeds may occur before the onset of labour.

Prednisolone (4 mg/kg/day) may be given to the severely affected neonate but the condition is transient, lasting at most 12 weeks. Treatment of severe thrombocytopenia includes fresh whole blood or platelet transfusion (10 mL/kg). Serious neonatal haemorrhage does not occur if the platelet count is above 50 000/mm³.

HAEMORRHAGIC DISEASE OF THE NEWBORN

Classic haemorrhagic disease of the newborn is caused by a deficiency of the vitamin K-dependent clotting factors, and its decline in incidence is due to the routine administration of vitamin K_1 (1 mg intramuscularly (i.m.) or by mouth) at birth. Vitamin K is produced by the bacterial flora of the gastrointestinal tract, but as the newborn infant has a sterile bowel at birth there is little production from this source in the first weeks of life.

Clinical features

Spontaneous bleeding can occur from any site but is usually gastrointestinal, producing haematemesis or melaena, umbilical or associated with circumcision. It occurs late in the first week of life, especially in the breastfed infant owing to the low vitamin K levels in human milk.

Gastrointestinal bleeding in the infant must be differentiated from swallowed maternal blood from antepartum haemorrhage, episiotomy or cracked nipples.

The Apt's test, which depends on the resistance of haemoglobin F (fetal red cells) to denaturation by sodium hydroxide, will distinguish the infant's blood (predominantly fetal) from maternal blood (adult blood).

Investigations

The diagnosis is confirmed by a prolonged PT but a normal PTT.

Treatment

Vitamin K_1 1 mg i.m. or intravenously (i.v.) is given after blood has been obtained for investigations. Whole-blood transfusion (30 mL/kg) will be indicated for hypovolaemic shock.

Vitamin K prophylaxis

Routine administration of intramuscular vitamin K to all newborn babies will prevent bleeding from vitamin K deficiency. Concerns about the safety of intramuscular vitamin K, in particular the risk of cancer, were raised in the early 1990s and although there are few data to support this, a small risk of leukaemia cannot be excluded. In order to avoid the potential risk of intramuscular injection a number of countries have recommended oral administration of vitamin K in all healthy full-term infants. Unfortunately, it appears that the protection this policy provides for the development of late-onset haemorrhagic disease of the newborn is not ideal, and approximately 2/100 000 cases of late-onset bleeding have been reported.

There is no doubt that the only certain way to prevent serious late-onset vitamin K deficiency bleeding is to give intramuscular vitamin K. If this is not acceptable to the parents, then oral administration can be used, but in exclusively breastfed babies, who constitute the highest risk for this condition, three doses are necessary to give full protection. Konakion MM paediatric drops are licensed in the UK for use in healthy neonates of 36 weeks' gestation and older. The recommended dosage regimen is 2 mg orally shortly after birth, a further 2 mg at 4–7 days and, if the baby is exclusively breastfed, a third dose of 2 mg should be given at 1 month of age. Failure to give a complete dosage regimen appears to be the reason for the re-emergence of serious late-onset vitamin K deficiency haemorrhage.

DISSEMINATED INTRAVASCULAR COAGULATION

DIC is an acquired coagulation disorder characterized by the intravascular consumption of platelets and clotting factors II, V, VIII and fibrinogen. Widespread intravascular coagulation results from the deposition of thrombi in small vessels and the consumption of clotting factors, with consequent haemorrhage. DIC is recognized as a complication of an increasing variety of neonatal conditions, including:
1 septicaemia;
2 severe shock;
3 severe perinatal asphyxia;
4 hyaline membrane disease in very low birthweight (VLBW) infants;
5 severe rhesus disease;
6 TORCH infections;

7 hypothermia;

8 maternal DIC with a transplacental effect. This occurs secondary to antepartum haemorrhage, a dead twin fetus or amniotic fluid embolism.

Investigations

1 Blood film shows haemolysis with fragmented and distorted red cells.
2 Thrombocytopenia.
3 Prolonged PT, PTT and thrombin time.
4 Low fibrinogen.
5 Increased FDPs.

Not all these features are necessary to make the diagnosis, but the presence of three or more makes DIC very likely.

Treatment

This is a complex disorder and haematological consultation will often be necessary. Treatment consists of:
1 treating the underlying disease process;
2 treatment of the haematological abnormality, including exchange transfusion with fresh whole blood and/or replacement of clotting factors with fresh frozen plasma, platelet concentrates and cryoprecipitate. Heparinization is unlikely to be of any benefit.

IMMATURITY OF CLOTTING MECHANISMS

Liver immaturity may result in prolonged PT and PTT. This, in addition to birth trauma, soft skull bones and lack of supporting tissue for the cerebral circulation, explains the high incidence of haemorrhage in the preterm infant. Thus, the haemorrhagic tendency in the preterm infant may not be entirely prevented by the administration of vitamin K_1 at birth.

INHERITED DISORDERS OF COAGULATION

Coagulation factors are not transferred from the maternal circulation to the fetus. Severe forms of haemophilia A (factor VIII deficiency) and Christmas disease (factor IX deficiency)

account for the majority of haemorrhagic problems of the newborn caused by congenital coagulation abnormalities. Bleeding in these X-linked recessive diseases occurs when male infants are subjected to surgical procedures such as circumcision, or from either birth trauma or routine sampling of capillary blood. The diagnosis is confirmed by a prolonged PTT, normal PT and decreased factor VIII assay.

Management

A specific diagnosis may be difficult to make at birth because in the healthy infant many of the clotting factor assays are low. Treatment consists of transfusion with fresh blood, and sometimes cryoprecipitate when a specific diagnosis can be made.

REFERENCES

Liley, A.W. (1961) Liquor amnii analysis in management of pregnancy complicated by rhesus sensitization. *American Journal of Obstetrics and Gynecology* **82**, 1359.

Oski, F.A. & Naiman, J.L. (1982) *Haematologic Problems in the Newborn*, 3rd edn. W.B. Saunders, Philadelphia.

Queenan, J.T., Tomai, T.P., Ural, S.H. & King, J.C. (1993) Deviation in amniotic fluid optical density at a wavelength of 450 nm in Rh-immunised pregnancies from 14 to 40 weeks gestation: a proposal for clinical management. *American Journal of Obstetrics and Gynecology* **168**, 1370–1376.

Rennie, J.M., Gibson, T. & Cooke, R.W.I. (1985) Micromethod for bleeding time in the newborn. *Archives of Disease in Childhood* **60**, 51–53.

Scott, F. & Chan, F.Y. (1998) Assessment of the clinical usefulness of the 'Queenan' chart versus the 'Liley' chart in predicting severity of Rhesus isoimmunization. *Prenatal Diagnosis* **18**, 1143–1148.

FURTHER READING

Lanzkowsky, P. (1995) *Manual of Paediatric Haematology and Oncology*, 2nd edn. Churchill Livingstone, New York.

Lilleyman, J.S. & Hann, I.M. (eds) (1992) *Paediatric Haematology*. Churchill Livingstone, Edinburgh.

Smith, H. (1996) *Diagnosis in Paediatric Haematology*. Churchill Livingstone, New York.

19 Neurological disorders

There is a continuum of brain development from the time of conception right through gestation and until the end of the first decade of life. The pattern of brain growth and development is illustrated in Fig. 19.1.

Neuronogenesis. The first neural tissue appears at about 18 days with the neural crest, from which the neural tube develops. There is a phase of rapid neuronogenesis occurring from 4 to about 18 weeks of gestation.

Differentiation. The primitive neural cells differentiate into the different populations of cells, both neurons and glia, which make up the mature brain. This process occurs mainly from weeks 4 to 18.

Proliferation. There is a vast increase in the number of neuronal cells up to about 18 weeks of life, most of which die off as part of the neuronal regression process (see below).

Neuronal migration. Neurons are produced deep in the brain and migrate to the cortex and other sites. Final migration of neurons has been achieved by 25 weeks of gestation.

Neuronal regression. The process of apoptosis ensures that only neurons which have achieved a functional capacity within the nervous system survive. Most neurons, during the course of migration, do not effect this function and regress as part of normal brain development.

Synapse development. Full function in the brain depends on the dendrites of each neuron developing and making many connections (on average each neuron is in contact with 10 000 other neurons). These connections are called synapses. Establishing new synaptic contact is part of the process of development and learning.

Myelination. Glial cells are associated with the process of myelination and there is rapid growth of these cells from 24 weeks as they migrate to their final sites. Myelination is not complete until about 12 years.

Factors adversely influencing brain growth and development may operate at different times. Community-based studies of disabled children, relating the timing of the brain insult to either prenatal, perinatal or postnatal events, show that prenatal insults account for more disability than perinatal and postnatal

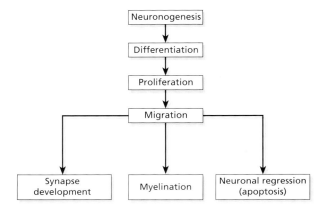

Fig. 19.1 The sequence of brain development.

Table 19.1 Estimated timing of events which cause neurological handicap in a community

Prenatal	70–75%	
Perinatal	20%	Premature 60% Full-term 40%
Postnatal	5–10%	

causes together. The approximate proportions for neurological handicap in a community are shown in Table 19.1.

Table 19.2 lists the relatively common insults which may cause prenatal, perinatal or postnatally acquired disability.

The brain is not a homogeneous organ. Specific areas of the brain grow at different times and rates. Thus, growth restriction at any one time (e.g. due to malnutrition) distorts the general growth of the brain and may selectively affect a particular area. Unlike general body growth, the brain has only one opportunity to develop properly and thus interference with growth at a particular time in development may be irreversible.

MALFORMATIONS OF THE CENTRAL NERVOUS SYSTEM

Abnormalities of the brain can be classified as malformations (a developmental defect in which the brain was never normal) and deformations, where an external insult has affected normal brain development causing an abnormality in subsequent structure.

The incidence of major central nervous system (CNS) abnormalities in the UK has fallen more than 10-fold in the last 30 years and in 1996 was less than 0.5/1000 live births. In Australia the incidence is approximately 1.2/1000.

Malformations of the CNS apparent at birth result from abnormalities in CNS development. These can be divided into two groups:
1 disorders of dorsal induction; and
2 disorders of ventral induction.

Dorsal induction refers to the formation and migration of the neural tube, with subsequent development of the anterior tube into the primitive brain structures. These processes occur during the third and fourth weeks of gestation. Disorders occurring at this time include anencephaly, encephalocoele, myelomeningocoele and meningocoele. These are collectively known as neural tube defects, and the incidence of babies born with these disorders has fallen markedly over the last 10 years.

Ventral induction refers to development at the ventral end of the neural tube, and particularly cleavage into bilateral hemispheres and ventricles, with thalamic and hypothalamic growth. These processes occur mainly in the fifth and sixth weeks of gestation. The commonest disorder occurring at this time is holoprosencephaly, which may be associated with abnormalities in facial development.

Table 19.2 Causes of neurological disability related to the timing of onset of the insult

Prenatal	Perinatal	Postnatal
Down syndrome	Birth asphyxia	Hypothyroidism
Neural tube defects	Intracranial haemorrhage	Meningitis
Other chromosomal disorders	Periventricular leukomalacia	Inborn errors of metabolism
Viral infection	Ototoxic drugs	Trauma
Intrauterine growth restriction	Kernicterus	
Toxins and drugs	Hypoglycaemia	

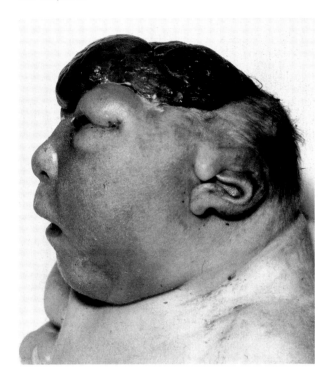

Fig. 19.2 Anencephaly.

Neural tube disorders

Aetiology

These conditions in general, and spina bifida in particular, have become much less common than they were previously. There are two main reasons for this: periconceptual folate and antenatal fetal screening. In some women the risk of a baby with neural tube disorders (NTDs) is increased. This includes families with a history of an affected child, or where the mother herself has the condition. A number of anticonvulsant drugs administered to the mother (particularly sodium valproate) are associated with a considerably increased risk.

It is now known that folic acid is an important substrate for normal early neural tube development, and periconceptual supplementation of at-risk women with folic acid reduces the incidence of this condition by approximately 75%. As it is not possible to know which women are at increased risk until their first baby is born with spina bifida, it is now recommended that all women intending to become pregnant take regular folate for 3 months prior to conception.

The second factor in the falling incidence of NTDs is early fetal ultrasound to detect congenital spine or brain abnormalities. In many developed countries virtually all pregnant women are screened at about 18 weeks of gestation. The detection of a seriously abnormal fetus offers the opportunity for the parents to consider terminating the pregnancy.

ANENCEPHALY

In this condition the forebrain is absent (Fig. 19.2); it occurs as the result of an insult before 24 days' gestation. With routine fetal scanning and termination of pregnancy this condition is now rarely seen at birth. Anencephaly is incompatible with life and results in stillbirth or neonatal death.

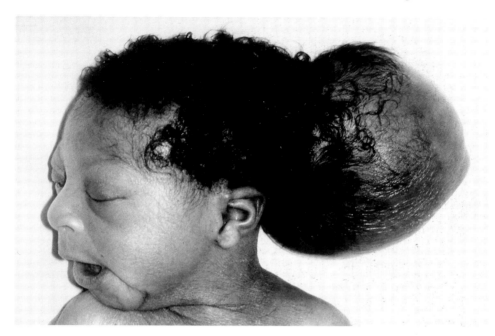

Fig. 19.3 Occipital encephalocoele. This infant was operated on. Although he has severe visual impairment, at 2 years he is otherwise normal.

ENCEPHALOCOELE

In this condition there has been failure of midline closure of the skull, usually with herniation of the brain. Up to 80% of cases occur in the occipital region (Fig. 19.3). This lesion occurs about 28 days after conception. The prognosis depends on the amount of brain in the sac. If the infant is microcephalic with a large encephalocoele, the prognosis is very poor. Neurosurgery is necessary to close the defect.

SPINA BIFIDA

This is a developmental failure of fusion of the vertebral column, often with an external protrusion of the meninges and cord. A meningeal sac of cerebrospinal fluid (CSF) with normal underlying spinal cord is referred to as a meningocoele, and if there is associated abnormality of the cord it is a meningomyelocoele. The abnormalities produced may be classified according to their severity.

Spina bifida occulta

The vertebrae are bifid but there is no meningocoele or myelomeningocoele sac (Fig. 19.4). This abnormality is seen in 10% of the population and is usually of no clinical significance. In a small proportion the spinal cord may be tethered and with growth becomes stretched, causing irreversible neurological signs in the lower limbs and bladder. This condition should be suspected if there are lesions over the midline of the lower back. Such lesions include:

1 a deep sinus;

2 a naevus;

3 a tuft of hair;

4 a soft fatty swelling referred to as a lipomyelomeningocoele. This is particularly likely to be associated with later neurological signs.

All newborn infants with any of these clinical features should be investigated with real-time ultrasound and, if spinal cord tethering is suspected, referred to a neurosurgeon. The prognosis is much better with early repair prior to the onset of neurological symptoms.

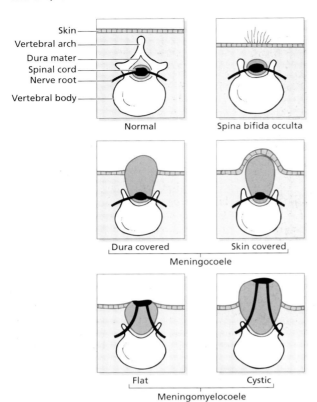

Fig. 19.4 The varieties of spina bifida.

Spina bifida cystica

This includes meningocoeles and myelomeningocoeles (Fig. 19.4). The incidence of this lesion in live born infants is now about 1/10 000 births, but is considerably higher in some parts of the world.

Meningocoeles account for 20% of spina bifida cystica lesions. In this condition there is no herniation of nervous tissue, and consequently no neurological deficit. There is a risk of meningitis if the sac leaks CSF.

Meningomyelocoeles (Fig. 19.5) account for 80% of spina bifida cystica lesions. They are associated with herniation of nervous tissue and permanent neurological deficit.

Clinical features

The antenatal features and diagnosis may be similar to those seen with anencephaly, as the spinal abnormality is obvious at birth; clinical examination should assess the following features:

1 *site of lesion.* About 70% are lumbosacral;
2 *covering of sac.* Usually meninges, but occasionally the sac is ruptured, leading to CSF leakage and consequent risk of meningitis;
3 *clinical assessment*:
   (a) motor loss: this is generally lower motor neuron in type and the extent depends on the site of the lesion;
   (b) sensory loss: this depends on the position of the lesion and the level is often asymmetrical;
   (c) neurogenic bladder: the patient usually dribbles urine constantly and has a distended expressible bladder;
   (d) patulous anal tone;
4 *hydrocephalus.* Ninety per cent of infants with meningomyelocoeles have an associated abnormality of the brain and skull base, re-

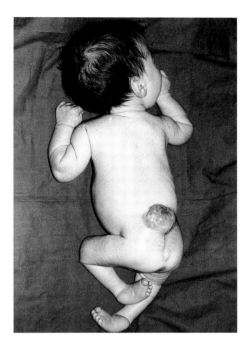

Fig. 19.5 Lumbosacral meningomyelocoele.

ferred to as the Arnold–Chiari type II malformation. This includes prolapse of the medulla, cerebellum and fourth ventricle through an abnormal foramen magnum into the cervical canal. Not all infants develop hydrocephalus, but most have ventricular dilatation on ultrasound scans. Progressive enlargement of the head may occur with advancing age;

5 *orthopaedic abnormalities*. These are common and include talipes, dislocated hips, kyphosis, scoliosis and contractures of the lower limbs;

6 *miscellaneous abnormalities*. These include renal, cardiac and visceral defects and chromosome disorders.

Investigations

The neural arches of the vertebrae are poorly mineralized at birth and spinal radiography is of little value except for the assessment of scoliosis. Ultrasound examination of the spine in the newborn period allows visualization of the spinal cord: if it does not move with respiration, this suggests that there may be tethering.

Management

A careful assessment of the newborn infant by appropriate specialists is necessary before a definite treatment plan can be formulated. Treatment is always discussed with the parents, whose wishes should be considered. Many centres use Lorber's (1971) criteria for conservative treatment. Lorber followed a large number of babies with meningomyelocoele during the period when all babies were energetically treated, and identified the following bad prognostic criteria:

1 total paralysis of the legs;
2 thoracolumbar or thoracolumbosacral lesions;
3 severe kyphoscoliosis;
4 hydrocephalus at birth;
5 other major congenital malformations, e.g. Down syndrome, congenital heart lesion.

If one or more of these features are present at birth, he recommended conservative management. This consists of nursing care only, but does not rule out subsequent reappraisal of the need for neurosurgery.

If active treatment is indicated, the following approach would be adopted:

1 *early neurosurgery*. Closure of the sac within 24 h of birth, with ongoing assessment for hydrocephalus and insertion of a shunt, usually ventriculoperitoneal, if indicated;

2 *orthopaedic assessment and treatment* as necessary;

3 *general surgical*. Urinary incontinence is a major problem and girls usually require an ileal conduit, whereas boys may be managed at least initially with a penile collecting system or intermittent catheterization. The aim of treating faecal incontinence is to produce a firm stool to prevent soiling and faecal impaction;

4 *supportive care*. Pressure sores need to be prevented by careful positioning and skin care. Psychological and social problems are common and parents need careful support and counselling. Schooling and employment also present difficult problems;

5 *genetic counselling*. This will be necessary for future pregnancies.

SCREENING FOR NEURAL TUBE DEFECTS

1 *α-Fetoprotein (AFP).* Blood is taken from the mother at 14–18 weeks' gestation and AFP measured. AFP in the first trimester normally increases with gestational age, and an accurate assessment of the duration of pregnancy is essential in assessing the significance of the AFP level. Those women with high serum levels should have repeat samples taken 1 week later. Only 10% of pregnancies complicated by a high serum AFP level are associated with NTDs. Multiple pregnancies, exomphalos and other abnormalities may cause high levels. AFP is raised in 90% of cases of anencephaly, and in most cases of open myelomeningocoele. A skin-covered lesion will not have raised levels.
2 *Ultrasound screening.* Various abnormalities are assessed, including careful examination of the lower spine for a skin defect and examination of the skull base for the 'banana' sign, which is a feature of the Arnold–Chiari malformation.

Disorders of ventral induction

HOLOPROSENCEPHALY

This is a rare condition where there is a failure of midline fusion of the CNS, resulting in a single cerebral vesicle. There may also be midline defects of the eyes, lips and palate.

Chromosome analysis should be carried out, as half of these lesions are associated with abnormal chromosomal patterns, most often trisomy 13. The prognosis for normal development is hopeless.

Holoprosencephaly may present in partial forms, referred to as lobar or semilobar, and the diagnosis is made on ultrasound or computed tomography (CT) examination. The appearances of agenesis of the corpus callosum and septo-optic dysplasia may be confused with holoprosencephaly if care is not taken.

MICROCEPHALY

Microcephaly occurs as the result of a variety of brain insults. It is defined as an occipitofrontal head circumference more than two standard deviations below the mean for the infant's gestational age. The child may show microcephaly in proportion to his weight and length (generalized growth retardation), or more ominously have a small head but a normally grown body. Microcephaly may be primary or secondary. Secondary implies normal growth up to a point when a major insult has occurred, after which brain growth fails. Table 19.3 lists various causes of microcephaly.

The underlying cause should be diagnosed and treated wherever possible. The prognosis is usually poor and treatment is supportive.

Table 19.3 Causes of primary and secondary microcephaly

Primary	Secondary
Familial	Intrauterine growth retardation
Autosomal recessive	Meningitis
X-linked recessive	Hypoglycaemia
Chromosomal	Asphyxia
Trisomy 13	Periventricular leukomalacia
Trisomy 18	
TORCH infections	
Maternal phenylketonuria	
Lissencephaly	
Fetal alcohol syndrome	

CRANIOSTENOSIS (CRANIOSYNOSTOSIS)

In this condition the skull sutures fuse prematurely, with resultant cranial distortions. The most common form of craniostenosis is premature closure of the sagittal suture, giving a scaphocephalic head shape. Premature closure of the coronal suture leads to a brachycephalic head and closure of both sagittal and coronal sutures gives an oxycephalic head. Autosomal dominantly inherited craniofacial deformities include:
1 Apert syndrome (acrocephalosyndactyly);
2 Crouzon syndrome (craniofacial dysostosis);
3 Carpenter syndrome (acrocephalopolysyndactyly).

Management

Skull X-rays are necessary to confirm the clinical suspicion. Surgery is indicated for cosmetic reasons or, rarely, if premature fusion of the sutures causes raised intracranial pressure.

Hydrocephalus

Hydrocephalus is caused by an imbalance between the production and the absorption of CSF, with resultant dilatation of the cerebral ventricles. Later a rapid increase in head size can occur as a result of progressive ventricular dilatation. The term 'hydrocephalus' has often been used inappropriately to describe an exces-

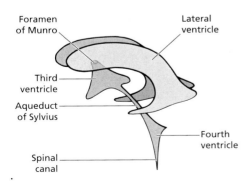

Fig. 19.6 Diagram to show intracerebral drainage of cerebrospinal fluid. (Reproduced from Levene 1986, with permission of Churchill Livingstone.)

sively large head without ventricular enlargement. The term megalencephaly is more appropriate under these circumstances. Babies can have considerable ventriculomegaly but at least in the early stages have normal head size.

CLASSIFICATION

Non-obstructive

In this extremely rare type there is no interference with CSF flow. The excessive production of CSF is usually due to a papilloma of the choroid plexus.

Obstructive (see Fig. 19.6 for site of obstruction)

Obstructive hydrocephalus can be divided into non-communicating and communicating.

Non-communicating. There is little or no communication between the ventricles and the subarachnoid space. There are three common sites of obstruction:
1 aqueduct of Sylvius (due to stenosis or atresia);
2 occlusion of the foraminae of Luschka and Magendie as a result of basal adhesions. This is the commonest site of blockage and is usually due to intraventricular haemorrhage;
3 Arnold–Chiari type II malformation secondary to spina bifida cystica.

Communicating. CSF can escape from the intracranial system via the foramina of Luschka and Magendie, but cannot be absorbed at the arachnoid granulations situated over the surface of the brain. This is usually due to arachnoiditis following either meningitis or intracranial haemorrhage (ICH). Ventricular dilatation occurring following intraventricular haemorrhage (IVH) is due to non-communicating causes in only 15%; in 85% of cases it is communicating.

CLINICAL FEATURES

Hydrocephalus due to congenital abnormalities may be present at birth or diagnosed *in*

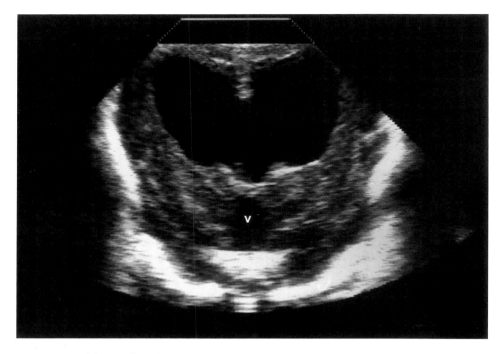

Fig. 19.7 Coronal ultrasound scan showing massive dilatation of both lateral and third ventricles (v).

utero by ultrasound examination. Follow-up studies have shown that about 50% of babies born with apparently isolated fetal ventriculomegaly (no other congenital malformation detected) are normal (Gupta *et al.* 1995). The prognosis is poor if the ventriculomegaly is associated with spina bifida.

Ventricular dilatation occurring after IVH can be detected by cranial ultrasound examinations (Fig. 19.7). Ventriculomegaly may be quite advanced before abnormal head growth is noted. A 'sunset' appearance of the eyes is a late sign in neonatal hydrocephalus and may be seen in infants without dilated ventricles.

INVESTIGATIONS

It is recommended that all infants with IVH have weekly ultrasound scans to detect ventricular dilatation. Accurate measurement of the occipitofrontal circumference at weekly intervals is essential in all infants, especially those with intracranial pathology.

MANAGEMENT

This depends on the underlying cause and the degree of ventriculomegaly.

Congenital hydrocephalus

If treatment of the general condition (e.g. spina bifida) is thought to be appropriate, then ventriculoperitoneal shunting is the treatment of choice. If the infant is unfit for surgery, then medical management with drugs such as isosorbide or acetazolamide may be used. These drugs do not prevent the need for shunting but may delay its timing.

Posthaemorrhagic ventricular dilatation

The management of posthaemorrhagic ventricular dilatation (PHVD) remains controversial. There is no convincing evidence that infants who develop ventricular dilatation following ICH are at greater risk

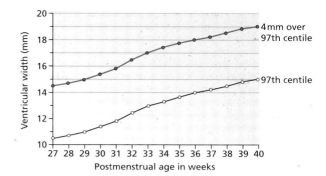

Fig. 19.8 Indication for significant ventriculomegaly. The lower line is the 97th centile for normal ventricular size. The upper line defines ventricular dilatation severe enough to require treatment (Kaiser & Whitelaw 1985).

of adverse neurodevelopmental outcome than those with haemorrhage of the same size but without ventriculomegaly. It is the extent of the haemorrhage that carries the major adverse risk, rather than posthaemorrhagic hydrocephalus *per se*.

Research into the management of posthaemorrhagic hydrocephalus has not suggested that early or aggressive therapy is advantageous to the baby. The European multicentre study (Ventriculomegaly Study Group 1990) on the management of PHVD showed that early treatment (lumbar puncture taps) to prevent further ventriculomegaly gave no benefit in terms of reducing subsequent disability, compared with conservative treatment started when the head circumference exceeded the 97th centile. The use of acetazolamide and frusemide treatment in established posthaemorrhagic hydrocephalus is associated with a worse prognosis than babies not treated with these drugs (International PHVD Drug Trial Group 1998). Recent evaluation of the direct instillation of thrombolytic agents into the ventricles of babies with early posthaemorrhagic hydrocephalus has not been promising for the safe treatment of this condition.

The important factors in the management of PHVD are probably the extent of the initial haemorrhage and the intraventricular pressure (Levene 1986).

A management protocol is as follows:

1 twice weekly ultrasound measurement of ventricular size;

2 if there is progressive ventricular dilatation, then careful measurement of occipitofrontal head circumference should be performed on alternate days;

3 measurement of CSF pressure if:

(a) there is a progressive increase in ventricular size on ultrasound to a point 4 mm above the normal ventricular index (Fig. 19.8);

(b) there is a progressive increase in occipitofrontal head circumference above the 97th centile;

(c) there are symptoms of raised intracranial pressure (apnoea, poor feeding, irritability, etc.).

CSF pressure can most safely be measured by lumbar puncture. Pressure is measured either by a fluid manometer and measuring the height of a column of CSF in cmH_2O, or by a non-fluid displacement technique by attaching a pressure transducer to the hub of the needle. Two important criteria must be applied to these measurements:

1 there is free flow of CSF. If less than 5 mL of fluid is obtained, it suggests that the obstruction is non-communicating and that the pressure can only be measured by ventricular tap;

2 the infant is lying quietly when the pressure measurement is made. If the infant is agitated or crying, the measurement is unreliable. Sometimes it will be necessary to sedate the infant to make accurate measurements.

In infants with non-communicating ventricular dilatation, or those who are very unstable and in whom the handling involved in lumbar puncture is unacceptable, ventricular tap is the alternative (see 30.15, p. 322).

If the pressure is elevated (> 10 cmH_2O, > 7.5 mmHg), then further treatment is warranted. If the CSF protein is < 1 g/L, then a ven-triculoperitoneal shunt should be inserted. If the protein is > 1 g/L, a ventricular reservoir or access device will be necessary to prevent raised intracranial pressure from being maintained. This can be later converted to a shunt. Drug treatment for posthaemorrhagic hydro-cephalus should be avoided.

PROGNOSIS

Complications of surgery include shunt obstruction, ventriculitis and the need for shunt revision. The long-term outlook depends on the cause and severity of the hydrocephalus and any subsequent complications.

Hydranencephaly

In this condition there has been almost total loss of all brain substance owing to an early massive insult *in utero*. The skull is entirely filled with fluid and at birth the head may be normal or enlarged. There is no treatment and the prognosis is hopeless.

Porencephaly

Porencephaly is the name given to cystic cavities in one or both cerebral hemispheres which may or may not communicate with the lateral ventricles. They can be congenital or acquired following meningitis, ICH or cerebral atrophy. The commonest cause is following an intra-parenchymal haemorrhage (see p. 228).

Diagnosis is made by ultrasound or CT/magnetic resonance imaging (MRI) examination. Rarely 'expanding porencephaly syndrome' is seen, in which the porencephalic cavity progressively enlarges. This may require ventriculoperitoneal shunting.

INTRACRANIAL HAEMORRHAGE

ICH in the newborn is a common finding at autopsy and 70% of infants who die have evidence of some degree of ICH. Subdural haem-orrhage, which 50 years ago was the most

common type of ICH, is now rare, and IVH has replaced it as the commonest ICH seen in the newborn infant. There are five important types of neonatal ICH:

1 subarachnoid;
2 subdural;
3 intraventricular;
4 intracerebral;
5 intracerebellar.

Subarachnoid haemorrhage

Blood in the subarachnoid space is most commonly secondary to IVH which tracks through the ventricular system.

Primary subarachnoid haemorrhage (SAH) is a common, and usually benign, condition and is seen in both premature and full-term infants. It occurs as a response to hypoxia or trauma, and is usually seen as a discrete area over the convexity of the brain.

CLINICAL FEATURES

SAH is usually asymptomatic, but when symptoms do occur seizures and apnoea are most commonly seen in full-term infants on the second day of life. Between seizures the infant is neurologically normal.

DIAGNOSIS

Ultrasound is very unreliable in detecting SAH and CT/MRI are much more sensitive for this diagnosis. The CSF is usually heavily bloodstained and does not clear in successive tubes.

PROGNOSIS

A good prognosis can be predicted if there are minimal neurological signs in the neonatal period and if the predisposing traumatic or hypoxic injury is mild.

In approximately 90% of cases infants with seizures as the primary manifestation of the haemorrhage are normal on follow-up. Rarely the patient dies or is left with serious neurological sequelae, such as hydrocephalus, which presents weeks to months after the initial insult.

TREATMENT

There is no specific treatment. Bleeding disorders should be excluded and, if present, treated appropriately (see Chapter 18). Posthaemorrhagic hydrocephalus may occur.

Subdural haemorrhage

Subdural haematoma used to be relatively common but is now extremely rare, owing to a reduced incidence of birth trauma associated with a reduction in the use of high and mid-cavity forceps deliveries, prolonged labours and a concurrent increase in caesarean section births. It is classically due to rapid changes in head shape during labour and delivery.

PATHOGENESIS

There are three basic origins of subdural haemorrhage:
1 tentorial laceration with rupture of the straight sinus, resulting in an infratentorial haematoma;
2 falx cerebri laceration and rupture of the inferior sagittal sinus, giving rise to a haematoma of the longitudinal cerebral fissure;
3 rupture of superficial cerebral veins with a subdural haematoma over the temporal lobe. Usually unilateral and accompanied by subarachnoid blood.

PREDISPOSING FACTORS

1 Rigid birth canal—primipara, elderly multipara, small pelvis.
2 Infant with large head.
3 Labour—precipitous, prolonged.
4 Presentation—breech, foot, face, brow.
5 Delivery—difficult forceps, difficult rotation.

CLINICAL FEATURES

Subdural haematomas may present as a recognizable symptom complex including tense fontanelle, hypotonia, lethargy and facial palsy. If the haemorrhage involves the posterior fossa, then apnoea, irregular sighing respiration, fixed bradycardia, opisthotonus and skew deviation of the eyes may occur. If there is only a minor haemorrhage, the baby may be asymptomatic. Signs of hydrocephalus may develop.

INVESTIGATIONS

Subdural haemorrhage over the brain convexity or associated with tentorial tears may be seen on ultrasound, particularly if large. A midline shift may be the only clue to a convexity subdural collection. A CT/MRI scan is more sensitive to the diagnosis than ultrasound.

TREATMENT

In convexity subdural haemorrhage subdural taps through the anterior fontanelle under strict aseptic conditions are necessary. Repeated taps may be required (see p. 322).

Intraventricular haemorrhage

IVH is a description of blood within the ventricular system and may be due to:
1 germinal matrix haemorrhage; or
2 choroid plexus haemorrhage. This is usually a relatively benign condition occurring in an asphyxiated full-term infant.

IVH is usually assumed to have arisen from the rupture of capillaries within the germinal matrix of the caudate nucleus. The condition occurs in premature infants and its incidence is approximately 33% in infants of 1500 g birthweight and below. In some infants the bleeding may be massive, with involvement of the cerebral parenchyma (Fig. 19.9). The initial bleeding occurs into the germinal matrix (also called the subependymal plate), which lies over the head of the caudate nucleus. The germinal matrix is present between 24 and 34 weeks of gestation and rapidly involutes after this time. Rupture into the ventricles (hence the term IVH) occurs in 80% of cases of germinal matrix haemorrhage. Rarely IVH is seen in

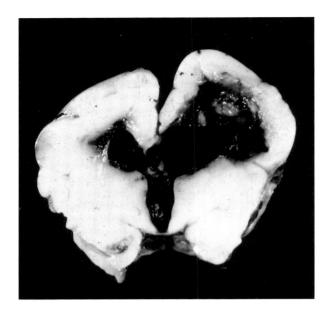

Fig. 19.9 Bilateral intraventricular haemorrhage with massive parenchymal extension into the right hemisphere.

full-term infants. Changes in cerebral blood flow probably precipitate the bleeding, and infants with respiratory distress syndrome (RDS) are most likely to have an unstable cerebral circulation. The following are the most important clinical features associated with IVH:
1 prematurity;
2 RDS;
3 intermittent positive-pressure ventilation;
4 hypercapnia;
5 metabolic acidosis;
6 birth outside a perinatal centre;
7 coagulation disorder.

CLINICAL FEATURES

1 *Minimal signs*. Approximately 60% of infants with IVH have no major clinical symptoms. Neurological examination (see p. 31) reveals subtle changes in tone, including a tight popliteal angle, and roving eye movements (slow nystagmus) for some weeks after the haemorrhage has occurred.
2 *Intermittent deterioration* over a period of days, with increasing signs of apnoea, bradycardia, metabolic acidosis and seizures.
3 *Massive collapse* with neurological signs

(seizures, coma), shock and anaemia. This is a rare clinical presentation and is more likely to occur as the result of other neonatal complications, including infection and metabolic disorders.

DIAGNOSIS

Real-time ultrasound is the method of choice. There is no generally agreed method for grading the severity of IVH. The two most commonly used schemes are:
Grade 1—subependymal and/or minimal IVH (Fig. 19.10);
Grade 2—intraventricular clot within the lateral ventricle;
Grade 3—intraparenchymal involvement. This is usually unilateral and occurs as a result of venous infarction. In this case the intraventricular clot reduces venous drainage in the periventricular white matter of one hemisphere, causing stasis with infarction (periventricular haemorrhagic infarction). If the parenchymal 'haemorrhage' is bilateral, then it is more likely to be due to bleeding into a primary ischaemic area of the brain, and this is referred to as *periventricular leukomalacia (PVL)* (see below).

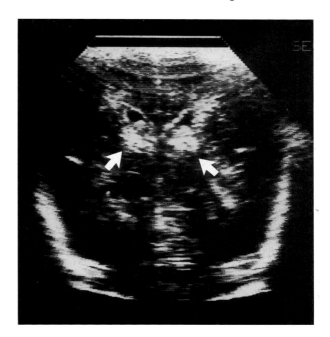

Fig. 19.10 Coronal ultrasound scan showing bilateral haemorrhage in the region of the germinal matrix (arrowed).

Papile classification:
Grade 1—subependymal germinal matrix haemorrhage;
Grade 2—IVH with no ventricular dilatation;
Grade 3—IVH with ventricle distended by blood; and
Grade 4—intraparenchymal haemorrhage.

COMPLICATIONS

1 PHVD. This occurs in up to 40% of infants with IVH (see section on hydrocephalus above).
2 Porencephaly (see p. 226).

TREATMENT

There is no specific treatment once IVH has occurred. Careful attention to respiratory management, coagulation disturbances and blood pressure is important in ill infants in an attempt to reduce the likelihood of IVH.

PREVENTION

A variety of drugs have been evaluated to assess their effect in preventing IVH when given shortly after birth. Only two, indomethacin and ethamsylate, have been shown on the basis of randomized controlled trials to reduce the incidence and severity of IVH. To date very few studies have reported follow-up data to show that these drugs reduce disability rather than just haemorrhage, and neither has been shown convincingly to demonstrate a reduction in adverse outcome. In our view the currently available evidence does not suggest that any drug should be routinely administered in all very premature babies to reduce the incidence of IVH.

Intracerebral haemorrhage

In 80% of cases this is due to secondary extension of IVH or to rebleeding into periventricular ischaemic areas of the brain. Other causes of primary intracerebral haemorrhage include:
1 coagulation disturbances;
2 cerebral artery occlusion;
3 TORCH (toxoplasmosis, other, rubella, cytomegalovirus, herpes simplex type II) infection;

4 thalamic haemorrhage;
5 arteriovenous malformation (very rare);
6 tumour (very rare).

Diagnosis is made by ultrasound examination or CT/MRI.

Intracerebellar haemorrhage

This type of haemorrhage occurs predominantly in preterm infants. It may be associated with hypoxic insults, a traumatic breech delivery or head compression caused by strapping techniques for nasal continuous positive airway pressure (CPAP) prongs.

Periventricular leukomalacia

PVL literally means softening of the white matter around the ventricles, and is now recognized as a major risk factor for the subsequent development of cerebral palsy. The lesion is thought to be due to underperfusion in the watershed region of the periventricular white matter and infection may be an important underlying factor in its development. The periventricular white matter is particularly vulnerable to ischaemic insults between 28 and 35 weeks of gestation. Diagnosis is made by real-time ultrasound, which initially shows areas of echodensity in the white matter which may resolve spontaneously or progress to cystic degeneration. Multiple cavities or cavities in the occipital region are known to carry a high risk of less severe cerebral palsy, and small or single cavities predispose the baby to a greater risk of adverse outcome. The prognosis for babies who show persistent echodensity ('flare') is uncertain.

NEONATAL CONVULSIONS

The terms convulsion, fit and seizure are used interchangeably to describe clinically evident, episodic events occurring in the neonatal period and arising from a brain disorder. The incidence of neonatal seizures is 5–8/1000 liveborn infants. It may be difficult to decide whether movements made by the sick neonate are abnormal or not. In addition, jitteriness must be distinguished from the infant having convulsions. Table 19.4 lists important differences between these two conditions.

Irritability. This is due to CNS depression and the infant behaves in an abnormal manner, lying quietly until disturbed when he cries excessively. The cry may be high pitched, the baby is difficult to console and takes longer to settle than normal.

Jitteriness. The jittery infant shows exaggerated responses to stimuli, with an exaggerated startle to noise or handling, and has exaggerated fine tremulous movements.

The essential difference between irritability and jitteriness is that the former is non-stimulus sensitive, whereas the latter occurs in response to minor stimulation.

Seizure type

The five basic descriptive types of convulsions in the newborn are subtle, tonic, multifocal clonic, focal clonic and myoclonic. The preterm infant with a less well-organized

Table 19.4 Important features in distinguishing the jittery infant from one who is having convulsions

	Jitteriness	Convulsions
Stimulus provoked	Yes	No
Predominant movement	Rapid, oscillatory	Clonic, tonic
Movements cease when limb is held	Yes	No
Conscious state	Awake or asleep	Altered
Eye deviation	No	Yes

immature CNS is more likely to show subtle convulsions.

SUBTLE

These may be difficult to distinguish from jitteriness. There are a number of recognized types:
1 horizontal deviation of the eyes with or without jerking;
2 chewing or sucking movements;
3 bicycling movements;
4 rhythmic or dancing movements of the eyes;
5 apnoea, which may be the only feature of seizures.

TONIC

Extensor spasms of the trunk and limbs with opisthotonic posturing. They may occur predominantly in preterm infants.

MULTIFOCAL CLONIC

There is a non-ordered progression of clonic movements of the limbs. These occur predominantly in term infants.

FOCAL CLONIC

Well-localized clonic jerking of a limb or jaw. They are sometimes associated with a convexity haemorrhage (e.g. subdural).

MYOCLONIC JERKS

Occasional myoclonic jerks may be normal in the newborn but multiple myoclonic jerks are usually pathological. They may be difficult to distinguish from jitteriness.

It is now recognized that these clinical patterns are not always associated with abnormal electrical seizure activity on the electroencephalogram (EEG). Good correlation exists between electroconvulsive activity on the EEG and focal tonic, focal clonic and some myoclonic movements. Poor correlation is found between electrical activity and subtle and generalized tonic 'seizures'. These are better referred to as 'brainstem release phenomena', and are often seen in neonates with global brain damage and are most likely to have the worst long-term outlook. It is also recognized that abnormal electroconvulsive activity can occur with no clinical signs of seizure activity.

It is unresolved whether electroconvulsive seizure activity recognized on EEG causes cerebral injury and requires treatment. Studies on the efficacy of drug treatment for neonatal fits have been based mainly on clinical seizures rather than EEG abnormalities. At present it is probably inappropriate to try and abolish all electroconvulsive seizure activity, as the dosage of anticonvulsant medication may cause significant compromise.

Aetiology

The major causes of neonatal convulsions depend on the time of onset and whether the infant is term or preterm. Table 19.5 lists the commoner causes of neonatal seizures and indicates their time of onset.

PERINATAL ASPHYXIA

This accounts for the aetiology of 50% of cases and is the commonest cause of neonatal seizures. They usually present on the first day of life as subtle in type, progressing to multifocal clonic and tonic seizures. They usually improve and cease within 4–5 days. Status epilepticus may occur with severe hypoxic ischaemic encephalopathy. This condition is discussed fully in Chapter 3.

INTRACRANIAL HAEMORRHAGE

All types of ICH may present with fits. The infant who convulses as a result of SAH usually appears to be neurologically normal between fits. Seizures secondary to cerebral contusion, especially a convexity subdural or subarachnoid collection, may exhibit predominantly focal features. All full-term infants with convulsions should have an ultrasound scan to exclude this as the cause.

Table 19.5 Causes of neonatal convulsions indicating whether they occur early or late. The overall frequency of convulsions is indicated by the number of ' +' signs shown

	Time of onset and relative frequency	
	0–2 days	2–10 days
Asphyxia	+++	–
Intracranial haemorrhage	++	+
Hypocalcaemia	++	+
Hypoglycaemia	++	+
Infection	+	++
Developmental abnormalities	+	+
Drug withdrawal	+	
Inborn errors of metabolism	+	+
Pyridoxine deficiency	++	
Fifth-day fits	–	++

INFECTIONS

Intracranial bacterial and non-bacterial infections account for a significant number of neonatal convulsions. The most common infecting organisms are the Gram-negative bacilli, group B β-haemolytic streptococcus and the TORCH group.

DRUG WITHDRAWAL (NARCOTICS AND BARBITURATES)

Over 65% of the babies of opioid-dependent women will show withdrawal symptoms in the first 3–5 days after birth. Symptoms of the neonatal abstinence syndrome include irritability, hypertonia, tremors and hyperactivity in over 70% of affected infants. Convulsions occur in less than 10% of cases. Other common symptoms include yawning, snuffliness, sweating, sneezing, diarrhoea, vomiting and poor feeding.

Management of the drug-addicted infant is discussed in Chapter 14 (p. 150).

Cocaine is becoming a commonly abused drug in pregnancy. It may cause fetal cerebral artery infarction, which may cause neonatal convulsions.

INBORN ERRORS OF METABOLISM

These are individually very rare and include maple syrup urine disease, urea cycle defects, organic acidaemias and galactosaemia. They often present once the baby is on full milk feeds and there may be a family history. Screening investigations when inborn errors of metabolism are suspected include urinary amino acids and organic acids, serum lactate and ammonia.

PYRIDOXINE DEFICIENCY

This is very rare but must be considered where there is a history of very early convulsions and where the convulsions are resistant to standard anticonvulsant medication.

FIFTH-DAY FITS

This is almost certainly not a single entity, but rather a group of benign conditions with unrecognized causes. The baby develops seizures on the fourth or fifth day of life, and these are self-limiting. Between seizures the infant appears to be entirely normal. The diagnosis is made by excluding other causes for the convulsions.

Diagnosis

Newborn infants with convulsions need a diagnostic evaluation, consisting of a careful history and examination and laboratory investigations. It is unusual not to find a cause for the convulsions as idiopathic epilepsy rarely, if ever, commences in the newborn period.

An approach to diagnosis is:

1 *history*. Family history of neonatal convulsions, maternal drug ingestion, antenatal and intrapartum infections, perinatal asphyxia, birth trauma;

2 *examination*. Developmental anomalies, signs of sepsis;

3 *metabolic*. Test for hypoglycaemia. Blood is obtained for assay of calcium, magnesium, phosphate and sodium;

4 *lumbar puncture*. Meningitis, haemorrhage;

5 *septic work-up and TORCH serology*. Meningitis, encephalitis;

6 *ultrasound scan of the brain*. Intracranial haemorrhage, developmental anomalies of the brain.

Additional investigations include:

1 urinary and serum amino acids;

2 urine for organic acids;

3 serum lactate;

4 serum ammonia;

5 galactose-1-phosphate uridyl transferase activity.

Treatment

Neonatal convulsions represent a neonatal emergency and require immediate treatment and investigation. With frequent convulsions feeding should be discontinued, an intravenous line inserted and regular observations commenced.

SPECIFIC TREATMENT

The underlying cause of the convulsion is treated if possible.

Hypoglycaemia. If the infant is hypoglycaemic (see p. 164), 25% dextrose (2 mL/kg) should be given intravenously followed by an infusion of 10% dextrose.

Hypocalcaemia. If serum calcium is less than 1.5 mmol/L, the baby is given 200 mg/kg of 10% calcium gluconate intravenously with electrocardiogram (ECG) monitoring. If convulsions are recalcitrant to calcium and serum magnesium level is low, 50–100 mg/kg of 50% magnesium sulphate heptahydrate should be administered by slow intravenous infusion under ECG control.

Asphyxia. This is discussed fully in Chapter 3.

Infection. The management of meningitis is discussed in Chapter 7.

Inborn errors of metabolism. Exchange transfusion may be helpful in some cases, and megavitamin therapy is also recommended (Wraith 1995).

ANTICONVULSANT DRUG TREATMENT

If the underlying cause of the convulsions is not known or cannot be treated specifically, or if specific treatment of the underlying cause does not stop the convulsions, anticonvulsant drug therapy will be necessary.

Phenobarbitone

This is the initial drug of choice. A loading dose of 20 mg/kg is administered intravenously. The maintenance dose is 6 mg/kg in two divided doses per day. A second loading dose of 10 mg/kg may be used in intractable seizures. Serum levels should be monitored with long-term therapy (therapeutic range 15–30 µg/mL). Dosing beyond 40–50 mg/kg with serum levels exceeding 50 µg/mL is unlikely to achieve additional seizure control.

Paraldehyde

This is a useful short-acting anticonvulsant to treat fits occurring after a loading dose of phenobarbitone or phenytoin. The dose is 0.15 mg/kg given by deep intramuscular injection every 4–6 h as required. Provided the drug is given soon after drawing up, it is safe to use in a plastic syringe.

Table 19.6 The chance of normal outcome depending on the cause of the neonatal seizure

Cause of seizures	Chance of normal development (%)
Hypoxic–ischaemic encephalopathy	50
Subarachnoid haemorrhage	90
Other intracranial haemorrhage	50
Hypoglycaemia	50
Hypocalcaemia	90
Bacterial meningitis	20–50
Developmental abnormality	0
Fifth-day fits	100
Idiopathic	75

Phenytoin

If the seizures are not controlled by phenobarbitone, phenytoin 20 mg/kg is frequently administered. The maintenance dose is 5 mg/kg/day in two divided doses. This drug is not recommended for long-term maintenance in neonates because of its unpredictable pharmacokinetics. Phenytoin must not be given intramuscularly and side-effects are commonly seen in very low birthweight (VLBW) infants.

Diazepam (Valium)

This drug is generally not used in the newborn infant for convulsions because of the problems of respiratory depression, jaundice and shock. Moreover, it is less effective than phenobarbitone.

Clonazepam (Rivotril)

Use in a dose of 0.15 mg/kg. Continuous intravenous infusion may be of value for intractable seizures.

Stopping anticonvulsant drugs

Only about 10% of babies with neonatal seizures will have convulsions in the first year of life after discharge from the hospital. It is therefore advisable to stop all anticonvulsant medication in the newborn, provided the baby is showing no abnormal neurological signs.

Prognosis

The prognosis for infants who have sustained neonatal convulsions depends on the underlying cause. A summary of the outcome following neonatal convulsions is given in Table 19.6.

NEONATAL HYPOTONIA

There are a large number of causes of neonatal hypotonia (see Heckmatt & Dubowitz 1995 for review). Hypotonia is a very significant symptom and should never be ignored. Generalized floppiness may be due to abnormalities in a variety of anatomical sites:

1 brain (asphyxia);
2 spinal cord (trauma);
3 anterior horn cell (spinal muscular atrophy);
4 nerve root (brachial plexus injury). This causes hypotonia only of the affected limb;
5 peripheral nerve (trauma);
6 neuromuscular junction (myasthenia gravis);
7 muscle (congenital dystrophy).

CLINICAL FEATURES

These infants are lethargic, show little movement and lie in the classic 'frog' posture with the hips abducted and external rotation of the limbs (Fig. 19.11). This posture must be differentiated from the normal posture of a preterm infant.

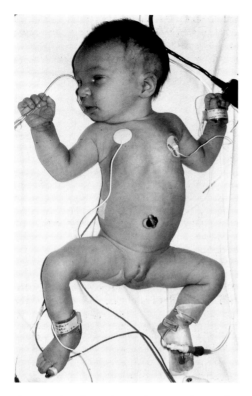

Fig. 19.11 An infant with severe hypotonia showing the characteristic 'frog' posture.

There are two main groups of infants in this category:

1 *non-paralytic*—weak infant with hypotonia and normal muscles, e.g. cerebral hypoxia. (This form may progress to cerebral palsy with increased tone.);

2 *paralytic*—weak infant with hypotonia and muscular disease, e.g. spinal muscle atrophy (Werdnig–Hoffman disease).

The two groups can be distinguished by the ability of the infant to move his limbs against gravity, either spontaneously or following a stimulus. The paralytic infant is unable to maintain the posture of an elevated limb, and has a poverty of spontaneous movement. Table 19.7 lists causes of paralytic and non-paralytic hypotonia.

Spinal muscular atrophy (Werdnig–Hoffman disease)

This is caused by an abnormality of the anterior horn cells in the spinal cord and is an autosomal recessive disorder. The infant presents with profound weakness and hypotonia, although the face is usually striking by its expressiveness as the facial muscles are not involved. Congenital contractures are sometimes present. Diagnosis is made by muscle biopsy. There is no treatment and the infant dies before the first birthday.

Myasthenia gravis

Ninety per cent of cases occur as a result of maternal disease but are transient and last 6–12 weeks, with complete recovery. Rarely a congenital form occurs without maternal disease. Infants show intermittent hypotonia responsive to Tensilon or neostigmine (0.5 mg/kg).

Congenital muscular dystrophy

A condition of unknown cause but inherited as an autosomal recessive, this may present in the newborn period with generalized hypotonia and the infant is often born with severe

Table 19.7 Causes of hypotonia in the newborn

Paralytic	Non-paralytic
Spinal muscular atrophy (Werdnig–Hoffman)	Birth asphyxia
Congenital muscular dystrophy	Down syndrome
Congenital myopathy	Prader–Willi syndrome
Congenital myotonic dystrophy	Skeletal and connective tissue disorders
Myasthenia gravis	Drugs
	Benign congenital hypotonia

contractures. The prognosis may be reasonably good, as improvement in the weakness may occur. Diagnosis is by muscle biopsy.

Congenital myotonic dystrophy

The disease is transmitted in an autosomal dominant manner but the mother is the affected parent in 90% of cases of neonatal disease. The mothers of all floppy infants should be screened for clinical evidence of myotonia or weakness (inability to close the eyelids tightly and bury her eyelashes).

Benign hypotonia

This is a diagnosis of exclusion and cannot be made in the neonatal period.

INVESTIGATIONS

In all infants with significant weakness or hypotonia the following investigations should be performed:
1 creatinine phosphokinase (CPK). This is often high in the first week of life in normal children. Blood for CPK should only be taken after 2 weeks of life for high levels to be significant;
2 electromyography;
3 motor nerve conduction velocities;
4 muscle biopsy only if the pathology department has adequate facilities for sophisticated histochemical staining techniques.

PROGNOSIS

This depends on the underlying cause of the hypotonia. In many cases the prognosis is poor and for this reason establishing a reliable histological diagnosis is very important.

REFERENCES

Gupta, J.K., Bryce, F.C. & Lilford, R.J. (1995) Assessment and management of fetal ventri-culomegaly and other associated congenital abnormalities. In: *Fetal and Neonatal Neurology and Neurosurgery* (senior eds, M.I. Levene, R.J. Lilford; associated eds, M.J. Bennett, J. Punt), pp. 215–230. Churchill Livingstone, Edinburgh.

Heckmatt, J. & Dubowitz, V. (1995) Neuromuscular disorders. In: *Fetal and Neonatal Neurology and Neurosurgery* (senior eds, M.I. Levene, R.J. Lilford; associated eds, M.J. Bennett, J. Punt), pp. 623–641. Churchill Livingstone, Edinburgh.

International PHVD Drug Trial Group (1998) International randomised controlled trial of acetazolamide and furosemide in posthaemorrhagic ventricular dilatation in infancy. *Lancet* **352**, 433–440.

Kaiser, A. & Whitelaw, A. (1985) Cerebrospinal fluid pressure in infants with post-haemorrhagic ventricular dilatation. *Archives of Disease in Childhood* **46**, 783–787.

Levene, M.I. (1986) *Current Reviews in Neonatal Neurology.* Churchill Livingstone, Edinburgh.

Lorber, J. (1971) Results of treatment of myelomeningocoele. *Developmental Medicine and Child Neurology* **13**, 279–289.

Ventriculomegaly Study Group (1990) Randomised trial of early tapping in neonatal posthaemorrhagic ventricular dilatation. *Archives of Disease in Childhood* **65**, 3–10.

Wraith, J.E. (1995) Inborn errors of metabolism—postnatal diagnosis and management. In: *Fetal and Neonatal Neurology and Neurosurgery* (senior eds, M.I. Levene, R.J. Lilford; associated eds, M.J. Bennett, J. Punt), pp. 511–524. Churchill Livingstone, Edinburgh.

FURTHER READING

Chasnoff, I.J. (1991) Chemical dependency and pregnancy. *Clinics in Perinatology* 18(1). W.B. Saunders, Philadelphia.

Levene, M.I., Williams, J.L. & Fawer, C-L. (1984) *Ultrasound of the Infant Brain.* Spastics International Medical Publications. Lavenham Press, Suffolk.

Levene, M.I., Lilford, R.J., Bennett M.J. & Punt, J. (1995) *Fetal and Neonatal Neurology and Neurosurgery.* Churchill Livingstone, Edinburgh.

Volpe, J.J. (1994) *Neurology of the Newborn*, 3rd edn. W.B. Saunders, Philadelphia.

20 The special senses: hearing and vision

Profound hearing and visual impairments are major causes of severe disability arising from the neonatal period. Assessment of both hearing and vision in high-risk infants is usually possible before the child leaves the neonatal unit, and early diagnosis is essential for optimal management.

HEARING

Hearing impairment takes one of the following forms:

1 *conductive*. This involves abnormalities of the external auditory meatus, the tympanic membrane or the ossicles within the middle ear. This can rarely be congenital if the meatus has not yet canalized, but much more commonly it is due to infection or serous exudate within the middle ear;

2 *sensorineural*. Abnormalities or damage to the cochlea or brainstem nuclei cause 'nerve' deafness. These conditions are considered below;

3 *mixed*. Not uncommonly children with sensorineural deafness may also develop infection, which may further impair hearing as a result of conductive loss.

Incidence

Deafness remains a common cause of disability, with approximately 2–3/1000 children requiring hearing aids and a considerably larger number having a permanent mild bilateral impairment or significant unilateral deafness.

The prevalence of deafness in the UK is 1/1000 children, and moderate or severe hearing loss is due to sensorineural causes in almost 90% of deaf children. Deafness is, however, much more common in infants who have received intensive care, and studies on this high-risk group report an incidence of moderate or severe hearing impairment of the order of 30/1000, a marked increase compared to the general population.

Although conductive deafness is an uncommon cause of permanent hearing loss, it is a common condition. In a study of infants receiving intensive care, 25% were found to have evidence of otitis media while on the neonatal unit (Berman *et al*. 1978). In many of these infants there were clear signs of systemic sepsis, but middle ear disease was never considered as the cause. Babies intubated and receiving ventilatory support are most at risk of otitis media. If this condition is recognized and adequately treated, it is unlikely to lead to long-term hearing impairment.

Aetiology

There are a large number of causes of sensorineural hearing loss affecting the newborn. The most important are detailed below.

GENETIC CAUSES

With the reduction in incidence of rubella embryopathy, genetically determined conditions are now the commonest cause of sensorineural deafness in the Western world. These are usually inherited as autosomal recessive conditions. Hearing impairment due to genetic causes can be divided into those where hearing loss is part of a recognized syndrome, and non-syndromic.

Syndromic

1 Pendred syndrome: goitre and deafness.
2 Waardenburg syndrome: white forelock, different-coloured eyes and deafness.
3 Usher syndrome: retinitis pigmentosa and deafness.

Non-syndromic

Genetic deafness is the commonest cause of sensorineural hearing loss. It is often late in onset and is frequently progressive. The age of onset of hearing loss is not useful in distinguishing environmental from genetic loss.

CONGENITAL INFECTION

A variety of prenatally acquired viruses can cause permanent deafness.

Rubella

The full-blown syndrome (now very rarely seen) includes microcephaly and cataracts in addition to deafness, but hearing impairment may be the only abnormality. Active infection may continue well after birth and deafness inapparent in the newborn period may develop later in childhood.

Cytomegalovirus

In infants with evidence of cytomegalovirus (CMV) infection at birth 30% will have hearing impairment (Pass *et al.* 1980), and in those with asymptomatic infection almost 20% will subsequently develop hearing loss.

BILIRUBIN TOXICITY

Sensorineural deafness is part of the clinical spectrum of kernicterus, which includes mental retardation, choreoathetosis and failure of upward gaze. It is due to the penetration of unconjugated bilirubin into the brain, with staining and damage to the basal ganglia. Deafness may be the only neurological manifestation. The sicker the infant, the more likely he is to develop kernicterus. This is presumably because penetration into the brain of unconjugated bilirubin is more likely to occur in sick immature infants. There is evidence (although not conclusive) that it is the free (non-protein-bound) bilirubin that causes the neural toxicity. It has been suggested that damage to the blood–brain barrier allows the entry of

bilirubin into the brain, thereby predisposing the infant to deafness.

Unfortunately, there are no adequate guidelines as to what levels of bilirubin are dangerous. It is clear that the sick premature infant is more liable to this complication, and treatment should be commenced earlier in this group than in more mature babies. de Vries *et al.* (1985) suggested that sensorineural hearing loss only occurred in very low birthweight (VLBW) infants whose total serum bilirubin exceeded 240 µmol/L (14 mg/dL). The recommended charts for the treatment of hyperbilirubinaemia are shown on p. 140.

DRUGS

Aminoglycoside antibiotics (gentamicin, amikacin, netilmicin, tobramycin and kanamycin) are potentially ototoxic but the risk of deafness in neonates treated with these drugs is probably overestimated. Provided that the appropriate dosages and intervals between doses are used together with measurements of trough and peak drug levels, these drugs are unlikely to contribute significantly to the numbers of deaf neonates. Peak serum levels (1 h after drug administration) and trough levels (immediately before the next dose) are used to calculate the drug regimen. High peak levels indicate too high a dosage, and high troughs indicate that the interval between dosages should be lengthened. Recent studies have suggested that combined use of aminoglycosides and frusemide increases the risk of sensorineural hearing loss in LBW infants.

INCUBATOR NOISE

It has been suggested that noisy incubators are an important cause of neonatal deafness, but there are few data to support this in the present era of relatively quiet incubators. Unnecessary environmental noise should always be avoided in the neonatal nursery.

HYPOXIA

It is extremely difficult to evaluate the importance

Table 20.1 Indications for routine auditory assessment

Family history of hearing impairment

Congenital perinatal infection, particularly rubella, CMV, syphilis

Anatomical malformations:
  Cleft palate
  Ear anomalies
  Syndromes (e.g. Down, Treacher–Collins')

Hyperbilirubinaemia:
  > 340 µmol/L for full term infants
  > 240 µmol/L for infants < 1500 g

Bacterial meningitis

Severe perinatal asphyxia

High aminoglycoside serum levels

---

of hypoxia as an independent variable in causing neonatal deafness. Hypoxia usually indicates that an infant is sick, and there is little evidence that auditory pathways are more sensitive than other areas of the brain to hypoxia.

Diagnosis

The importance of early diagnosis in hearing-impaired children is obvious, as appropriate sound amplification and the provision of skilled educational facilities will enable the deaf child to realize his maximal potential. Speech in children is much better if hearing aids are fitted in the first 6 months of life. Table 20.1 lists the indications for auditory assessment in the neonatal period.

There are approximately 840 children a year in the UK born with significant permanent hearing impairment and at present the currently available screening (mainly Health Visitor Distraction Testing) misses about 400 of these (Davis *et al.* 1997). It has been suggested that neonatal screening is likely to have a considerably higher diagnostic yield and would have a lower cost per case diagnosed.

There are a number of different neonatal screening tests available.

1 *Behavioural responses.* These cradle-like devices detect an infant's behavioural response to a 70–80 dB sound delivered via an earphone.

The cradle monitors the baby's gross motor responses to the stimuli and gives a pass or fail after a number of stimuli.

2 *Auditory brainstem responses (ABRs).* This technique measures evoked electrical signals detected by surface electrodes from within the hearing pathways of the brain in response to sounds at predetermined frequencies. This technology was initially cumbersome and required considerable expertise in analysis, but more recently automated screening devices have been developed and have been shown to have a very high sensitivity (98%) and specificity (96%).

3 *Otoacoustic emissions (OAEs).* This technology detects the physiological response from the cochlea in response to a wide-band click stimulus. The normal ear will produce transient evoked OAEs and these are not apparent in babies with cochlear abnormalities. This method is also computerized and has been assessed for mass screening, with good results.

Strategy for screening

Two strategies suggest themselves for screening neonatal populations: mass screening of all babies and targeted screening for at-risk babies. Table 20.1 lists the indications for auditory assessment in at-risk babies in the neonatal period.

In Britain mass screening is very limited in its availability, but studies have shown that screening by OAE reaches 90% of babies born in a district, although it is less specific when done in the first 24 h of life. This method was, however, significantly better than the Health Visitor Distraction Testing in detecting children with severe hearing impairment. The auditory response cradle (ARC) has also been shown to be a good screening test for large unselected populations (Davis *et al.* 1997).

There are logistical difficulties in attempting to test all babies born as increasingly babies are discharged home with their mothers within hours of birth. For this reason, targeting a high-risk population only for hearing screening has been attempted. Most studies attempt to assess the hearing of all babies discharged from a neonatal intensive care or special care baby unit, and some also test those with a family history of hearing impairment. Studies utilizing this strategy have shown that ARC screening is less effective than OAE or ABR, and that both the latter have a potential yield of about 60% in all cases of moderate to severe hearing impairment.

The median age of identification of deafness using neonatal screening (either mass or targeted) is 2 months, compared to 12–20 months when Health Visitor Distraction Testing is the only form of screening. It is clear that neonatal screening is likely to be a valuable innovation in neonatal medicine.

VISION

Retinopathy of prematurity

Retinopathy of prematurity (ROP), formerly known as retrolental fibroplasia, is a relatively common condition affecting the most immature infants. Studies in the 1950s proved a direct association between oxygen dosage and the development of retinal abnormalities. The controlled use of oxygen reduced the incidence of this condition in mature neonates. More recently, it has been noted that the relationship between oxygen and ROP is more complex than was originally thought, particularly in preterm babies. Some infants develop ROP despite never having received supplemental oxygen, and others sustain high levels of oxygen without developing retinal changes.

INCIDENCE

The reported incidence of acute ROP derived from high-risk infants born in the 1980s varies from 2.8% to 42%. These figures must be analysed with caution, as inevitably patient selection occurs in larger centres and methods for diagnosis differ. Phelps estimated in 1979 (Phelps 1981) that 1.5% of VLBW infants born in the USA will become blind as a result of ROP. The incidence increases with decreasing birthweight. Phelps estimated an incidence of

5–11% in infants below 1.0 kg and 0.3–1.1% in infants with birthweight 1–1.5 kg. In Australia Yu et al. (1982) reported an incidence of 13.3% for ROP developing in infants admitted to a neonatal intensive care unit.

The incidence of ROP in the UK has been investigated in a geographically based cohort of infants weighing 1700 g and below (Ng et al. 1988). Of these, 50% developed ROP of some degree, but severe forms occurred in less than 5% of cases. The incidence is almost 90% in babies of < 1000 g. Approximately 70–80% of infants with acute proliferative ROP show complete regression of the retinal changes, but it is the remaining 20–30% that fail to do so who are most at risk of visual handicap.

RISK FACTORS

Immaturity

This is the most consistently recognized risk factor. The more immature the infant the more likely he or she is to develop ROP.

Oxygen

The risk of ROP developing is in general related to both oxygen concentration and the duration of oxygen therapy. Respiratory complications such as respiratory distress syndrome (RDS), pneumothorax, chronic lung disease and patent ductus arteriosus, which are all related to the development of ROP, probably just reflect the severity of the lung disease and therefore the oxygen exposure. In very immature infants oxygen is probably not the major aetiological factor.

Blood transfusions

Top-up transfusions with adult blood cause a shift in the oxygen dissociation curve (see p. 115), so that more oxygen is given up for a particular Pao_2, thus exposing the retina to higher oxygen levels. Recently, it has been suggested that Fe^{2+} in the transfused blood generates oxygen free radicals, which predisposes to ROP.

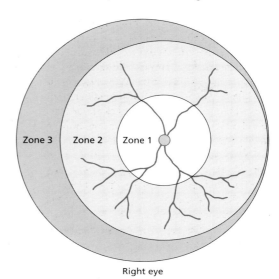

Right eye

Fig. 20.1 The three zones shown on the right retinal field.

DIAGNOSIS

The diagnosis of ROP is made clinically by means of indirect ophthalmoscopy after prior pupillary dilatation with 0.5% cyclopentalate eyedrops. The examination is best performed by a paediatric ophthalmologist, as considerable expertise is required, particularly for the diagnosis of less severe forms of retinopathy. The most recent international classification of the staging of ROP is as follows (Anonymous 1984):

stage 1 (demarcation line). A thin white line of demarcation in the periphery of the retina separating the avascular retina anteriorly from the vascularized retina posteriorly;

stage 2 (ridge). The line is more extensive and forms a ridge;

stage 3 (proliferation). Vascular proliferation immediately posterior to the ridge;

stage 4. Retinal detachment—subtotal;

stage 5. Retinal detachment—total.

Stages 1 and 2 usually regress completely to normal and it is only stage 3 that may require treatment.

'Plus' disease

'Plus' is added to any stage of ROP if the following signs of activity are seen:

1 tortuosity and engorgement of retinal vessels;
2 vascular engorgement and rigidity of the iris;
3 vitreous haze;
4 pupil rigidity.

Location by zone

The location of ROP is described by the zone involved (Fig. 20.1). The zones are centred on the optic disc.

Zone 1. Extends from the optic disc to twice the disc–foveal distance.

Zone 2. From the periphery of the nasal retina in a circle around the anatomical equator.

Zone 3. This is anterior to zone 2 and is present temporally, inferiorly and superiorly, but not in the nasal retina.

ONSET OF ROP

ROP only affects the immature retina and does not occur once the retina is fully vascularized. It develops between 30 and 45 weeks of postmenstrual age (PMA = gestational age + postnatal age). There is therefore little point in screening for this condition before the baby reaches a PMA of 30–32 weeks. If the retina is normal at 40 weeks' PMA, then the baby is safe from developing ROP.

PREVENTION

1 *Monitoring of oxygen in sick newborn infants.* The Po_2 of such infants should be maintained at 6–8 kPa (45–60 mmHg).
2 *Vitamin E.* It has been shown that early supplementation with vitamin E reduces the severity and incidence of ROP (Hittner & Kretzer 1985). Some neonatal units have a policy routinely to supplement babies of birthweight < 1500 g with 100 mg/kg/day of α-tocopherol.

SCREENING FOR ROP

There is now effective treatment for severe acute ROP and screening is a necessary clinical procedure in all at-risk infants. The aim of screening is to detect severe ROP (stage 3 disease). The following screening guidelines are recommended by the Royal College of Ophthalmologists and the British Association of Perinatal Medicine (Joint Working Party on Retinopathy of Prematurity 1995):
1 all infants ≤ 1500 g birthweight or ≤ 31 weeks' gestational age;
2 the first examination should be between 6 and 7 weeks' postnatal age;
3 examinations should be undertaken every 2 weeks;
4 if stage 1 or 2 disease is present, regular examinations are necessary until the process of resolution is well under way. In those with no evidence of ROP, screening may cease once the vessels have entered zone 3;
5 signs of 'plus' disease are ominous.

TREATMENT OF ACUTE ROP

The Multicentre Trial of Cryotherapy for ROP (Cryotherapy for ROP Cooperative Group 1988) has shown that cryotherapy saves vision in infants with severe disease. Therapy should be started within days of the identification of threshold disease, and although both cryotherapy and laser therapy have been shown to be effective there is no good evidence that one is better than the other. Treatment should be confined to centres with special expertise in their use.

Cataracts

Cataracts account for blindness in 20% of children with severe visual handicap. The causes of cataracts seen in the neonatal period include:
1 congenital rubella syndrome (see p. 65);
2 other prenatal viral infections (CMV and toxoplasma) less commonly;
3 prematurity: cataracts may be due to trauma rather than prematurity *per se*, and are usually transient requiring no treatment;
4 galactosaemia (see p. 183);
5 hypocalcaemia;
6 Lowe syndrome (oculocerebrorenal syndrome): an X-linked condition;
7 Down syndrome: 5–10% of these children have cataracts at birth;
8 inherited: usually as an autosomal dominant condition;
9 idiopathic: accounts for up to 50% of cases.

DIAGNOSIS

Cataracts should always be looked for at the routine neonatal examination. Normally, on shining a light directly into the infant's eye, a red reflex is seen. If a white reflection is seen, then this is suggestive of a cataract, although retinoblastoma will give a similar appearance. If there is any doubt, careful ophthalmic examination should be performed under anaesthetic by an experienced person.

TREATMENT

Urgent referral to an ophthalmologist is essential. Unless most of the pupil is occluded by the cataract, it can be left and observed. If surgical treatment is necessary, the lens is removed and contact lenses are placed.

Glaucoma (buphthalmos)

Congenital glaucoma occurs in 1/10 000 births and is usually bilateral. It may be a familial condition. The eye appears large (buphthalmos) in only one-quarter of infants with congenital glaucoma. The commonest presentation is the observation of a cloudy cornea. The treatment is surgical.

REFERENCES

Anonymous (1984) An international classification of retinopathy of prematurity. *British Journal of Ophthalmology* **68**, 690–697.

Berman, S.A., Balkany, T. & Simmons, M. (1978) Otitis media in the neonatal intensive care unit. *Pediatrics* **62**, 198–203.

Cryotherapy for ROP Cooperative Group (1988) Multicentre trial of cryotherapy for retinopathy of prematurity results. *Archives of Ophthalmology* **106**, 471–479.

Davis, A., Bamford, J., Wilson, I. *et al.* (1997) A critical review of the role of neonatal hearing screening in the detection of congenital hearing impairment. *Health Technology Assessment* **1**, 10.

Hittner, H. & Kretzer, F. (1985) Retinopathy of prematurity. Pathogenesis, prevention and treatment. In: *Recent Advances in Perinatal Medicine*, Vol. 2, (ed. M.L. Chiswick), pp. 145–163. Churchill Livingstone, Edinburgh.

Joint Working Party on Retinopathy of Prematurity (1995) *Guidelines for Screening and Treatment.* The Royal College of Ophthalmologists and the British Association of Perinatal Medicine.

Ng, Y.K., Fielder, A.R., Shaw, D.E. & Levene, M.I. (1988) Epidemiology of retinopathy of prematurity. *Lancet* **ii**, 1235–1238.

Pass, R.F., Stagno, S. & Myers, G.J. (1980) Outcome of symptomatic congenital CMV infection. Results of a long-term longitudinal follow-up. *Pediatrics* **66**, 758–762.

Phelps, D.L. (1981) Retinopathy of prematurity. An estimate of vision loss in the United States. *Pediatrics* **67**, 924–926.

de Vries, L.S., Lary, S. & Dubowitz, L.M.S. (1985) Relationship of serum bilirubin levels to ototoxicity and deafness in high risk low birth weight infants. *Pediatrics* **76**, 351–354.

Yu, V.Y.H., Hookham, D.M. & Nave, J.R.M. (1982) Retrolental fibroplasia—controlled study of four years' experience in a neonatal intensive care unit. *Archives of Disease in Childhood* **57**, 247–252.

21 Congenital postural deformities and abnormalities of the extremities

It is convenient to discuss these conditions together. In some cases there may be an obvious cause for the deformity, such as posture in the uterus, but in others there may be a mixed aetiology, including chromosomal abnormalities and genetic factors. Sometimes no obvious cause can be found. It is not unusual for an infant to show several postural abnormalities, for example facial asymmetry, talipes and congenital dislocation of the hip. For predisposing factors see Chapter 14.

ABNORMALITIES OF THE EXTREMITIES

Malformations of digits

These are common and frequently inherited as autosomal dominant disorders. They are usually symmetrical.
1 Syndactyly: fusion of the fingers or toes.
2 Polydactyly: extra digit.
3 Ectrodactyly: 'lobster claw' deformity.

Limb malformations

These may be symmetrical but occasionally affect only one joint.

1 Amelia: absence of a limb or limbs.
2 Ectromelia: gross hypoplasia or aplasia of one or more limbs.
3 Phocomelia: partial deficiency of the proximal segment with preservation of distal parts ('seal-like' limbs).
4 Hemimelia (reduction malformation): rudimentary formation of the distal part of a limb with normal development of the proximal part.
5 Amputations *in utero*: thought to be due to amniotic bands.

MANAGEMENT

Orthopaedic or plastic surgery will be necessary to achieve maximal function and acceptable cosmetic appearance.

Abnormalities of the lower limbs

These are common and may vary from a mild postural problem to more marked intrauterine compression leading to talipes calcaneovalgus or equinovarus. These may be severe and there may be associated muscle wasting. These abnormalities are illustrated in Fig. 21.1.

Talipes equinovarus (clubfoot) occurs in

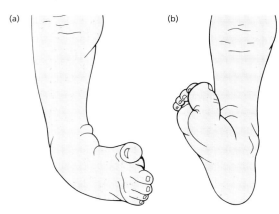

(a) (b)

Fig. 21.1 Talipes: talipes equinovarus (a) and talipes calcaneovalgus (b).

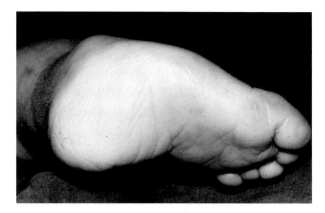

Fig. 21.2 Metatarsus varus.

1/1000 births and is 10 times more common than severe calcaneovalgus. Minor degrees of postural calcaneovalgus deformity are common. When either of these conditions is seen, other associated congenital abnormalities should be sought (e.g. dislocation of the hip and myelomeningocoele).

Metatarsus varus is a common disorder affecting the feet (Fig. 21.2). It may be present as an isolated finding or seen in conjunction with talipes.

MANAGEMENT

If the foot can be passively corrected to the position opposite the deformity, it is considered to be mild. Mild positional deformities will require simple passive exercise treatment by a physiotherapist and the parents. More severe deformities will require explanation, physiotherapy, splinting, and possibly surgical correction under orthopaedic supervision.

The parents of children with metatarsus varus should be strongly reassured that the disorder is usually self-correcting.

Genu recurvatum

This is a rare disorder in which the knees are hyperextensible. In severe cases there may be dislocation of the knee joint, and splinting may be necessary.

Femoral retroversion

This is a common condition seen at the follow-up examination of infants leaving the neonatal unit. The child lies or stands with his legs externally rotated at 90° ('Charlie Chaplin' gait). There is little or no internal rotation when in extension, but good external rotation. This condition often causes distress to the parents but they should be strongly reassured as it rapidly corrects within a year of the child learning to walk. It is, however, important to exclude congenital dislocation of the hip as the cause of the external rotation.

CONGENITAL DISLOCATION OF THE HIP

Congenital dislocation of the hip (CDH) is an important asymptomatic neonatal congenital condition that should be detectable during the routine screening examination at birth. Examination of the hip should start with observation for signs of established dislocation, such as unequal leg length and asymmetry of the thighs. The physical examination should be undertaken in two parts.

Ortolani's (reduction) test

This test assesses whether the hip is already dislocated. With the baby relaxed on a firm

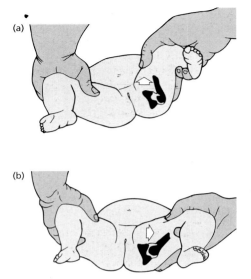

Fig. 21.3 Ortolani's test. The hip cannot be abducted because of posterior dislocation of the femoral head. The hip is pulled upwards (a) and the head clunks into the acetabulum, permitting abduction (b).

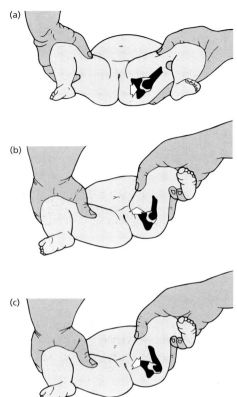

Fig. 21.4 Barlow's test. The hip is abducted to establish that it is not dislocated (a). The adducted hip is then pulled upwards (b) and the femoral head pushed downwards and laterally to see whether it is dislocatable (c).

surface the hips and knees are flexed to 90°. The examiner grasps the baby's thigh with the middle finger over the greater trochanter and lifts it to bring the femoral head from its dislocated posterior position to opposite the acetabulum. Simultaneously, the thigh is gently abducted, reducing the femoral head over the posterior lip of the acetabulum. In a positive finding the examiner senses reduction by feeling a 'clunk', and there is a movement forward of the head of the femur (Fig. 21.3).

Barlow's (dislocation) test

This test assesses whether the hip is dislocatable and is really a reversal of Ortolani's test. With one hand fixing the pelvis with the thumb anteriorly over the symphysis pubis and the other fingers posteriorly over the coccygeal region, the other hand grasps the baby's thigh and adducts it gently downwards. Dislocation is palpable as the femoral head slips over the posterior lip of the acetabulum (Fig. 21.4).

It is known that infants may have normal hips at birth which may subsequently dislocate some time later. For this reason, the hips should be examined at a 6-week assessment. Failure to abduct a hip is a very significant sign. Shortening of the leg, and asymmetric skin creases in the newborn period, may not be reliable clinical signs of a dislocated hip.

Aetiology

Hip dislocation diagnosed in the neonatal period was reported to occur in 19/1000 births (Dunn *et al.* 1985). The left hip is dislocated four times more commonly than the right, and this is due to the fetal position causing the left hip to be more adducted than the right. The following associations are described with CDH:

1 *polygenic or multifactorial condition*. This condition recurs in families at a rate of about 1/30;

2 *presentation*. Breech/vertex ratio 10 : 1. The incidence of CDH in singleton breech deliveries is 14% (Dunn *et al*. 1985);

3 *sex*. Female/male ratio 6 : 1;

4 *race*. Incidence increased in some countries (Italy) and reduced in others (China);

5 *abnormalities producing muscular imbalance around the joint*, e.g. spina bifida, hypertonia, congenital hypotonia, arthrogryposis congenita multiplex;

6 *syndromes*: e.g. trisomy 13, trisomy 18;

7 *multiple congenital abnormalities*.

Terminology

A variety of terms are used to describe abnormal hips. At the newborn examination the hips are carefully examined using both the Ortolani and the Barlow manoeuvres. The hips are then described as follows.

Stable. There is no abnormal movement of the joint.

Clicking. The hips are stable but a click is heard or felt during examination. This is probably normal if there is no excessive movement of the femoral head in the joint. Some paediatricians recommend that the hip should be examined again at 6 weeks of age. Clicking occurs as a result of ligamentous laxity and is found in up to 10% of newborn infants.

Dislocatable joint. The femoral head is in the joint (the hip can be fully abducted), but when Barlow's test is attempted on adduction the hip dislocates posteriorly.

Dislocated joint. The hip is out of joint at birth and cannot be abducted. It is detected on Ortolani's test.

Imaging

Ultrasound is the best method for imaging the hips. There is no place for X-ray examination for the assessment of hip dislocation until ossification occurs in the femoral epiphysis at about 3–4 months of age.

Ultrasound clearly defines the hip anatomy and allows evaluation of the shape of the acetabulum. In some centres routine ultrasound examination of the hips of all babies has been recommended, but this is expensive and probably unnecessary. Ultrasound examination of the hips is indicated in the following cases:

1 clinical instability;

2 family history of unstable hips;

3 associated lower limb abnormality.

Management

There are many ways to treat this condition in the newborn period. The principle is to keep the hip immobilized in an abducted position for 2–3 months to allow the acetabular rim to develop and the hip ligaments to strengthen. Several varieties of splint are used, including the Aberdeen, the Von Rosen and the Pavlik Harness. There is no place for treatment with 'double nappies'. After 3 months the splint may be removed and, if the hip is clinically stable, check X-rays are taken usually at 6 and 12 months of age. Fixed dislocations of the hip, failure to respond to treatment and late-diagnosed dislocated hips will require individual orthopaedic consideration.

SCOLIOSIS

Severe curvature of the spine (scoliosis) is usually due to vertebral defects, whereas milder cases may be caused by abnormal posture in the uterus.

Management will depend on the severity and cause, and orthopaedic consultation with regular follow-up is necessary.

MANDIBULAR ASYMMETRY, TORTICOLLIS, PLAGIOCEPHALY

These deformities may be due to abnormal posture of the fetus in the uterus. They usually correct either spontaneously during the first year of life or with the assistance of physiotherapy. Torticollis may also be associated with a sternomastoid tumour (see Chapter 15).

ARTHROGRYPOSIS MULTIPLEX

This term describes multiple joint deformities involving more than one limb (Fig. 21.5). It is caused by restriction of joint movement *in utero* and there may be a variety of underlying causes:
1 neuromuscular—congenital dystrophy, spinal muscular atrophy;
2 oligohydramnios;
3 bicornuate uterus.

All infants with this disorder require orthopaedic referral and vigorous physiotherapy. An underlying neuromuscular problem should be considered and creatinine phosphokinase levels measured. Other investigations are described in Chapter 19.

NEONATAL DWARFISM

Dwarfism may be classified as either primordial or chondrodystrophic.

Primordial

This generic term is used to cover a wide variety of different syndromes associated with dwarfism and which have a variety of characteristic features, including mental retardation. These children are severely growth retarded at birth (intrinsic group) but there is no selective shortening of the limbs. Examples of these dwarf syndromes include Russel–Silver, Cornelia de Lange, Conradi, Seckel's bird head, Cockayne, leprechaunism and progeria.

Chondrodystrophic (skeletal dysplasia)

An underlying skeletal dysplasia should be sus-

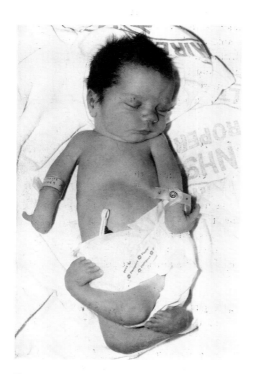

Fig. 21.5 Arthrogryposis multiplex.

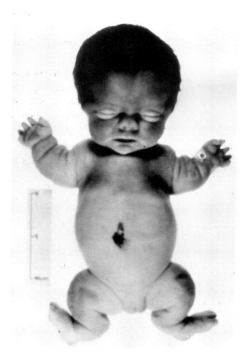

Fig. 21.6 Thanatophoric dwarf.

pected in any baby who is small for gestational age with other congenital abnormalities and who has disproportionate shortening of the limbs and trunk.

Skeletal dysplasias may present simply as short stature or disproportionate body habitus, but a variety of other anomalies, such as hydrocephalus, craniostenosis, cleft lip and palate, polydactyly, syndactyly, dislocated hips and dysmorphic facial features, may coexist.

There are many classifications of the more than 100 distinct syndromes. The most commonly recognized syndromes in the newborn are:

1 achondroplasia;
2 osteogenesis imperfecta: types I–V;
3 asphyxiating thoracic dystrophy;
4 thanatophoric dwarf (Fig. 21.6);
5 osteopetrosis (marble bone disease);
6 diastrophic dwarf;
7 Ellis–van Creveld syndrome.

REFERENCES

Dunn, P.M., Evans, R.E., Thearle, M.J., Griffiths, H. & Witherow, P.J. (1985) Congenital dislocation of the hip: early and late diagnosis and management compared. *Archives of Disease in Childhood* 60, 407–414.

FURTHER READING

Graham, J.M. (ed.) (1988) *Smith's Recognizable Patterns of Human Deformation: Identification and Management of Mechanical Effects on Morphogenesis*, 2nd edn. W.B. Saunders, Philadelphia.

Hutson, J.M., Beasley, S.W. & Woodward, A.A. (eds) (1992) *Jones' Clinical Paediatric Surgery: Diagnosis and Management*, 4th edn. Blackwell Scientific Publications, Melbourne.

Jones, K.L. (1997) *Smith's Recognizable Patterns of Human Malformation*, 5th edn. W.B. Saunders, Philadelphia.

22 Renal disorders in the newborn

The fetus does not depend on the kidney to excrete waste products as the placenta performs this function. The fetal kidney does, however, produce very dilute urine, and this is the major contribution to the volume of amniotic fluid. An absence of fetal urine as a result of severe renal impairment is usually associated with severe lung hypoplasia (see below).

Renal function in the newborn depends on both gestational and postnatal age. Renal function rapidly matures within the first week after birth.

Glomerular filtration rate

The newborn infant has a very low glomerular filtration rate (GFR) compared to the older child. This is partly related to a relatively fewer number of nephrons. For this reason, the neonate cannot excrete a water load as well as older children. After 34 weeks of gestation and in response to birth there is a marked increase in GFR. The measurement of serum creatinine is the most convenient index of GFR in immature infants, but plasma urea is unreliable as it increases with catabolism even in the presence of normal renal function. The normal limits of creatinine are shown in Table 22.3 (see p. 254).

Tubular function

The concentrating ability of the developing kidney increases throughout gestation and improves rapidly after birth. This is due partly to elongation of the collecting tubes and partly to a hormonal effect (see below).

Tubular function can most easily be assessed by measuring the fractional excretion of sodium (FES):

$$FES = \frac{urine\ Na}{serum\ Na} \times \frac{serum\ creatinine}{urine\ creatinine} \times 100$$

In the newborn FES_{Na} should be $< 2.5\%$.

Sodium conservation

The fetus has a very poor ability to conserve (reabsorb) sodium. The stress of birth rapidly matures the tubules' ability to conserve sodium, and this is related to the renin–aldosterone response. Sodium conservation is closely related to gestational age as well as postnatal age. All babies born < 30 weeks of gestation have a negative sodium balance when fed standard formulas, but this improves with increasing gestational age.

Hormonal function

The kidney is influenced by a variety of hormones.
1 *Antidiuretic hormone (ADH)*. This increases water reabsorption from the collecting ducts. It is present from early in fetal life but the fetal kidney is relatively insensitive to it. After birth the collecting ducts become more sensitive and ADH is active in very premature infants, and even the most immature infant is capable of concentrating the urine to a remarkable extent within days of birth.
2 *Renin–aldosterone*. Renin levels are higher in newborn infants than in adults and increase in response to sodium loss. However, the adrenal does not respond with high aldosterone levels and consequently sodium retention is poor, but matures in response to birth.

Presentation of renal disease

Genitourinary disease in the newborn may present in a number of different ways. These are discussed separately.

1 Potter syndrome.
2 Obstructive uropathy.
3 Acute renal failure.
4 Infection.
5 Renal mass.
6 Haematuria.
7 Congenital abnormalities.

POTTER SYNDROME

Potter syndrome refers to the association of dysmorphic clinical features and bilateral renal agenesis. The incidence of this condition is 1/4000 births, with a male predominance. Failure of renal development is associated with oligohydramnios and retardation of lung development. These infants usually have severe lung hypoplasia, which is incompatible with life. The oligohydramnios also gives rise to characteristic facial features, including a beaked nose, low-set abnormal ears, prominent epicanthic folds and an antimongolian slant to the eyes (Fig. 22.1). The fetal surface of the placenta often shows *amnion nodosum*, which is small white plaques of fibrinoid necrosis.

Facial features identical to those seen in Potter syndrome are seen in other causes of oligohydramnios due to urinary outflow obstruction, sometimes referred to as pseudo-Potter syndrome. In these cases large kidneys are usually palpable.

Infants with Potter syndrome are severely asphyxiated at birth and, although often resuscitated, die within several hours owing to their lung hypoplasia. Prenatal or postnatal ultrasound may be particularly helpful in assessing either kidney size or pathology, but large adrenals (common in this condition) may be confused with normal kidneys. After birth a

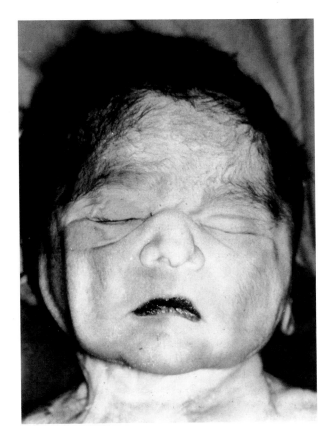

Fig. 22.1 Potter syndrome. Note the beaked nose as if the face has been pressed up against a windowpane, and the prominent epicanthic folds.

renal angiogram, performed by injecting contrast material through the umbilical arterial catheter, will display any renal tissue present. The syndrome is usually considered to be sporadic, but may be polygenic with a recurrent risk of unilateral or bilateral renal agenesis of approximately 1%.

OBSTRUCTIVE UROPATHY

Causes of urinary obstruction are listed in Table 22.1. These usually occur in males, but the commonest cause (pelviureteric junction obstruction) occurs equally in both males and females.

Clinical features

Infants may present with an abdominal mass (bladder and/or kidney) or dribbling urine. Oligohydramnios may have been reported by the obstetricians. If obstruction has been severe, the infant may be born with the facial appearances of Potter syndrome and lung hypoplasia. Prune-belly syndrome should be obvious from the wrinkled appearance of the abdomen. The penis should be examined carefully for a normal meatus. The spine should be inspected for meningomyelocoele.

Prune-belly syndrome (triad syndrome)

This occurs mainly in males. There is an absence of the musculature of the anterior abdominal wall, with bladder neck obstruction in 25%, dilatation of the ureters and unde-

Table 22.1 Causes of obstructive uropathy in the newborn

Posterior urethral valves
Urethral meatal stenosis in males
Neurogenic bladder
Ureterocoele
Prune-belly syndrome

scended testicles. It is probably due to degeneration of the abdominal musculature as a result of a distended bladder.

Treatment is directed towards draining the bladder and preventing infection. Cosmetic surgery for the abdominal wall deficiency may be necessary.

Posterior urethral valves

This condition occurs only in male infants and successful treatment depends on early diagnosis, which is often made on fetal ultrasound scanning. Urine dribbling from the penis is always an ominous sign and should alert the clinician to the presence of urethral valves. There is proximal obstruction of the urethra, owing to mucosal folds arising from the verumontanum producing a valve-like obstruction. This causes hypertrophy and dilatation of the urethra, bladder, ureters and kidneys.

On examination of the abdomen, a hard muscular bladder is felt arising from the pelvis. In addition, both kidneys are easily palpable.

Ultrasound will confirm the presence of a hypertrophied bladder and establish the degree of upper tract involvement. The bladder should be drained by a urethral or suprapubic catheter. A micturating cystourethrogram will confirm the diagnosis.

MANAGEMENT

If the lesion is mild, surgical resection of valve cusps through a cystoscope is all that is necessary. Antenatal diagnosis and the insertion of a vesicoamniotic catheter into the fetal bladder are indicated in highly selected cases of severe obstruction. If renal impairment has occurred, urinary drainage via bilateral cutaneous ureterostomies or vesicostomy will be necessary before resection of the valves.

Ureterocoele

This is a ballooning of the intravesical portion of the distal ureter into the bladder, which obstructs the drainage of the kidney on that side. Investigation is by ultrasound, cystogram or cystoscopy. The ureterocoele should be excised and the ureter reimplanted to avoid urinary reflux.

Pelviureteric junction obstruction

This is usually unilateral, but in 25% of cases is bilateral. It presents as a unilateral mass in the loin, which may become massive. If the kidney is grossly hydronephrotic with less than 20% function as shown by a functional MAG3 scan, then nephrectomy is the best treatment. In milder or bilateral cases plastic repair of the pelvi–ureteric junction may be all that is necessary.

ACUTE RENAL FAILURE

Acute renal failure may occur as the result of many disease processes, many of which are detected on antenatal ultrasound (Fig. 22.2); these can be divided into prerenal, renal and postrenal causes (Table 22.2). Prerenal failure is the commonest variety and usually occurs with severe respiratory disease or as a postoperative complication.

Clinical features

The baby develops oliguria (urine output < 1.0 mL/kg/h), a rising serum creatinine and blood urea, electrolyte disturbances in which

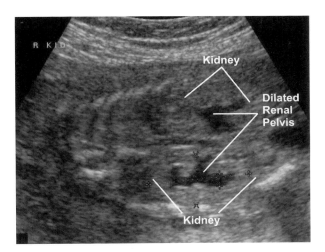

Fig. 22.2 Longitudinal ultrasound view of fetal abdomen showing bilateral renal pelvocalyceal dilatation. (Courtesy of Dr R. Cincotta.)

Table 22.2 Causes of renal failure in the neonate

Prerenal	Renal	Postrenal
Dehydration	Cystic disease	Obstructive uropathy (see Table 22.1)
Hypotension due to:	Acute tubular necrosis	
Haemorrhage	Cortical necrosis	
Infection	DIC	
Cardiac dysrhythmia	Infection (pyelonephritis)	
Asphyxia	Haemolysis	
Hypothermia	Venous thrombosis	
	Congenital nephrotic syndrome	
	Drugs (aminoglycosides)	

potassium and phosphate are increased, and the calcium and magnesium are often decreased. Metabolic acidosis commonly develops. Fluid retention with oedema commonly occurs, and cardiac dysrhythmias may develop as a result of hyperkalaemia.

Oliguria may be difficult to detect early in the infant's life as the passage of urine may have occurred unnoticed or may not have been recorded. Over 90% of normal infants pass urine in the first 24 h of life, and 98% have voided by 48 h from birth. If oliguria is suspected, then a urinary catheter will determine whether urine is present in the bladder and allow assessment of the volume. Abdominal ultrasound may also be useful in showing whether there is urine in the bladder.

In oliguric infants there may be difficulty in distinguishing prerenal from renal failure. FES_{Na} may be used in such cases. In prerenal failure the urine is concentrated and the serum and urinary creatinine measurements are high. If doubt still exists, an infusion of blood or plasma (20 mL/kg) with a dose of frusemide (3 mg/kg) should resolve the issue. Postrenal causes of acute renal failure must be excluded (see p. 252).

Pathological examination of the kidneys of infants dying with acute renal failure shows acute tubular necrosis, acute cortical necrosis or bilateral renal vein thrombosis. With renal vein thrombosis, loin masses are generally palpable and the baby has haematuria.

Creatinine

The most important index of renal function in the newborn is serum creatinine. The plasma urea is unreliable as it increases with catabolism even in the presence of normal renal function. The normal limits of creatinine are shown in Table 22.3.

Management

In established renal failure the following management regimen should be carried out under the direction of a nephrologist. The underlying cause should be treated wherever possible.

Table 22.3 Upper limit for normal serum creatinine levels (µmol/L) in neonates: the figure represents the 95th centile of normality for gestational age. (Reproduced from Rudd *et al.* 1983, with permission)

Gestational age (weeks)	Age of infant (days)				
	2	7	14	21	28
28	220	145	118	104	95
30	192	132	107	95	87
32	175	119	97	86	78
34	158	109	88	78	71
36	143	98	80	71	64
38	130	89	72	64	59
40	118	81	66	57	53

FLUID RESTRICTION

Water intake is necessary to replace insensible water loss as well as the urinary loss. These are calculated separately. Insensible loss depends on the infant's birthweight and gestational age. In the first week of life the following approximate figures apply:

< 1250 g   60 mL/kg/24 h;
1250–1750 g   30 mL/kg/24 h; and
> 1750 g   20 mL/kg/24 h.

For all infants over 1 week of age the insensible water loss is approximately 20 mL/kg. The volume of urine voided by the infant every 12 h should be added to the input over the next 12 h. Daily weighing is an accurate way of assessing fluid balance, and no change in weight is to be aimed for.

PROTEIN AND POTASSIUM RESTRICTION

Potassium should not be given unless the infant is hypokalaemic. To avoid endogenous protein breakdown, a high carbohydrate infusion (15% dextrose) should be given. The volume depends on the infant's output (see above).

CORRECTION OF ELECTROLYTE IMBALANCE

Hyponatraemia is usually due not to sodium

depletion but rather to fluid overhydration. Water should be restricted until this is corrected.

METABOLIC ACIDOSIS

Sodium bicarbonate is carefully administered if the pH falls below 7.25. Care is necessary to avoid hypernatraemia.

ANAEMIA

Fresh blood (10 mL/kg) is given if the haemoglobin falls below 8 g/dL.

These measures are usually sufficient to maintain homeostasis until renal function recovers.

Constant attention should be paid to life-threatening complications, including:
1 hyperkalaemia (> 7.5 mmol/L). Calcium resonium enemas should be given when hyperkalaemia occurs. Insulin and dextrose may also be necessary to drive potassium into the cells;
2 severe metabolic acidosis (pH < 7.20);
3 fluid overload with severe oedema and congestive cardiac failure;
4 hypertension, usually due to fluid overload;
5 severe uraemia with central nervous system (CNS) depression.

Under these circumstances peritoneal dialysis may be indicated (see p. 324).

INFECTION

The incidence of symptomatic urinary tract infection in the neonatal period is 1%. The symptoms of urinary tract infection in the newborn are generally non-specific, with jaundice, vomiting, failure to thrive, temperature instability, lethargy and poor feeding. Specific symptoms of dysuria, frequency and abdominal discomfort are rarely seen. Urinary tract infections in the newborn are more common in the male and may be bloodborne, ascending or secondary to an abnormality of the urinary tract. In the neonatal period pyelonephritis is usually due to bloodborne infection.

Urinary tract infection should be suspected in infants with non-specific symptoms. A 'clean voided' bag sample of urine is used only as a screen and is never the basis for a definitive diagnosis. If the bag sample suggests a urinary tract infection or if the baby is sick and in need of urgent treatment, either a 'clean catch', suprapubic aspiration (see p. 323) or a urinary catheter sample will be necessary. The following interpretations can be made on an adequately collected urine sample.

Microurine. A pus cell count of more than 30 000/mL suggests infection and a count of less than 10 000/mL is probably normal. Some normal newborn infants have up to 30 000 pus cells/mL, even on a bladder tap aspirate of urine. Pus cell counts in urine specimens from collecting bags are high and should be interpreted carefully, and only in conjunction with colony counts.

Culture. More than 100 000 organisms/mL indicates a significant infection, less than 10 000/mL or mixed organisms suggests contamination, and counts between 10 000 and 100 000/mL indicate that the urine sample should be repeated. If any growth of organisms is obtained on bladder tap, this is significant. The infecting organisms are usually coliform bacteria or rarely Gram-positive cocci.

Treatment

Antibiotics which are excreted in the urine should be started immediately in an infant with a strong clinical suspicion of urinary tract infection. This is particularly important in pyelonephritis. In the presence of severe or suspected infection, therapy is usually commenced with an intravenous aminoglycoside (e.g. gentamicin 5 mg/kg in two divided doses) and ampicillin (150–200 mg/kg in two divided doses). Once cultures and sensitivities are known, an inappropriate antibiotic may be deleted. Less severely affected infants may be treated with oral amoxycillin (50–100 mg/kg). Cotrimoxazole (Septrin 0.3 mL/kg) may be used after the first week of life. Other suitable antibiotics include cephalexin, ceftriaxone or cephotaxime. Treatment is continued for 10 days, when repeat microurine and culture are performed.

Routine diagnostic imaging for urinary tract infection remains controversial (Dick & Feldman 1996). Radiographic studies consisting of ultrasound examination together with a micturating cystourethrogram (MCU) are indicated in all neonates with urinary tract infection. A dimercaptosuccinic acid (DMSA) radionuclide scan may further delineate renal scarring or dysplasia and aids in assessing renal function; a diethylenetriaminepentaacetic acid (DTPA) renal scan followed by frusemide gives valuable information on the severity of the obstructive uropathy. Severe reflux may be associated with renal scarring even in the absence of infection. Specimens of urine should be regularly checked during the first year of life to ensure that reinfection does not occur.

RENAL MASS

Normal kidneys, especially the right, may be just palpable in the newborn infant. If a renal mass is easily felt, the kidney is probably pathologically enlarged. Differentiation of the mass can be achieved using ultrasound, computed tomography (CT) scanning or intravenous pyelography. The causes of a renal mass are listed in Table 22.4.

Cystic disease of the kidneys

There are a great variety of cystic conditions of the kidney in the newborn. Congenital renal cystic diseases are a genetically and clinically

Table 22.4 Causes of a renal mass in the newborn period

Hydronephrosis (bilateral)
Pelviureteric junction obstruction (unilateral)
Cystic disease of the kidneys
Renal vein thrombosis
Wilms' tumour (nephroblastoma)
Adrenal haemorrhage

diverse group of disorders with the common pathologic finding of diffuse bilateral cystic structures without dysplasia. Many hereditary malformation syndromes are associated with renal cysts. They may be classified as follows (Becker & Avner 1995).

1 *Polycystic kidney disease.* Linkage analysis and positional cloning have led to advances in the isolation of the genes and gene products responsible for these conditions.

(a) Autosomal dominant polycystic kidney disease (ADPKD). This is the commonest inherited renal disease, with an incidence of 1/200–1/1000. It was originally known as 'adult-onset PKD' because of the usual clinical presentation in the third to fifth decades, although the disease can manifest itself *in utero* or at any time thereafter. It may be diagnosed on perinatal ultrasound with the finding of enlarged or cystic kidneys. Clinically the disease can present along a spectrum, from the severe neonatal form with renal failure and Potter syndrome to the asymptomatic unilateral renal cyst found on renal ultrasound.

(b) Autosomal recessive polycystic kidney disease (ARPKD). Originally known as 'infantile PKD' because of its more common perinatal presentation, ARPKD can present at any time from *in utero* to adulthood. It is characterized by cystic dilatation of the renal collecting ducts and hepatic biliary dysgenesis with periportal fibrosis.

2 *Glomerular cystic kidney disease (GCKD).* Primary GCKD can be sporadic or inherited in an autosomal dominant pattern. It may present in the newborn with palpable enlarged cystic kidneys.

Cystic dysplasia of the kidneys

1 *Cystic dysplastic (multicystic) kidneys.* This is a sporadic condition producing a nonfunctioning kidney and may be unilateral. The kidney shows multiple large and small cysts. There is little or no renal function on the affected side and a unilateral cystic dysplastic kidney should be surgically excised in infancy. If bilateral, it is incompatible with life.

Table 22.5 Neonatal renal disorders associated with haematuria

Acute tubular necrosis
Infection
Renal vein thrombosis
Bleeding disorders
Cystic renal disease
Obstructive uropathy
Tumours

2 *Cysts secondary to obstruction.* This condition occurs as a result of obstruction to urinary outflow (e.g. posterior urethral valves).

HAEMATURIA

In the first few days of life the presence of red cells in the urine is not uncommon, but after this haematuria is an important finding and must be further investigated. Table 22.5 lists causes of haematuria. Investigations include urinalysis, clotting studies, creatinine, ultrasound examination and intravenous urography. Treatment depends on the underlying cause. Haematuria must be differentiated from the presence of urates in the urine, a benign condition which produces pink staining of the diaper.

CONGENITAL ABNORMALITIES

Hypospadias

In this condition the urethral meatus opens on to the undersurface of the glans penis, the penile shaft or the perineum. It is one of the most common abnormalities of male infants, with an incidence of 1/350 male births. It may be classified as glandular, penoglandular, penile, penoscrotal or perineal, depending on the site of the urethral opening. Frequently there is a dorsal hood to the penis and a ventral curvature of the glans (chordee). Chromosome studies are indicated with undescended testes and severe penoscrotal or perineal lesions. Epispadias refers to the urethra opening on the dorsal surface of the penis.

TREATMENT

The infant must not be circumcised, otherwise definitive surgical treatment will be made more difficult. Mild types are repaired in a one-stage procedure in the first 6 months, but severe types require several staged operations.

Ectopia vesicae (bladder exstrophy)

This is a complex disorder of the abdominal wall, bladder and pelvis. The mucosa of the bladder herniates through a deficient lower abdominal wall. There is a deficient pelvic floor and wide separation of the pubic symphysis. It is commoner in male than in female infants. In the male there is total epispadias, undescended testes and a deficient penis. In the female the two halves of the clitoris are separate and the vagina is duplicated.

The surgical management of this complex disorder is extremely difficult and continues over many years. Urinary continence is rarely achieved.

REFERENCES

Becker, N. & Avner, E.D. (1995) Congenital nephropathies and uropathies. *Pediatric Clinics of North America* **42**, 1319–1329.

Dick, P.T. & Feldman, W. (1996) Routine diagnostic imaging for childhood urinary tract infections: a systematic overview. *Journal of Pediatrics* **128**, 15–22.

Rudd, P.T., Hughes, E.A., Placzek, M.M. & Hodes, D.T. (1983) Reference ranges for plasma creatinine during the first months of life. *Archives of Disease in Childhood* **58**, 212–215.

FURTHER READING

Barrett, T.M., Avmer, E.D. & Harmon, W.C. (eds) (1998) *Pediatric Nephrology*, 4th edn. Williams & Wilkins, Baltimore.

Edelmann, C.M. (ed.) (1992) *Paediatric Kidney Disease*, 2nd edn. Little, Brown & Co., Boston.

Gilbert-Barness, E. (ed.) (1997) *Potter's Pathology of the Fetus and Infant*. 2 vols. Mosby, St Louis.

23 Gastrointestinal disorders

Development

The gastrointestinal tract develops 4 weeks after conception as a tube from mouth to cloaca. Part of the foregut differentiates into trachea and oesophagus, and disorders of development at this stage cause oesophageal atresia, usually with tracheo-oesophageal fistula. The lower bowel initially opens into the yolk sac and later forms the vitello-intestinal duct. The midgut forms a loop, which protrudes from the abdominal cavity and then re-enters the abdomen after turning through 270°. Failure of the bowel to re-enter the abdomen causes exomphalos, and failure to twist leads to malrotation. During the sixth week of gestation a septum separates the cloaca into rectum and urogenital sinus. The gut then ruptures through the perineum to form an anus. The liver and pancreas develop from the gut endoderm at the same time as the duodenum is formed. The gut is fully differentiated by 20 weeks.

Function

The bowel develops functionally as follows.

MOTILITY

Bowel motility is present from 16 weeks' gestation but is not fully functional until 36 weeks, and the passage of meconium *in utero* is rare under 34 weeks. Disorganized bowel motility in the last trimester makes functional intestinal obstruction or paralytic ileus not uncommon in premature infants.

SWALLOWING

In the second trimester the fetus begins to swallow, and hydramnios often occurs if the upper gastrointestinal tract is not patent by midpregnancy. Gastro-oesophageal reflux is common, especially in the preterm infant, because of low gastro-oesophageal sphincter pressures.

CARBOHYDRATE ABSORPTION

Disaccharidase activity in the small bowel is low at term and gradually increases to mature levels by 10 months of age. In the preterm baby maltase is the first disaccharidase to reach reasonable activity, followed by sucrase and then lactase. Lactase deficiency is common prior to 30 weeks' gestation, with consequent lactose intolerance in these infants.

FAT ABSORPTION

Bile salts are essential for fat absorption but are themselves not readily absorbed. Fat malabsorption in the newborn may occur because of reduced bile salts. In infants below 1300 g birthweight, 70–75% of dietary fat is absorbed. Premature infants are better able to absorb polyunsaturated fats (as are present in excess in human milk) than saturated fats. Some degree of physiological steatorrhoea is therefore normal in preterm infants. Premature infants cope better with the absorption of medium-chain triglyceride fats than long-chain fatty acids.

SECRETIONS

Gastric acid secretion does not occur to any significant degree before 32 weeks' gestation. Pancreatic secretions of lipase are adequate for dietary needs by full term, but trypsin is often deficient, resulting in relative protein malabsorption.

MALFORMATIONS

Cleft lip

Cleft lip, with or without cleft palate, occurs in 1/1000 births. It is usually of polygenic inheritance (rarely autosomal dominant) and has a higher frequency in some families. The risk of recurrence in subsequent pregnancies is about 5%. It is more common in the pregnancies of older mothers. It may be unilateral (70% on left side) or bilateral. Severe midline facial clefts are associated with intracranial anomalies, including holoprosencephaly (see p. 222), and are a feature of trisomy 13. Cleft lip and palate have been associated with maternal anticonvulsant therapy, and also occur in the fetal alcohol syndrome.

MANAGEMENT

The infant has an unattractive appearance and time must be spent with the parents talking to them about the condition. Photographs of treated cases showing the preoperative and postoperative appearances are particularly helpful in allaying parental anxieties (Fig. 23.1). There may be feeding difficulties, particularly if there is an associated cleft palate (see below).

Surgical treatment

Most surgeons prefer to repair the lip in the first 6–12 weeks of life, but very early closure in the first week is recommended by some.

Cleft palate

In 70% of cases this is associated with a cleft lip. The palate forms by fusion of the bilateral maxillary processes and the midline premaxilla. A variety of clefting abnormalities occur:
1 complete cleft of the hard and soft palate, which may involve the alveolar margin. It may be unilateral, bilateral or involve the midline. Cleft palate may be associated with the Pierre Robin syndrome;

2 submucous cleft. There is a bony defect completely covered by mucosa. There is often a bifid uvula;
3 simple cleft of the soft palate.

Pierre Robin sequence. This is the association of cleft palate (hard or soft) with micrognathia (Fig. 23.2). The small jaw allows the tongue to prolapse backwards, thereby obstructing the airway and leading to cyanotic spells. The infant should be nursed prone to prevent airway obstruction, and a special nursing frame to keep the head in the midline may be required. The jaw usually grows rapidly and the infant can then be fed with a bottle and gradually sat up. The cleft palate is treated surgically.

CLINICAL FEATURES

1 Feeding is usually a problem because the baby is unable to achieve adequate suction, with resultant regurgitation of milk through the nose.
2 Aspiration of milk, causing recurrent pneumonitis.

TREATMENT

If feeding is difficult, a special teat may be required. These include a lamb's teat (longer than usual), a flanged (Great Ormond Street) teat or a Maws' teat. The rubber flange acts as an artificial palate. The careful use of a squeeze bottle aids suction in many infants. In some cases the fitting of an acrylic dental obturator around the edges of the palate is helpful.

The surgical management of cleft palate requires the services of a plastic surgeon, an orthodontist, an ear, nose and throat (ENT) surgeon and a speech therapist. If the alveolar ridge is involved, an orthodontist may make a series of plates to encourage appropriate bone growth. Surgical closure of the palate is attempted at 9–12 months before speech has developed.

PROGNOSIS

The following problems are to be anticipated.

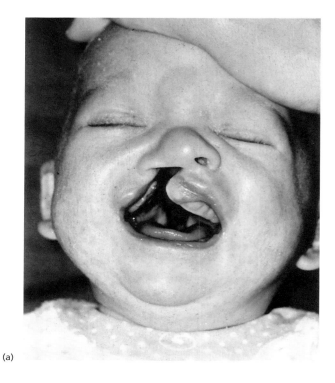

(a)

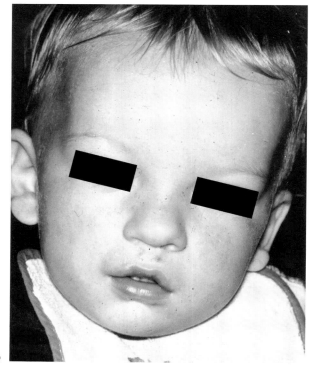

(b)

Fig. 23.1 Cleft lip. At birth the infant has a right-sided cleft lip (a). The same infant following repair (b).

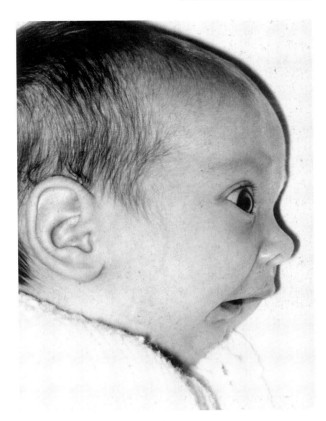

Fig. 23.2 Pierre Robin syndrome
showing micrognathia.

Speech and language

These problems include nasal escape and ar-
ticulation. A speech therapist should always be
closely involved in the management of these
children.

Hearing

Eustachian tube function is usually impaired,
predisposing the child to middle-ear infections.
Regular hearing assessment and ENT supervision are essential.

Dental

Dentition is often delayed and there may be
malocclusion.

Local ulceration

This may be due to poorly fitting acrylic plates.

INTESTINAL OBSTRUCTION

Intestinal obstruction occurs in about 1/1000
babies and may be associated with maternal
hydramnios. If more than 25 mL of fluid is
aspirated from the stomach after birth, intestinal
obstruction should be suspected. Occasionally,
bile-stained amniotic fluid from intrauterine
vomiting may be confused with meconium-
stained liquor. There are a variety of types of
congenital bowel obstruction (Table 23.1).
Oesophageal atresia is discussed in Chapter 10.

CLINICAL FEATURES

The infant presents with some or all of the following features:
1 bile-stained vomiting. This is a very important sign which must not be ignored. A history
of bile-stained vomiting demands immediate
investigation;

Table 23.1 Types of intestinal obstruction in the newborn

Oesophageal atresia
Duodenal atresia
Jejunal atresia
Volvulus neonatorum
Meconium ileus
Colon atresia
Stricture secondary to NEC
Hirschsprung's disease
Meconium plug syndrome
Imperforate anus

2 abdominal distension. This may not be prominent with a high obstruction;
3 visible peristalsis;
4 delayed passage of meconium. In cases of low obstruction there may be no passage of meconium at all. With a high obstruction meconium may be passed for a day or two. A changing stool is never seen with congenital bowel obstruction. Anal atresia should be recognized early at routine examination;
5 dehydration. The infant may present with dehydration and collapse as the result of excessive vomiting.

CLASSIFICATION OF INTESTINAL OBSTRUCTION

The causes of obstruction may be classified depending on the site of blockage (large or small bowel) or whether it is anatomical or functional. On occasions it is impossible to be sure of the diagnosis or even the level of obstruction, and laparotomy may be the only way of making a diagnosis in order to treat the condition effectively.

Anatomical obstruction

PYLORIC STENOSIS

This occurs very rarely as a cause of obstruction in the first week of life, but is an important condition in slightly older infants who develop persistent vomiting. The vomitus contains partially digested milk but no bile. Gastric peristalsis may be seen. The condition is due to hypertrophy of the pylorus and a definite tumour can be felt on palpation. There is often a family history, and boys are affected three times more often than girls. The cause of the hypertrophy is not known, but may be related to stress in a genetically susceptible infant.

Diagnosis is made by palpation of the upper abdomen during a test feed. Ultrasound examination reveals a characteristic 'doughnut' ring corresponding to the hypertrophied pylorus. Only rarely should radiological contrast studies be necessary.

Treatment is surgical following adequate restoration of electrolyte and fluid balance. At surgery the muscle fibres of the hypertrophied pylorus are incised down to the mucosa. This is known as Ramstedt's procedure.

DUODENAL OBSTRUCTION

Complete duodenal obstruction presents early with vomiting, which will be bile stained if the obstruction is below the second part of the duodenum. Partial duodenal obstruction, such as occurs with malrotation, may be more difficult to diagnose, as vomiting may be intermittent and stools are passed (see below). Duodenal atresia may be due to either intrinsic or extrinsic obstruction.

Intrinsic causes

1 Duodenal atresia—50% are associated with Down syndrome.
2 Duodenal stenosis—septum or membrane.

Extrinsic causes

Malrotation may cause the second part of the duodenum to be obstructed by Ladd's peritoneal bands. Annular pancreas may also cause extrinsic obstruction to the duodenum.

Diagnosis

A plain X-ray of the abdomen classically shows a 'double-bubble' appearance (Fig. 23.3) in

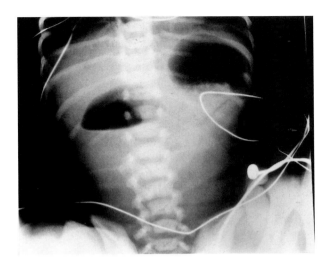

Fig. 23.3 Duodenal atresia. Abdominal radiograph showing the 'double-bubble' appearance.

duodenal atresia. If there is no air beyond this double bubble, then the diagnosis of duodenal atresia is certain and no further investigations are required. Small bubbles of air beyond the second part of the duodenum suggest an incomplete bowel obstruction and must be investigated further for malrotation.

Treatment

After resuscitation with fluids and electrolytes definitive surgical repair is performed. Postoperatively these infants often require prolonged total parenteral nutrition because of poor peristaltic activity across the anastomosis.

MALROTATION (VOLVULUS NEONATORUM)

This results from incomplete fixation and rotation of the bowel after it returns to the fetal abdominal cavity from the yolk sac early in the third month of gestation. The three features of malrotation are:

1 the duodenojejunal junction is at or to the right of the vertebral column;
2 the ileocaecal junction is near the midline and higher than normal;
3 it is abnormally fixed by avascular bands (Ladd's bands) which cross the second part of the duodenum.

These abnormalities cause the small bowel mesentery in which the superior mesenteric artery lies to be abnormally mobile and to twist around its axis, leading to a volvulus with rapid impairment of gut blood flow. This may cause intestinal obstruction in one of two ways:

1 strangulation obstruction: the superior mesenteric artery supplying blood to the bowel is occluded;
2 Ladd's bands obstructing the second part of the duodenum.

Diagnosis

This lesion characteristically produces episodic obstruction with abdominal distension, bile-stained vomiting, pallor and a vague abdominal mass in an infant who was previously tolerating feeds well. The baby may rapidly proceed to shock.

Plain X-ray of the abdomen in the erect position may show a characteristic double bubble, but gas is seen beyond the duodenum. Contrast studies may show a corkscrew duodenum or an abnormally situated subhepatic position of the caecum. Ultrasound scan may show an abnormal relationship between the superior mesenteric artery and vein strongly suggestive of malrotation.

Treatment

Laparotomy needs to be performed urgently to

Table 23.2 International classification of anorectal malformations (Stephens & Smith 1986)

	Female	Male

High	Anorectal agenesis
	  Rectovaginal fistula
	  No fistula
	  Rectal atresia
		Anorectal agenesis
		  Rectoprostatic fistula
		  No fistula
		  Rectal atresia

Intermediate	Rectovaginal fistula Rectovestibular fistula Anal agenesis	Bulbar fistula Anal agenesis
Low	Anovestibular fistula Anocutaneous fistula Anal stenosis	Anocutaneous fistula Anal stenosis
Persistent cloaca		

untwist and relieve the volvulus. It may be difficult to exclude volvulus clinically and, in view of the rapidity with which bowel infarction occurs, an early laparotomy is advisable in suspected cases.

JEJUNAL ATRESIA

This is the commonest site for intestinal atresia and is probably due to bowel ischaemia in early fetal life. The atretic segment may be isolated or multiple. The diagnosis is often made on prenatal ultrasound examination. After birth the infant rapidly develops marked abdominal distension and X-ray shows loops of dilated bowel with multiple fluid levels. Treatment is by resection of the atretic segment, but sacrifice of grossly dilated bowel above the stricture may be necessary before primary anastomosis is possible.

COLONIC ATRESIA

This is very rare and when it does occur is probably due to a vascular accident in the mesentery during early pregnancy. The infant presents with low obstruction, but diagnosis can only be made for certain at laparotomy.

ANORECTAL MALFORMATIONS

An imperforate anus is a perineum without an anal opening. The commonest classification of anorectal malformations is shown in Table 23.2. The arrested development of the anus and rectum may be divided into high lesions (rectal deformities), intermediate or low lesions (anal deformities).

The incidence is 1/5000 live births. There is a slight preponderance of male infants, in whom there is a higher incidence of the more serious rectal deformities, whereas in females the anal type is more common, with a stenotic ectopic orifice.

Clinical features

This condition should be obvious on examination. Other anomalies, such as genitourinary, vertebral, alimentary tract (especially oesophageal atresia), cardiac and central nervous system, must be carefully excluded. Anal atresia may be one of the features of the VACTERL association (Vertebral, Anal, Cardiac, Tracheal, Esophagus, Renal and Limb defects).

Defecation and micturition should be observed in these infants. In the female all orifices must be carefully examined and probed for evidence of additional fistulous tracts. Most female infants will decompress their bowel spontaneously via a vaginal fistula. In the majority of males meconium will be seen in the urine owing to a rectovesical or rectourethral fistula.

Investigations

X-Rays of the spine and sacrum will detect any vertebral or sacral anomalies. An invertogram is performed after 24 h of age, when adequate gas should have passed to the end of the bowel. This is an X-ray of the pelvis in an exact lateral projection, with a radio-opaque marker on the anal skin, while the baby is held upside down. A line drawn between the pubic symphysis and the sacrococcygeal junction constitutes the pubococcygeal line. Gas cranial to this line indicates a high rectal anomaly, whereas gas caudal to this line indicates an anal anomaly.

An intravenous pyelogram or ultrasound examination will reveal a renal anomaly in 25% of cases. A micturating cystourethrogram will demonstrate a rectovesical fistula and vesicoureteric reflux. Low lesions have a good prognosis and can usually be managed with local reconstructive surgery of the anus.

Management and outcome

High lesions will require a colostomy in the neonatal period to decompress the bowel, followed by rectoplasty at 6–12 months of age. High lesions are generally associated with rectal incontinence after treatment.

The results of surgery in intermediate or low atresia are somewhat better. Generally, about one-third will have normal anal continence, one-third will have acceptable continence with some soiling, and one-third will be totally incontinent. The avoidance of repeated urinary tract infections in males with rectovesical fistula is important. Long-term constipation is a common complication of this disorder.

Functional obstruction

HIRSCHSPRUNG'S DISEASE (AGANGLIONOSIS)

This condition results from the absence of ganglion cells in the plexus of Auerbach, which prevents orderly peristaltic activity through the bowel. It is the commonest cause of large bowel obstruction in the newborn and has an incidence of 1/5000. It is more common in Down syndrome (5%) and in babies with congenital cardiac defects. It is inherited as a polygenic disease with a recurrence risk within families of 12.5%, and the RET gene has been implicated as the cause in 10–20% of patients (Cass 1996). There are two distinct types:

1 *short aganglionic segment*. This is the most common type, with a male to female ratio of 5 : 1. It usually affects the rectum and sigmoid colon;

2 *long aganglionic segment*. This is rarer and has an equal male to female ratio. This type is more commonly inherited in families.

Diagnosis

The most common presentation in the newborn period is with acute obstruction. The infant vomits and has a distended abdomen, with failure to pass meconium. Rectal examination may reveal an explosive gush of meconium, to be followed by progressive constipation and further signs of obstruction. In older infants chronic constipation may develop with 'spurious diarrhoea', which is not seen in the neonate. It may be difficult to distinguish Hirschsprung's disease from cystic fibrosis and meconium plug syndrome.

The meconium plug syndrome may occur with intrauterine growth restriction, Hirschsprung's disease, meconium ileus, or as an isolated condition. The infant fails to open his bowels in the first 24 h and may develop clinical and radiological signs of obstruction. A white plug of meconium is passed and the signs of obstruction settle spontaneously. These infants require careful follow-up in order to detect those with Hirschsprung's disease or cystic fibrosis.

Necrotizing enterocolitis (NEC; see p. 267) may develop acutely in infants with Hirschsprung's disease. This diagnosis must be considered in all infants with NEC.

Investigations

A plain X-ray of the abdomen may show

dilated bowel loops and fluid levels, and lateral X-ray of the pelvis may show the air-filled cone. Contrast studies using barium or other agents may show the dilated normal bowel above a tapering transitional zone with distal microcolon. The definitive diagnosis is made by biopsy. This may be either a suction biopsy of the rectal mucosa and submucosa (less invasive), or a formal full-thickness strip biopsy of the bowel under a general anaesthetic. Histology reveals the absence of ganglia in the nerve plexus. Some centres use cholinesterase staining techniques to confirm the histological findings.

Treatment

In the neonate a colostomy is performed just above the site of transition, together with a biopsy to confirm that the stoma has been fashioned in normally innervated bowel. Rectosigmoidectomy is performed 3–6 months later, with closure of the colostomy at that time or at a third operation.

MECONIUM ILEUS

Ten to 15 per cent of infants with cystic fibrosis present with meconium ileus owing to pancreatic insufficiency with inspissated meconium. In about half, meconium ileus is complicated by ischaemia, stenosis and malrotation, or meconium peritonitis with intraperitoneal calcification secondary to intrauterine perforation. Ninety per cent of infants with meconium ileus have cystic fibrosis.

Diagnosis

Cystic fibrosis may present with an acute bowel obstruction, a meconium plug syndrome, or the infant may become acutely ill with sepsis and cardiovascular collapse.

A plain X-ray of the abdomen shows multiple fluid levels and typically a foamy pattern of air bubbles trapped around inspissated meconium. A Gastrografin enema shows a microcolon. The first specimen of meconium can be tested chemically for albumin with a Boehringer–Mannheim screening test, but this is unreliable.

In the first month of life measurement of immunoreactive trypsin (IRT) on a heel-prick blood specimen is a very sensitive method for diagnosing cystic fibrosis, and can be used as a screening test. Unfortunately, after operation for meconium ileus the IRT level may rapidly fall despite the child having cystic fibrosis. For this reason, all neonates with signs of bowel obstruction should have an IRT measurement prior to surgery. Eighty per cent of children with cystic fibrosis have the δ F508 gene, which should be determined in all cases of meconium ileus. Definitive diagnosis of cystic fibrosis is by genetic probes as soon as the condition is suspected, or by sweat testing at 1–3 months of age.

Treatment

The decision as to whether the bowel obstruction is to be managed medically or surgically will be made by the surgeon. Management with Gastrografin enemas under fluoroscopic control may be initially diagnostic and subsequently therapeutic by softening the meconium so that it can be passed normally. Surgical decompression is often necessary in complicated cases, and is done in conjunction with Gastrografin washouts of the bowel. The baby with cystic fibrosis will also require lifelong treatment with appropriate antibiotics, chest physiotherapy, salt replacement, pancreatic extracts and fat-soluble vitamins. Genetic counselling is essential for this autosomal recessive condition.

ABDOMINAL WALL DEFECTS

Exomphalos (omphalocoele) and gastroschisis are discussed together as they are both eviscerations of gastrointestinal contents: an exomphalos emerges through the umbilicus, whereas gastroschisis is through a right paramedian abdominal cleft.

EXOMPHALOS (OMPHALOCOELE)

Exomphalos occurs in 1/5000 births and is due to an embryological abnormality at 18 weeks of gestation, resulting in the bowel failing to re-enter the abdomen. The extra-abdominal bowel is covered by peritoneum and the umbilical cord is at the apex of the exomphalos. It is associated with other anomalies in 60–80% of cases, particularly when the defect is small. These include congenital heart disease, Beckwith–Wiedemann syndrome (exomphalos, large tongue and hypoglycaemia) or chromosomal disorders (trisomy 13, trisomy 18).

The diagnosis is often made on prenatal ultrasound examination and fetal chromosome analysis is essential, together with careful surveillance for other congenital malformations.

Management

Small lesions, with abdominal defects of less than 5 cm, can generally be treated surgically with primary closure. Larger defects may be amenable to primary closure, but if this is not possible the eviscerated bowel is protected by a Teflon silo which is progressively reduced in size to allow reduction of the hernia.

GASTROSCHISIS

In contrast to exomphalos, gastroschisis has no peritoneal covering and the bowel is loose within the amniotic cavity. Consequently, it becomes scarred and bound with adhesions, with resultant stenosis, strictures and atresias. There is often intrauterine growth failure, possibly associated with a short bowel syndrome, failure to thrive and steatorrhoea. Gastroschisis is less common than exomphalos, with an incidence of 1/20 000 and, unlike exomphalos, it is rarely associated with other congenital malformations. There is no satisfactory embryological explanation for gastroschisis.

Management

At birth the bowel must be handled very carefully to avoid further trauma. It should be placed in a sterile saline-filled plastic bag to avoid hypothermia. Primary repair is possible if the defect is small, but becomes more difficult when there is massive evisceration. A silo may be necessary before the abdomen can be fully closed. Following abdominal repair severe respiratory embarrassment may occur as the result of diaphragmatic splinting secondary to raised intra-abdominal pressure. Prolonged mechanical ventilation is often required postoperatively.

Unlike in exomphalos, the bowel tends to show prolonged dysfunction in the absence of any anatomical abnormality. This may require long-term total parenteral nutrition.

NECROTIZING ENTEROCOLITIS

NEC is the most important acquired bowel abnormality occurring in the newborn period. It is defined as an inflammatory disease with ulceration and sometimes perforation of the bowel. It most commonly affects the terminal ileum or sigmoid colon. The radiographic appearance of intramural gas (pneumatosis intestinalis) is generally considered confirmatory evidence of the disease. A definitive diagnosis can only be made at autopsy or on pathological examination of surgical specimens.

NEC is much commoner in very low birth-weight (VLBW) infants (approximately 5% of these), but is generally less commonly seen in the UK and Australia than in the USA. The incidence varies between 0.2 and 3/1000 births. It may rarely be seen in otherwise well full-term healthy breastfed infants.

Pathogenesis

The cause of NEC is unknown, but there are three main predisposing factors (Weaver 1997).
1 *Mucosal injury.* This may occur as a result of immaturity of the mucosal defences or as a complication of abnormal blood flow to the gut mucosa, as occurs in:

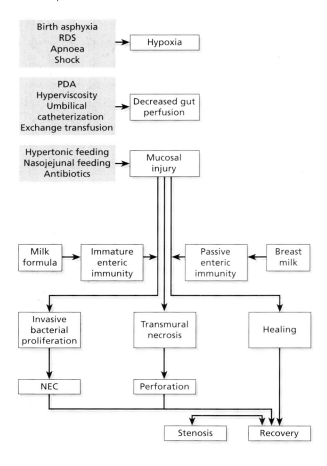

Fig. 23.4 Schema for the development of NEC.

(a) asphyxia;

(b) patent ductus arteriosus, which is twice as common in babies who develop NEC than in controls;

(c) polycythaemia;

(d) severe intrauterine growth restriction with evidence of compromised blood flow on antenatal Doppler studies (absent or retrograde diastolic flow);

(e) umbilical venous and arterial catheter use;

(f) cyanotic heart disease;

(g) a complication of Hirschsprung's disease due to local mucosal ischaemia.

2 *Enteral feeds.* NEC is very rare in babies who have received no enteral feeds. The risk of NEC may be due to milk's effect on bacterial proliferation, or the volume of feed. NEC is also more common where hyperosmolar feeds and formula feeds rather than breast milk are used. Although the leukocytes and immunoglobulins in breast milk are thought to protect an infant from this disease, NEC occasionally occurs in exclusively breastfed infants.

3 *Infection.* Although infection is probably not the direct cause, some enteric organisms predispose to the development of this condition. Many organisms have been implicated, including coliforms, staphylococci, *Clostridia* and rotavirus.

Mucosal injury by one of the above mechanisms allows secondary invasion of gas-producing bacteria, which causes pneumatosis coli. A schema to illustrate this process is shown in Fig. 23.4.

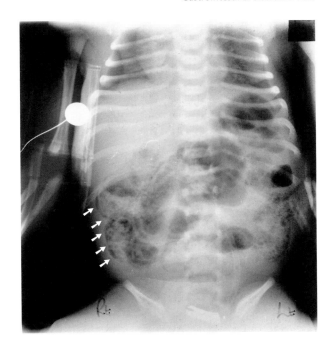

Fig. 23.5 Radiological appearance of NEC. The bowel shows extensive intramural gas (arrowed).

CLINICAL FEATURES

The early signs of NEC are often non-specific, with lethargy, apnoea, bile-stained aspirates and failure to maintain body temperature. These features are common in preterm infants, but the early cessation of feeding under these circumstances may prevent the progression to full-blown NEC. The signs may progress to include abdominal distension, blood and mucus in the stool, and circulatory collapse. Apnoea, bradycardia, shock, poor urine output and metabolic acidosis are commonly seen in severe cases. Complications of the disease include:

1 DIC (disseminated intravascular coagulation);
2 septicaemia in 33% of cases;
3 bowel perforation with a localized abscess or generalized peritonitis;
4 bowel obstruction;
5 gangrenous bowel;
6 lactose intolerance and malabsorption in the recovery period;
7 relapse after commencing oral feeds;
8 intrahepatic cholestasis relating to inflammatory bowel disease and total parenteral nutrition.

Investigations

1 *Erect and cross-table lateral abdominal X-rays* may show distension of bowel loops only. Later a foamy gas pattern (pneumatosis intestinalis, Fig. 23.5), portal vein gas, pneumoperitoneum, fluid levels or free peritoneal fluid may be seen on abdominal films.
2 *Full blood count.* This shows a neutropenia or neutrophilia, a shift to the left of the leukocytes, toxic granulations in the neutrophils and thrombocytopenia.
3 *Microbiological investigation.* Faeces and blood are examined and cultured. Many Gram-positive and Gram-negative organisms have been associated with NEC, but the most frequent isolates are *Clostridium* sp. and *Klebsiella* sp. Faeces should also be sent for viral studies and examination for rotavirus, as this agent has been incriminated in the pathogenesis of some cases of NEC.

MANAGEMENT

Prevention

Various strategies have been suggested to

reduce or eliminate the risk of NEC. These include:

1 antenatal steroids have shown a dramatic effect in reducing the risk of NEC. This is most likely to be related to the reduced risk of respiratory distress syndrome (RDS) and the lower likelihood of gut ischaemia secondary to this;

2 delay in milk feeding in high-risk babies. Babies delivered early because of severe intra-uterine growth restriction, particularly when there has been retrograde flow on antenatal Doppler assessment, appear to be at increased risk of NEC. Delaying the introduction of any milk feed for the first 5 days is advisable;

3 breast milk is also known to confer a reduced risk of NEC compared with formula feeds. In one controlled study, the risk of NEC was six times higher in the formula-fed group than in the breastfed premature infants (Lucus & Cole 1990). Small volumes of breast milk and breast milk mixed with formula also appear to lower the risk;

4 oral antibiotic therapy has been shown to reduce the risk of NEC in a number of small studies (McDonnell & Wilkinson 1997), but this is not recommended at present because of the risk of antibiotic resistance;

5 oral immunoglobulin (IgA and IgG) has been suggested to reduce the risk of NEC, but the results of larger randomized controlled studies are awaited before this can be recommended.

Therapy

A high index of suspicion should be exercised when the infant is given milk. At the first sign of gastrointestinal intolerance feeds are stopped in order to rest the bowel. Total parenteral nutrition is started for at least 10 days and broad-spectrum antibiotics given (gentamicin, ampicillin and metronidazole), or third-generation cephalosporins for 7–10 days. Fluid, electrolyte and acid–base disorders must be corrected. Transfusions with fresh whole blood may be necessary.

Infants with proven NEC are best managed conservatively. The indications for surgical intervention include:

1 free air in the peritoneum, indicating bowel perforation;

2 clinical deterioration during conservative management should be carefully assessed with a view to surgical intervention;

3 failure to improve on medical management.

Surgical intervention includes peritoneal drainage or formal laparotomy. The former may be done under general anaesthetic or in the newborn unit with a cannula under local anaesthesia.

Laparotomy is best done in a specialist neonatal surgical centre. Fashioning an ileostomy in a healthy bowel with peritoneal drainage is usually the best form of treatment, and necrotic bowel is often not resected as a primary procedure. A second laparotomy may be necessary when the baby has recovered from the acute NEC.

COMPLICATIONS

Short bowel syndrome

This is a major problem in babies with very extensive NEC. If the bowel is too short (< 40 cm in a full-term baby) or if the ileocaecal valve has been surgically resected along with a significant amount of ileum, then the baby may be left with too little bowel for normal absorption. Some centres undertake long-term total parenteral nutrition at home for this condition.

Stricture

This occurs in approximately 15% of infants following NEC and the descending colon is the most commonly affected site.

Lactose intolerance

This is caused by damage to the brush border of the mucosa, with sloughing of the disaccharidases. 5–10% of infants will develop this condition after NEC. Semielemental formulas are recommended when the gut is rechallenged after recovery from extensive disease.

Recurrence

This is uncommon, occurring in less than 5% of babies. If it does occur, Hirschsprung's disease must be considered as an aetiological factor.

RECTAL BLEEDING

Blood and mucus in the stool is a common finding in the neonatal period, but the sight of blood on the nappy of a newborn infant is alarming for a mother. It is important to distinguish whether the blood is fresh or altered, confined to the outside of the stool or mixed throughout. Other symptoms, such as constipation, abdominal distension or pain, may assist with the diagnosis.

Common causes of blood in the stools include:

1 swallowed maternal blood;
2 rectal or anal fissure from thermometer, rectal examination or severe constipation;
3 NEC;
4 malrotation, intussusception;
5 Meckel's diverticulum and bowel duplication with ectopic gastric mucosa;
6 gastroenteritis: human rotavirus, *Shigella* sp., *Salmonella* sp., enteropathogenic *Escherichia coli*;
7 rectal polyp;
8 haemorrhagic disease of the newborn;
9 benign haemorrhagic colitis. This is one of the commonest causes of blood in the stool. It is usually associated with mucus and occurs most commonly in formula-fed infants. It may be due to cows'-milk protein intolerance and recurs when cows'-milk protein is reintroduced in the feeds.

The clinical history and examination will elucidate many of the above causes. Apt's test will distinguish fetal from maternal blood.

Plain X-rays of the abdomen may confirm NEC or may suggest malrotation. Faecal cultures and examination of the stool for human rotavirus or other infectious agents will confirm the clinical diagnosis of gastroenteritis. The ectopic gastric mucosa in a bleeding Meckel's diverticulum or bowel duplication may be demonstrated with a technetium radioisotope scan. The bleeding and prolonged prothrombin time in an infant with haemorrhagic disease of the newborn are corrected by a dose of vitamin K, 1 mg intramuscularly.

Most infants with blood and mucus in their stool will settle spontaneously without any obvious cause being found on investigation.

REFERENCES

Cass, D.T. (1996) Unravelling the pathogenesis and molecular genetics of Hirschsprung's disease. *Seminars in Neonatology* **1**, 211–217.

Lucus, A. & Cole, T.J. (1990) Breast milk and neonatal necrotising enterocolitis. *Lancet* **336**, 1519–1521.

McDonnell, M. & Wilkinson, A. (1997) Necrotizing enterocolitis—perinatal approach to prevention, early diagnosis and management. *Seminars in Neonatology* **2**, 291–296.

Stephens, F.D. & Smith, E.D. (1986) Classification, identification and assessment of surgical treatment of anorectal anomalies. *Pediatric Surgery International* **1**, 200–205.

Weaver, L.T. (1997) Digestive system development and failure. *Seminars in Neonatology* **2**, 221–230.

FURTHER READING

Altman, P.R. & Stylianos, S. (1993) Paediatric surgery. *Pediatric Clinics of North America* **40**(6).

Lloyd, D.A. (1996) Neonatal surgery. *Seminars in Neonatology* **1**(3).

Wilkinson, A.R. & Tam, P.K.H. (1997) Necrotizing enterocolitis. *Seminars in Neonatology* **2**(4).

Cutaneous lesions are present at birth in 8% of newborn infants. They are immediately obvious, attract attention and may cause considerable concern. Sometimes they are part of a more systemic disorder, such as neuroectodermal dysplasia. Cutaneous lesions in the newborn can be classified in the following major groups:

1 vascular birthmarks;
2 epidermal naevi;
3 pigmented birthmarks;
4 ichthyotic disorders;
5 blistering and bullous disorders;
6 miscellaneous.

VASCULAR BIRTHMARKS

Vascular birthmarks may be classified as either haemangiomas or vascular malformations. Older descriptive terminology, such as 'cavernous', 'strawberry', 'naevus flammeus', should be avoided.

Haemangiomas

These vascular tumours are characterized by rapid endothelial growth followed by slow involution. Approximately 30% are present at birth as a blanched area or a telangiectatic patch. The majority appear during the first month of life, with rapid expansion of growth over the next 5 months (Fig. 24.1). Slow involution subsequently occurs over the next 5–10 years.

Superficial haemangiomas deep in the dermis, subcutaneous fat or muscle produce a bluish colour in the overlying skin.

The majority of haemangiomas do not require treatment. Oral corticosteroids commenced during the rapid growth phase in the first 5 months of life are very effective in slowing growth and hastening resolution. Indications for treatment include lesions that interfere with vital functions, 'edge structures' (e.g. eyelids, nares, philtrum, lips or pinnae), those associated with high cardiac output failure, and extensive facial lesions. Bleeding is rarely a problem, even after trauma, but large lesions around limb girdles may be associated with thrombocytopenia, intravascular coagulation and severe bleeding (Kassabach–Merritt syndrome).

Vascular malformations

These represent structural anomalies, are present at birth, grow in proportion to the infant's growth, and in general do not have a tendency to resolve.

CAPILLARY MALFORMATIONS

Fine capillary haemangiomas which are deep red in colour and blanch with pressure occur on the glabella, upper eyelids, upper lips and

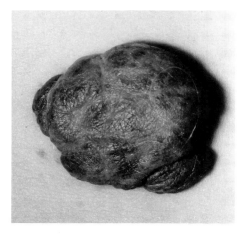

Fig. 24.1 Vascular haemangioma.

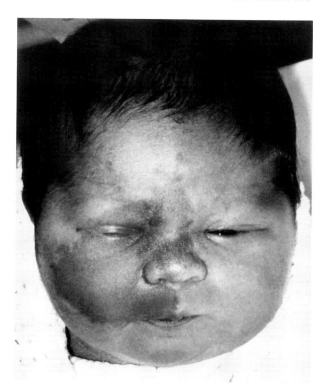

Fig. 24.2 Port-wine stain affecting the maxillary region.

nape of the neck. They are of no significance and tend to fade during the first 6 months.

Larger, flat, deep, purple/red ('port-wine') lesions may occur on any part of the body. Those in the distribution of the trigeminal nerve may be associated with retinal and intracranial haemangiomas, requiring ophthalmological follow-up (Fig. 24.2). Association of this type of lesion with vascular malformation of the ipsilateral meninges and cerebral cortex is termed the Sturge–Weber syndrome and requires neurological assessment. The skin manifestations may be treated with cosmetic cover creams or by pulsed dye laser in the second decade.

EPIDERMAL NAEVI

These birthmarks presenting at birth or in the first few months of life represent proliferation of keratinocytes or cells of the skin appendage.

They are rare lesions which may involve any area of the skin, including the oral cavity. On the scalp and face they are often yellowish because of a prominent sebaceous gland component. Trunk and limb epidermal naevi are scaly, flat or raised, varying in colour from black or brown to pale grey, with plaque or linear streak distribution. Treatment with topical retinoic acid or oral retinoids is unsatisfactory. Excision may be indicated for small and linear lesions and irritating and cosmetically troublesome naevi.

HYPERPIGMENTED AND HYPOPIGMENTED BIRTHMARKS

These must be differentiated from the skin lesions of generalized disorders, such as neurofibromatosis and tuberous sclerosis, which usually appear after birth.

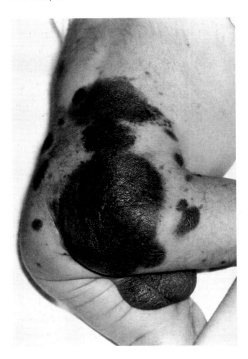

Fig. 24.3 Congenital melanocytic naevus involving the buttock and loin.

Congenital hyperpigmented patches

These common pale or dark-brown macular or flat hypermelanotic patches may be solitary or extensive, involving large areas of the trunk or limbs. They must be differentiated from the *café au lait* spots of classic neurofibromatosis, which are occasionally present at birth. Treatment consists of cosmetic cover creams, or plastic surgery for smaller lesions.

Congenital melanocytic naevi

These are collections of melanocytes in the epidermis, dermis or both. Most are not present at birth, but when present appear as raised verrucous or lobulated lesions of various shades of brown to black (Fig. 24.3). They vary in size and may have blue or pink components, often growing long black hairs. They grow in proportion to the infant's growth. Controversy exists about the risk of malignant change. Lesions over the lower spine may be associated

with a tethered spinal cord (see p. 219). Large or multiple lesions may be associated with benign or, rarely, malignant proliferation of melanocytes in the leptomeninges, demonstrated by magnetic resonance imaging (MRI). Small lesions are easily removed surgically; for larger lesions plastic procedures may be possible.

Mongolian spots

These are flat, blue or slate-grey lesions comprising collections of melanocytes in the dermis. They are seen in the majority of oriental and black infants. In white infants there is usually a background of Mediterranean origin. Single or multiple, they occur particularly in the lumbosacral area, less often on the shoulders, back or other areas, and tend to fade with age. No treatment is necessary.

Congenital hypopigmented patches

Pale areas of reduced cutaneous melanication varying in size from a few centimetres to large areas covering the trunk and limbs. They do not involute. Similar lesions occur in incontinentia pigmenti, a rare genetic condition in females associated with multiple abnormalities, especially of the eye, skeletal and central nervous systems.

ICHTHYOTIC DISORDERS

These are a rare group of skin disorders where the skin at birth resembles fish scales. There are several varieties.

Ichthyosis vulgaris

This is an autosomal dominant disorder and other members of the family may have a history of atopy. It rarely causes problems in the newborn period and is best treated with an aqueous ointment.

Recessive X-linked ichthyosis

This condition only affects males and is

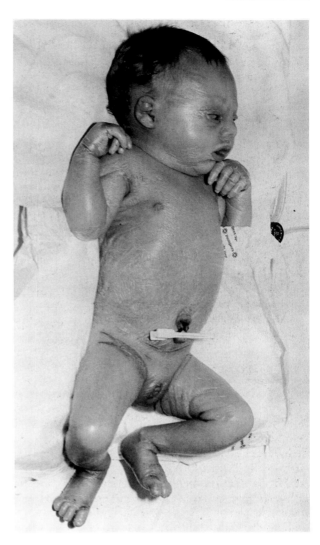

Fig. 24.4 Newborn infant with collodion skin. Six weeks later the skin appeared entirely normal.

associated with placental sulphatase deficiency. Unrecordable oestriol measurements during pregnancy should alert the clinician to this possibility in male infants.

Collodion baby

The most severe form of this group of disorders is the collodion baby (Fig. 24.4). At birth the infant looks as if he has a dry plastic-like membrane instead of skin, which cracks easily. These infants often later develop lamellar ichthyosis, but some may have no persistent skin abnormality. It is likely that the collodion baby, and the more severe harlequin fetus, represent a heterogeneous pathological group.

BLISTERING AND BULLOUS DISORDERS

This is a wide group of unrelated disorders characterized by blistering of the skin. They can be divided into transient and chronic (Table 24.1).

Table 24.1 Classification of blistering and bullous disorders affecting the neonate

Transient	Chronic
Erythema toxicum	Epidermolysis bullosa:
Congenital candidiasis	Non-scarring
	Scarring
Impetigo neonatorum	
Toxic epidermal necrolysis	

Transient

ERYTHEMA TOXICUM (URTICARIA NEONATORUM)

This appears in the first few days as multiple vesicles. They are differentiated from infection by a macular base and the presence of multiple eosinophils within the vesicular fluid. No treatment is necessary.

CANDIDA VESICLES

These are usually associated with oral candidiasis and may rarely be present at birth. Diagnosis is by the identification of hyphae or budding spores from the blister. Treatment is by topical nystatin or miconazole.

IMPETIGO NEONATORUM (PEMPHIGUS NEONATORUM)

This term is used to describe staphylococcal bullous lesions appearing on the second or third day of life. The pustules develop on an erythematous base and are often seen on the neck, axillae or groin. The infant may show signs of systemic infection. Intravenous flucloxacillin should be given while culture from the pustules is awaited, as the condition may spread quickly.

TOXIC EPIDERMAL NECROLYSIS (SCALDED SKIN SYNDROME OR RITTER'S DISEASE)

This condition is characterized by generalized erythema accompanied by fever and irritability, which is followed within a few hours by the formation of flaccid bullae filled with serous fluid. Sheets of epidermis can be stripped away, revealing a raw, oozing surface (Nikolsky's sign) (Fig. 24.5). This clinical picture is most commonly associated with a *Staphylococcus*

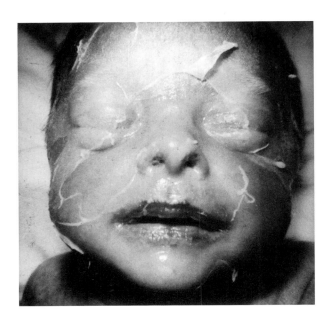

Fig. 24.5 Toxic epidermal necrolysis ('scalded skin syndrome').

aureus infection (phage type 50 or 71), although sometimes no infectious aetiology can be established.

Treatment is with systemic flucloxacillin. The large denuded areas of skin must be treated like a severe burn, requiring isolation to prevent secondary infection and careful fluid and electrolyte management.

Chronic

Epidermolysis bullosa includes a group of conditions in which blistering or bullous eruptions occur at birth or are seen in the first week of life in response to mechanical trauma. They can be divided into scarring and non-scarring forms.

NON-SCARRING (EPIDERMOLYSIS BULLOSA SIMPLEX)

This is a relatively mild form and is inherited as an autosomal dominant condition. The soles, toes and fingers are most often affected. Blisters may be present within minutes of delivery. A more severe form, inherited as an autosomal recessive condition, may heal to leave atrophic areas. Differentiation is only possible on electron microscopy. The non-scarring types tend to improve by puberty, but lesions frequently become secondarily infected.

SCARRING (DYSTROPHIC) FORMS

These conditions may be inherited as either autosomal dominant or recessive disorders. These blisters often occur early and are deep. The recessive form is usually more severe and the gastrointestinal tract may be involved. The scarring is often extremely destructive, with loss of nails, the formation of ugly scars and contractures, fusion of digits, and sometimes digit or limb amputations.

Management

This will depend on the individual case, but the parents should be encouraged to ensure that the child's lifestyle is as normal as possible.

Nevertheless, the avoidance of mechanical trauma, hot baths and high temperatures is important. Genetic counselling will be necessary.

MISCELLANEOUS

Cutis marmorata

This represents a normal physiological reaction to cold commonly seen in the neonate and young infant. The bluish mottling usually exhibits a characteristic reticulated pattern on the trunk and extremities. It is symptomless and transient, requiring no treatment.

Harlequin colour change

This refers to a differential colour change commonly seen during the first few days of life in preterm but also in term infants. It occurs with axial rotation: when the infant is lying on its side the upper part of the body is paler than the lower half, which is normal or reddish in colour. It may last for seconds or minutes and requires no treatment.

Acrodermatitis enteropathica

This is due to zinc deficiency. The classic tetrad consists of diarrhoea, apathy, alopecia and a vesicular bullous rash around the mouth and anus. Excellent results can be achieved with oral zinc therapy.

Neonatal eczema (atopic dermatitis)

Eczema is a common problem after 2 months of age but is unusual in the newborn. Management consists of avoiding potential allergens, including soap and cows' milk. Moisturizing creams and emulsifying ointment should be used in the bath. Severe cases may require 0.5% hydrocortisone cream in urea base, antipruritics, and occasionally hospitalization for intensive nursing care.

Seborrhoeic dermatitis

This is a chronic inflammatory disease of the

skin and scalp occurring in all paediatric age groups, especially early infancy. Crusting and scaling of the scalp (cradle cap) may be the initial and only manifestation. It may spread to the face, neck, behind the ears, axillae and napkin area. Treatment consists of the use of moisturizing creams, regular shampooing and steroid creams for severe cases.

Ectodermal dysplasia

This is an abnormality affecting the skin, sweat glands, hair and nails. It is divided into hidrotic and anhidrotic (sweating and non-sweating) forms.

HIDROTIC

Affected children have hyperkeratosis of the hands and feet, sparse hair and hypoplastic or absent nails. The teeth are usually normal. It does not present in infancy. In contrast to the anhidrotic form the infected child has the ability to sweat.

ANHIDROTIC

The most serious problem is inability to sweat, which may cause hyperpyrexia. The skin is thin, the hair is sparse, and when the first dentition appears the teeth are peg-like. It is usually inherited as an X-linked recessive trait and males are most severely affected.

FURTHER READING

Cohen, B.A. (1993) *Atlas of Paediatric Dermatology*. Wolfe, London.

Frieden, I.J. (1997) Special Symposium. Management of Haemangiomas. *Paediatric Dermatology* 14(1), 57–83.

Rogers, M. (1996) The significance of birthmarks. *Medical Journal of Australia* 164, 618–623.

Rudolf, A.J. (1997) *Atlas of the Newborn* Vol. 4. B.C. Decker, Hamilton, Ontario.

Schachner, L.A. & Hansen, R.C. (eds) (1995) *Pediatric Dermatology*, 2nd edn. Churchill Livingstone, Edinburgh.

Williams, M.L. (1983) The ichthyoses—pathogenesis and prenatal diagnosis: a review of recent advances. *Paediatric Dermatology* 1, 1–24.

25 Multiple births

The incidence of multiple births was first studied by Hellin in 1895. Following this work the Hellinic law was described, which stated that the incidence of twins was 1/89 and of triplets $1/89^2$ (1/7921) and quadruplets $1/89^3$ (1/704 969). Ovulation induction using drugs such as clomiphene and pituitary gonadotrophins, as well as new reproductive technologies (*in vitro* fertilization and gamete intrafallopian transfer), has dramatically modified these incidence figures. At the Mater Mother's Hospital in Brisbane the incidence of twins is 1/55 and that of triplets 1/770.

ZYGOSITY

Monozygous

Twins are monozygous (identical) when one ovum is fertilized which then splits during the first 14 days to produce two identical embryos. The monozygotic twinning rate is constant throughout the world at 3–4/1000 pregnancies, and is not influenced by heredity. The ensuing twins are identical and they usually share the same chorionic membrane.

Of all twins, 40% are monozygous, and 70% of monozygous twins have monochorionic placentas.

Dizygous

Dizygous (dissimilar) twins develop when two separate ova are fertilized, and their incidence is affected by fertility drugs. Dizygous (unlike monozygous) twins are much more likely to occur in families, or even to the same mother. Older and multiparous women are more likely to produce dizygous twins.

Taller, heavier women have a twinning rate 25–30% higher than short, nutritionally deprived women. Some spontaneous multiple ovulation is related to overstimulation by follicle-stimulating hormone and the surge of luteinizing hormone. Twinning rates vary between countries, from only 4.3/1000 in Japan to 12.4/1000 in Scotland, to a high of 57.2/1000 in Nigeria. Fertility and parity influence the rate of twinning.

Determination of zygosity

This may be extremely difficult, but may be determined by several factors (summarized in Fig. 25.1).

SEX

Twins of different sexes must be dizygous.

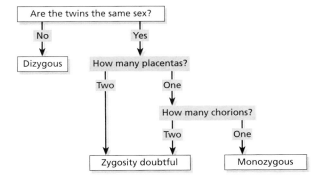

Fig. 25.1 Determination of the zygosity of twins.

PLACENTA

Monozygous twins who divide before the sixth day after fertilization have separate chorions. They may share the same placenta or have separate placentae. Those who divide later will always have only one chorion and either one or two amniotic cavities. Their placentae will be fused. If the twins are of like sex and have dichorionic placentae, then determination of zygosity is not possible without blood grouping.

BLOOD GROUPS

Monozygous twins will have identical blood groups, but up to 15 red cell antigens must be measured before 95% confidence of monozygosity can be assumed. Any blood group or antigen difference indicates dizygous twins.

COMPLICATIONS OF TWIN PREGNANCY

Discordant growth rates

Normally both twins will continue to grow at the rate of a singleton fetus until 30 weeks' gestation, after which growth retardation occurs. As the number of fetuses increases from twins to triplets to quadruplets, the gestational age at which birthweight first falls below that of a singleton fetus also decreases. Twins have birthweights similar to singletons up to 30 weeks, but thereafter are below singleton levels; similarly, birthweights in triplets deviate from the singleton curve at 27–28 weeks and in quadruplets at approximately 26 weeks. In addition, as the fetal number increases the rate of individual fetal growth in the third trimester decreases. Thus, the further the multiple gestation advances and the higher the fetal number, the more individual birthweights will differ from singleton values. Twins usually grow at nearly identical rates, the mean intertwin birthweight difference being 11%. Small for gestational age (SGA) infants have been reported in 24–40% of twin gestations. In one study, 13%

of twin gestations resulted in one SGA fetus and 9.4% in two. Monozygous twins grow less well than dizygous, and major discrepancies in weight are commoner in monozygous twins. Causes of discrepancy are poor insertion of the cord into the placenta in one twin, and in dichorionic twins poor placentation of one twin. The commonest cause is fetofetal transfusion (see below).

Disappearing twin phenomenon

Ultrasound studies in the first weeks of pregnancy have shown that up to 50% of pregnancies found to contain twins in the first 8 weeks of gestation absorb one conceptus and continue as singleton pregnancies. This has been referred to as the 'disappearing twin' phenomenon. Rarely, the dead twin is not resorbed and fetus papyraceous ensues. It is suggested that the disruption to the surviving twin as a result of the early fetal loss of the co-twin predisposes the baby to cerebral palsy, but there is little direct evidence for this at the present time.

Fetus papyraceous

This occurs if one twin dies early in the first trimester and becomes mummified. The other twin continues to grow normally. There is a high association with embolic phenomena (from the dead fetus) into the surviving twin. Multicystic encephaloleukomalacia and multiple cutis aplasia have been reported in the surviving twin.

Conjoined twins

This occurs in 1/100 000 pregnancies and is often incompatible with life (Fig. 25.2).

Prematurity

The incidence of premature delivery in twin pregnancies is 20–30% and is higher in more multiple pregnancies. Fifty per cent of twins weigh less than 2500 g at birth. Premature birth relates to increased intrauterine volume,

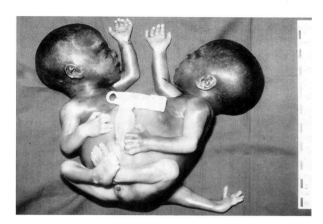

Fig. 25.2 Conjoined twins attached from chest to buttocks.

premature rupture of the membranes and third-trimester bleeding.

Malpresentation

Twins may present in the uterus in many ways, some of which predispose them to trauma:

Vertex and vertex	45%
Vertex and breech	40%
Breech and breech	10%
Vertex and transverse	3%
Breech and transverse	1.5%
Transverse and transverse	0.5%

Locked twins may occur as a result of unstable lies and cause obstruction to delivery.

Congenital malformations

The incidence of major malformation is 2% and minor malformation 4%. It is often stated that monozygotic twinning results from a chance teratogenic event. Malformations due to the event of twinning itself are conjoined twins, amorphous twins, sirenomelia, holoprosencephaly, neural tube defects and anencephaly. Other malformations result from vascular interchange between monozygotic twins, and include acardia in one twin, disseminated intravascular coagulation (DIC) from embolization, with defects such as microcephaly, hydranencephaly, intestinal atresia, cutis aplasia and limb amputation.

Postural deformities

Deformations such as talipes and hip dysplasia result from intrauterine crowding and are equally common in monozygotic and dizygotic twins.

Twin-to-twin transfusion

This occurs in monozygous twins with a shared placenta. The donor (anaemic) twin grows poorly if the transfusions have been occurring over a long period of time. In acute fetofetal transfusion the twins are similar in size but one is grossly anaemic and the other plethoric. Rapid treatment of the anaemic twin may be necessary (see p. 205) and the plethoric twin may require a dilutional exchange transfusion (see p. 211). An acute twin-to-twin bleed may cause severe hypotension in one twin, which may cause cerebral infarction and subsequent cerebral palsy.

Infection

This occurs much more commonly in the first twin and probably relates to premature rupture of the membranes of the first amniotic sac.

Asphyxia

The second twin is more vulnerable to

asphyxia than the first twin. This is related to delayed delivery, cord prolapse, placental separation and malpresentation. The second twin, if SGA, is also more at risk of respiratory distress syndrome (RDS) and hypoglycaemia. Asphyxia is more common in twins than singletons owing to increased rates of prematurity, operative delivery and malpresentation.

Respiratory distress syndrome

Overall, there is an 8.5% incidence of RDS in twins, with 29% of preterm twins being diagnosed as having RDS. The increased incidence in the second twin probably relates to birth asphyxia rather than a difference in lecithin to sphingomyelin (L/S) ratios.

Neurological morbidity

Twins are over-represented in populations with cerebral palsy (5–10% in most studies), particularly spastic diplegia. Probable antecedents are premature birth, growth retardation, birth trauma, asphyxia and intrauterine demise of one twin. The risk of a twin developing cerebral palsy is 5–6 times higher than in a singleton pregnancy, and the risk in a triplet is 17–20 times higher than in a singleton. This risk is particularly increased where there is the death of a monozygotic co-twin *in utero*. In all such cases the brain of the surviving twin must be carefully examined with ultrasound or magnetic resonance imaging (MRI) to detect evidence of cerebral infarction (most likely periventricular leukomalacia (PVL)). The mechanism for this is that the twins share a placental circulation. When a co-twin dies, the mixing of the blood supplies means that the falling blood pressure of the dying twin will cause the surviving twin to become transiently hypotensive, with resultant cerebral injury. It is estimated that the risk of cerebral palsy in a surviving monozygotic twin whose co-twin dies is 12 times greater than when both twins survive.

IMPACT OF ASSISTED REPRODUCTION ON MULTIPLE GESTATION

The past decade has seen an expansion in therapeutic options available to the 8–12% of couples who experience difficulty in conception. In 1978, Edwards and Steptoe pioneered *in vitro* fertilization and many technologies, including gamete intrafallopian transfer (GIFT), have followed. Associated with ovulation stimulation and the new technologies there has been a dramatic increase in multiple births—not just twins, but triplets and higher multiples —placing extraordinary demands on neonatal intensive care units.

PROGNOSIS

The perinatal mortality rate is much higher for multiple pregnancies than for singletons, with a 12–15-fold greater incidence of both stillbirth and neonatal death. Similarly, twinning is markedly over-represented in neonatal morbidity. The mortality rate for the second twin is considerably higher than that for the first. At the Mater Hospital, multiple births represent 3.8% of all births but contribute 18.8% of admissions to the intensive care nursery, and 29.6% of all neonatal deaths.

Parents need a great deal of support and advice with the care of their twins or triplets. The mother particularly needs encouragement to breastfeed her infants. Voluntary community groups, such as the Twins Club and Twins and Multiple Birth Association, may be helpful in providing support and counselling.

FURTHER READING

Bryan, E.M. (1983) *The Nature and Nurture of Twins*. Baillière Tindall, London.

Gall, S.A. (ed.) (1988) Twin pregnancy. *Clinics in Perinatology*, **15**(1), 1–162.

26 Neonatal transport and organization of perinatal services

TRANSPORT *IN UTERO*

The ideal time to transfer a potentially sick infant is *in utero*, if the problem can be anticipated. High-risk pregnancies should be transferred before delivery and a high-risk fetus should be transferred *in utero* to a unit with perinatal intensive care facilities. In all cases there must be consultation before transfer with the receiving hospital. Unfortunately, not all neonatal problems can be recognized from an at-risk pregnancy, and some women are unwilling to be transported before delivery.

The rationale for transporting sick or low birthweight (LBW) neonates to special care or intensive care nurseries is based on the premise that specialized units reduce mortality and improve outcome, and that these advantages outweigh the risk of transport. A number of studies have reported a lower incidence of IVH (intraventricular haemorrhage) in infants born in a referring hospital after *in utero* transfer than in a similar group of outborn babies (Cooke 1983).

ORGANIZATION OF PERINATAL CARE

Levels of neonatal care in the UK were proposed by the British Paediatric Association and the British Association for Perinatal Paediatrics and are divided into three categories (Categories of Babies Requiring Neonatal Care 1992). Similar levels of care have been defined by the Sub Specialty Services Subcommittee of the Australian Health Ministers Advisory Council (1990).

Description of neonatal services

Neonatal intensive care is a coordinated effort by healthcare providers in a defined geographical region to intervene in the reproductive process so as to make available to every neonate a level of medical care commensurate with the perceived risk of neonatal death or serious morbidity.

Integration of neonatal and obstetric services into a perinatal programme offers the best opportunity for prevention and treatment.

A neonatal intensive care unit should provide care for all babies born in a district or region, and babies requiring intensive care are referred to the intensive care nursery. Facilities for neonatal surgery and cardiology should be available in neonatal intensive care units.

1 *Neonatal units in Britain* are classified according to the intensity of the care they provide and are described as follows.

Level 1 intensive care (maximal intensive care): care given in an intensive care nursery which provides continuous skilled supervision by qualified and specially trained nursing and medical staff. Such care includes support of the infant's parents. This requires 5.5 nurses, qualified and trained, per cot.

Level 2 intensive care (high-dependency intensive care): an intensive or special care nursery which provides continuous skilled supervision by qualified and specially trained nursing staff who may care for more babies than in level 1 intensive care. Medical supervision is not so immediate as in level 1 intensive care. Care includes support of the infant's parents. This requires 3.5 nurses, qualified and trained, per cot.

Special care: care given in a special care nursery, transitional care ward or postnatal ward which provides care and treatment exceeding normal routine care. Some aspects of special care can be undertaken by a mother supervised by qualified nursing staff. Special nursing care includes support and education of the infant's parents. This requires 1.0 qualified nurse per cot.

Normal care: care given by the mother substitute, with medical or neonatal nursing advice if needed.

Level 1 intensive care should be provided for the following babies:

1 receiving assisted ventilation (including intermittent positive pressure ventilation (IPPV), intermittent mandatory ventilation (IMV) and continuous positive airway pressure (CPAP) and in the first 24 h after its withdrawal);

2 of less than 27 weeks' gestation for the first 48 h after birth;

3 with birthweight less than 1000 g for the first 48 h after birth;

4 who require major emergency surgery for the preoperative period and postoperatively for 48 h;

5 on the day of death;

6 being transported by a team including medical and nursing staff;

7 who are receiving peritoneal dialysis;

8 who require exchange transfusions complicated by other disease processes;

9 with severe respiratory disease in the first 48 h of life requiring a fractional inspiratory oxygen (FiO_2) of > 0.6;

10 with recurrent apnoea needing frequent intervention, for example over five stimulations in 8 h or resuscitation with IPPV two or more times in 24 h;

11 with significant requirements for circulatory support, for example inotropes, three or more infusions of colloid in 24 h, or infusions of prostaglandins.

Level 2 intensive care should be provided for the following babies:

1 requiring total parenteral nutrition;

2 who are having convulsions;

3 being transported by a trained, skilled neonatal nurse alone;

4 with an arterial line or chest drain;

5 with respiratory disease in the first 48 h of life requiring an FiO_2 of 0.4–0.6;

6 with recurrent apnoea requiring stimulation up to five times in an 8-h period or any resuscitation with IPPV;

7 who require an exchange transfusion;

8 who are more than 48 h postoperative and require complex nursing procedures;

9 with tracheostomy for first 2 weeks.

Special care should be provided for the following babies:

1 requiring continuous monitoring of respiration or heart rate or by transcutaneous transducers;

2 receiving additional oxygen;

3 with tracheostomy after first 2 weeks;

4 being given intravenous glucose and electrolyte solutions;

5 who are being tube fed;

6 who have had minor surgery in the previous 24 h;

7 who require terminal care but not on the day of death;

8 being barrier nursed;

9 undergoing phototherapy;

10 receiving special monitoring (for example frequent glucose or bilirubin estimations);

11 needing constant supervision (for example babies whose mothers are drug abusers);

12 being treated with antibiotics.

2 *Neonatal units in Australia* are classified according to the intensity of the care they provide and are described as follows.

Level 3 units provide the highest level of life support, which includes the mechanical ventilation of infants. Cots are divided into ventilator (1 : 1 or 1 : 1.5 nurse/patient ratio) and high-dependency non-ventilator (1 : 2).

The requirement for Level 3 cots is 1.1/1000 live births, with 0.7 ventilator and 0.4 non-ventilator cots.

Level 2 units (special care) are mainly for infants who require less intensive care than Level 3 and are used in a 'step-down' capacity. Cots are divided into Level 2A, high dependency (ratio 1 : 3), and Level 2B, low or medium dependency (ratio 1 : 5).

The requirement for Level 2 cots is 4.25/1000 live births.

Level 1 units care only for healthy infants and each obstetric bed is said to possess a Level 1 cot as well.

Level 4 is a term that has been used to describe services provided to neonates requiring paediatric subspecialty care (e.g. those with complex metabolic and/or cardiac conditions, and surgical cases). Units at paediatric referral centres provide Level 4 neonatal services.

The development of perinatal services and changes in clinical practice have included:

1 the development of specialist perinatal units to concentrate expertise and utilize high-cost services efficiently;

2 collaborative antenatal and perinatal management of high-risk pregnancies;

3 emphasis on *in-utero* transfer of high-risk pregnancies to tertiary-level hospitals to optimize perinatal management;

4 coordinated neonatal transport of sick and premature newborn from peripheral hospitals to Level 3 neonatal intensive care units;

5 application of technological developments in the areas of fetal monitoring, prenatal diagnosis and neonatal intensive care.

Normal care. This is care given in a postnatal ward, usually by the mother under the supervision of a midwife or doctor but requiring minimal medical or nursing advice.

All maternity units must provide normal care for babies. A district general hospital with a consultant obstetric unit should provide special care facilities and approximately 6% of infants will require this type of care.

NEONATAL TRANSPORT

Infants requiring transport

The decision to transfer a sick neonate will depend on the expertise of the intensive care nursery, the safety of travel and the facilities available at the hospital where the baby was born. Discussion with a neonatal paediatrician may obviate the need for transport or provide advice on the best methods of transfer. Personnel from the Neonatal Emergency Transport Service can assist with the decision on whether transfer is necessary.

Consideration should be given to the transfer of the following infants to special care or intensive care nurseries:

1 birthweight less than 1750 g;

2 respiratory distress of early onset or persisting more than 4–6 h;

3 oxygen requirement > 50% or associated apnoea, meconium aspiration or suspected pneumonia;

4 apnoeic episodes;

5 convulsions;

6 depression following birth asphyxia;

7 jaundiced infants in need of exchange transfusion;

8 bleeding;

9 surgical conditions;

10 congenital heart disease;

11 severe or multiple congenital abnormalities;

12 need for special diagnostic or therapeutic services;

13 'unwell' infants with lethargy, poor perfusion, oliguria, etc.

Preparation for transport

The infant should be resuscitated and his condition stabilized prior to transport. While awaiting transfer the referring hospital should provide the following care:

1 the infant is kept warm (ideally servo-controlled to a skin temperature of 36.5°C). Bubble plastic may help to reduce heat loss;

2 the infant is given sufficient oxygen to maintain a pink colour (cyanotic threshold test is useful). If blood-gas analysis is available, the arterial oxygen tension should be maintained at 50–80 mmHg (6.7–9.7 kPa). Oxygen saturation should be maintained > 90%;

3 ensure a clear airway by adequate suction;

4 ensure adequate respiration;

5 frequent observations of temperature, heart rate, respiratory rate, blood pressure and blood sugar by reagent stick;

6 procedures for surgical patients:
  (a) attention to fluids and electrolytes;
  (b) intravascular volume;
  (c) special requirements;

7 intravenous dextrose with maintenance of blood glucose > 2.5 mmol/L;

8 prostaglandin E (PGE) infusion if possibility of duct-dependent cyanotic heart disease (see p. 194).

Principles of stabilization

The amount of stabilization prior to departure depends on the baby's condition and the rate of progress of the disease. It is also influenced by the distance to be travelled, the time for transport and the mode of transport.

It is important not to waste time, power, oxygen or air. Always use the nursery or ambulance utilities where possible. Staff must be aware of the difficulties of detecting and correcting problems in transit, and must ensure appropriate stabilization before transport.

Important decisions to be made

1 Intubation.

2 Exogenous surfactant administration, by either referring or retrieval staff.

Individual Neonatal Emergency Transport Systems need to develop their own protocols.

Before leaving

The referring hospital should provide the following:

1 perinatal history sheet, completed in detail;

2 signed parental consent for the infant's transfer and treatment;

3 copies of relevant records and results of tests, including X-rays;

4 10 mL of clotted blood from the mother to allow accurate cross-matching prior to surgery or exchange transfusion;

5 cord blood if available;

6 placenta if available.

Choice of vehicle

On the UK mainland infants are generally transferred by the road ambulance service. Occasionally, a fixed-wing aircraft (civil or RAF) is necessary for transportation overseas or over longer distances. In Australia there is usually a range of options, including road ambulance (up to 100–150 km), helicopter (up to 250 km) and fixed-wing (> 200 km). The choice of vehicle depends on availability, distance, degree of urgency, weather conditions and other factors. Each transfer is considered individually on its merits.

Principles of transportation

These include:

1 complete resuscitation and stabilization of the infant prior to transport;

2 procedures such as insertion of an intravenous line or umbilical artery catheter, intubation, mechanical ventilation and Polaroid photography of the baby for the mother are performed prior to transport if indicated;

3 the baby is not fed during transport and the stomach is aspirated prior to leaving the referring hospital. Gastric tube remains *in situ*;

4 frequent gastric and pharyngeal suction is necessary to prevent aspiration;

5 an intravenous (i.v.) line with 10% dextrose is set up prior to transfer to prevent hypoglycaemia;

6 if oxygen is necessary, it should ideally be warmed and humidified;

7 the percentage of inspired oxygen should be measured with an oxygen analyser;

8 a headbox should be used if greater than 30% inspired oxygen is necessary;

9 oxygenation should be monitored continuously by either pulse oximetry or transcutaneous P_{O_2};

10 monitoring of temperature, heart rate and respiration rate is essential, and monitoring of blood pressure is desirable.

Who should accompany the baby?

A nursing sister should accompany babies over

1500 g who are not critically ill. The attending doctor, registrar or resident should escort babies with apnoea, convulsions, or spontaneously breathing infants with respiratory distress who require oxygen. A neonatal retrieval team is usually necessary for infants of birthweight less than 1500 g and those requiring mechanical ventilation. It is desirable, but not always practicable, that the mother should be transported with her baby to promote bonding. Careful monitoring of the baby's heart rate, respiratory rate, temperature and blood pressure should be continued during transport.

Surgical problems

Babies with surgical lesions may have special problems, including:

Diaphragmatic hernia. These babies must not receive bag-and-mask ventilation. If mechanical ventilation is necessary, it should be through a carefully positioned endotracheal tube. If possible, very high ambient oxygen environments are preferable to ventilation because of the risk of pneumothorax. The stomach must be frequently aspirated via a nasogastric tube. Correct acidosis before departure and consider paralysis if hypoxic.

Oesophageal atresia with tracheo-oesophageal fistula. Feeding is absolutely contraindicated in these infants. The infant is nursed prone with body elevated to 30° from the horizontal, and frequent suctioning with an indwelling nasopharyngeal tube is essential to empty the blind-ending upper pouch. Limit crying with the use of a pacifier.

Exomphalos/gastroschisis/myelomeningocoele. The eviscerated lesions should be wrapped in a sterile plastic bag to prevent heat and fluid losses from evaporation and excessive cooling. The infant is nursed on the surface opposite to the lesion. Reposition the bowel if it appears to have impaired blood supply. Assess perfusion and give colloid if necessary.

An indwelling open nasogastric tube is placed in the stomach and aspirated intermit-

tently. An intravenous infusion is desirable. Moist packs are contraindicated as they quickly become cold and lead to hypothermia.

Bowel obstruction. Fluid and electrolyte disturbances should be corrected prior to transport and continuous nasogastric suction maintained throughout. The infant should be nursed prone or lying on his right side with the head up.

Pierre Robin sequence/choanal atresia. In these conditions an adequate airway must be established for the infant, both while awake and when asleep. The infant is nursed in the prone position and an oropharyngeal airway strapped in place. In some cases a long nasopharyngeal tube is positioned just above the epiglottis. Continuous observation of respiratory pattern, skin colour and oxygen saturation is required.

Transport equipment

1 *Quantity.* A minimum of two sets of equipment is required for any one geographical area to allow for breakdown, maintenance, concurrent calls and twin transportation.

2 *Safety requirements.* The equipment should satisfy all areas of safety regulation and other statutory requirements.

3 *Transport incubators.* These must provide a neutral thermal environment under a wide range of external temperature and environmental conditions. There must be good lighting and visibility and easy access. Incubators must be capable of operation from a mains source, aircraft (24 V d.c.) and road vehicle (10–13 V d.c.) power. Most transport systems have an air compressor.

4 *Monitoring equipment.* Monitoring of temperature, heart rate, inspired oxygen concentration and oxygen partial pressure and/or saturation is essential. Blood pressure monitoring is desirable.

5 *Respiratory support.* Independent supplies of oxygen and medical air are required to provide controlled inspired oxygen concentrations from 21% to 100%. Ideally, inspired gases should be heated and humidified.

6 *A mechanical ventilator* able to provide IPPV and CPAP is required. A suitable hand-operated ventilator system, consisting of bag and mask with manometer, must be available as a back-up to mechanical ventilation.

7 *Suction.* Suction equipment must have an independent power supply, and negative pressure must be controlled and adjustable. Oral suction mucus traps must be available as back-up.

8 *Infusion pumps.* Infusion by constant-rate pump is required for intravenous and/or intra-arterial infusion. Battery-operated syringe infusion pumps are safer and lighter.

Emergency equipment

9 Equipment for emergency intubation: laryngoscope, endotracheal tubes with introducers, tape.

10 Equipment for emergency insertion of chest tube: intercostal catheter, Heimlich one-way flutter valve.

11 Equipment for emergency insertion of umbilical arterial catheter.

12 Drugs for resuscitation, such as adrenaline, sodium bicarbonate, calcium gluconate, plasma. Special drugs such as surfactant, PGE, anticonvulsants.

Other equipment

13 Polaroid camera.
14 Paediatric stethoscopes.
15 Blood glucose meter and strips.

Transport vehicles

Transport vehicles should be dedicated neonatal ambulance vehicles, and are desirable for large services where retrievals exceed 150 per annum. The vehicles must meet national passenger safety standards, and have adequate seating with safety restraints for staff. Adequate lighting and internal climate control are necessary. A fixed positive mounting system is required to restrain the transport system. Tolerable noise and vibration levels

are an essential prerequisite. External communication should be available to allow the team to be directly connected to any telephone number at any stage of the transfer.

Aerial transport

Transfer by aeroplane or helicopter has several unique problems.

1 Any air flight, even in a pressurized cabin, decreases ambient pressure with resultant expansion of gases in body cavities. This is particularly relevant in infants with pneumothorax, lung cysts or trapped gas in the bowel or the peritoneal cavity. Pain may occur as a result of expansion of air in the facial sinuses in larger infants.

2 Inspired oxygen is decreased owing to the rarefied atmosphere.

3 Noise and vibration may lead to loss of the gag reflex and promote vomiting, with resultant aspiration.

4 Difficulty with illumination, observation and especially auscultation of the heart and lungs.

The role of a neonatal transport service

An integral part of a successful neonatal transport programme is frequent communication with personnel in the referring nursery, and especially with the mother. The infant should be transferred back to the referring nursery at the earliest possible time.

A coordinated neonatal transport service organizes retrievals and return transfers of infants back to the base hospital, and is also involved with consultation services and education for outlying practitioners. It provides an active role in the coordination of all neonatal transport facilities, utilization of perinatal facilities and outreach education.

It plays a pivotal role in the coordination and utilization of perinatal facilities. The selection and standardization of transport facilities involves liaison with all transport providers. There is also a commitment to audit, research and quality assurance.

Care of parents

The transport team must be sensitive to the needs of the parents during this stressful period. They must introduce themselves to parents and explain the nature of the transport, treatment and likely prognosis. Parents are encouraged to touch their baby and are offered a Polaroid photograph. An information booklet about the tertiary hospital is provided and informed consent for transfer and care given.

Relationships with referring hospital and staff

The retrieval staff must be sensitive in relating to referral hospital personnel: never, either directly or by implication, criticize the referring doctor's management. Smooth communication and relationships between referring and receiving units are essential for effective regionalization of care. Staff should involve ambulance officers with equipment needs and educate them about the infant's condition. A debriefing with referring staff is an essential component of quality management improvement.

REFERENCES

Cooke, R.W.I. (1983) *In utero* transfer to specialist centres. *Archives of Disease in Childhood* 58, 483–484.

FURTHER READING

Australian Health Ministers Advisory Council. Sub Specialty Services Subcommittee (1990) *Guidelines for Level Three Neonatal Intensive Care*. Australian Institute of Health, Canberra.

Bowman, E.D., Levi, S.M., McLean, A.J. & Presbury, F.E. (eds) (1998) *Stabilization and Transport of Newborn Infants and At-Risk Pregnancies*, 4th edn. Newborn Emergency Transport Service, Melbourne.

Report of working group of the British Association of Perinatal Medicine and Neonatal Nurses Association on categories of babies requiring neonatal care (1992) *Archives of Diseases in Childhood* 67, 868–869.

Jaimovich, D.G. & Vidyasagar, D. (eds) (1996) *Handbook of Pediatric and Neonatal Transport Medicine*. Hanley & Belfus, Inc. Philadelphia; Mosby, St Louis.

Mir, N.A. (ed.) (1997) *Manual of Neonatal Transport*. Nisar A Mir, Liverpool.

Parents whose babies have had a prolonged stay in hospital will be anxious about the discharge of those babies. Ideally, the mother should 'room in' with her baby, or at least sleep in the hospital in close proximity to her baby for some days prior to discharge, so that she can gain confidence and learn to care for her previously sick infant. Prior to discharge the parents will need advice on feeding, iron, vitamins, introduction of mixed feeds, immunizations, etc. An information booklet on these subjects should be issued to the parents. A full discharge letter to the infant's general practitioner and referring paediatrician/obstetrician should be sent shortly after the discharge of all high-risk neonates.

FEEDING ADVICE

Feeding of the low birthweight (LBW) infant is discussed in Chapter 6. The frequency of feeds depends on the maturity and neurological integrity of the infant, but 3–4-hourly feeds are usually necessary on discharge from the neonatal unit. The mother should be encouraged to demand feed her baby, but feeds should not be more than 5 h apart during the day. It is recommended that infants should not be given undiluted cows' ('doorstep') milk until 12 months corrected age.

Iron

Term infants receive sufficient iron from breast milk until about 6–9 months of age. Although the iron content in breast milk is low (0.5 mg/L), the absorption is excellent. The term infant being fed on iron-fortified formula receives sufficient iron until 5–6 months, at which time iron-containing foods such as cereal, vegetables, egg and meat should be started. The term infant who receives unmodified cows' milk requires supplemental iron therapy during the first 6 months of life. Although the preterm infant needs supplemental iron from 3 months of age, whether breastfed or not, for convenience iron therapy is commenced in hospital on day 28, with 30–50 mg/day of ferrous sulphate or ferrous gluconate paediatric mixture.

Additional folic acid is only necessary if the infant has a haemolytic disease (particularly important for babies with rhesus isoimmunization).

Vitamins

Full-term infants probably receive adequate vitamins in their breast milk or vitamin-fortified breast-milk substitutes. However, preterm infants and other ill infants will require extra vitamins, especially D and C. Preterm infants with inadequate vitamin C intake often have an immaturity of the enzyme phenylalanine hydroxylase and may develop transient tyrosinaemia, which is potentially harmful to the brain. A multivitamin preparation such as Dalivit, Pentavite or Abidec (0.6 mL) should be commenced on day 7 of life and continued until 6–12 months in premature infants. Sick and extremely preterm infants receive multivitamins in parenteral nutrition infusion, and oral supplementation can wait until the baby is on full enteral feeding.

Fluoride

Fluoride drops are recommended in areas in which the water supply is not fluoridated. The dose is four drops per day in the first year of life, eight drops per day from 1 to 2 years and 15 drops per day or 1 tablet after 2 years of age. It is important to adhere to this dosage

Table 27.1 Recommended immunization schedule for the UK and Australia

	UK	Australia
Hepatitis B	0.1 and 6 months (selected infants)	
BCG	At birth (given only to selected infants, see text)	At birth (selected infants)
DPT and polio	2, 3 and 4 months	2, 4 and 6 months
HIB†	2, 3 and 4 months	2, 4 and 6 months
DPT	—	18 months
Booster DPT and polio	3–5 years 13–18 years	5 years 15 years
MMR	12–18 months	12 months
Booster MMR	3–5 years	
Rubella*	10–14 years	10–16 years

* Given to girls only if not given MMR earlier.
† *Haemophilus influenzae* B vaccine given at same time as DPT, but into opposite limb.

Table 27.2 Immunizations used in UK and Australia

Vaccine	Type	Dose	Route
BCG	Live attenuated	0.05 mL (for infants)	Intradermal
Pertussis*	Killed *B. pertussis*	0.5 mL	Deep i.m. injection
Diphtheria*	Toxoid	0.5 mL	Deep i.m. injection
Tetanus*	Toxoid	0.5 mL	Deep i.m. injection
Polio	Live attenuated virus (Sabin)	3 drops	Orally
Measles†	Live attenuated virus	0.5 mL (reconstituted freeze dried)	i.m.
Mumps†	Live attenuated virus	0.5 mL (reconstituted freeze dried)	i.m.
Rubella†	Live attenuated virus	0.5 mL (reconstituted freeze dried)	i.m.
Hepatitis B	Live attenuated virus	0.5 mL	i.m.

* These three are given as a single dose of triple vaccine.
† These three are given as a single dose as the MMR vaccine.

schedule as excessive fluoride may cause tooth staining as a result of fluorosis. Fluoride drops should preferably be given in water rather than milk to permit better absorption.

IMMUNIZATION

Details of the immunization schedules in the UK and Australia are shown in Tables 27.1 and 27.2. The current recommendations advise starting the immunization programme when the infant is 2 months of actual age, rather than age corrected for prematurity.

Contraindications to pertussis immunization

The following are the current contraindications given by the UK Department of Health:

Table 27.3 Milestones in development. It must be emphasized that these ages are very approximate and there are wide variations between normal babies

Age	Social	Speech and language	Gross motor	Fine motor
1 month	Quietens when talked to	—	Holds head up momentarily	Fists clenched at rest
2 months	Smiling with good visual interest	Listens to bell	Chin off couch when prone	Hands largely open
3 months	Follows objects through 180°	Vocalizes when talked to	Weight on forearms when lying prone	Holds objects placed in hands
4 months	Laughs aloud	—	Pulling to sit—no head lag	Hands come together
6 months	Imitates	Localizes sound	Lying prone, pushes up on hands	Reaches for objects
7 months	Feeds him/herself with biscuit	Makes 4 different sounds	Sits unsupported	Transfers from hand to hand
9 months	Waves bye-bye	Says 'mama'	Stands holding on	Pincer grasp
12 months	Plays 'pat-a-cake'	2–3 words	Walking unsupported	Gives objects
15 months	Drinks from a cup	4–5 words	Climbs up stairs	Tower of 2 cubes
18 months	Points to 3 parts of body	8–10 words	Gets up and down stairs	Tower 3–4 cubes
21 months	Dry (mostly) during day	2 word sentences	Runs	Scribbles circles
24 months	Puts on shoes	2–3 word sentences	Walks up and down stairs	Tower 6–7 cubes
2½ years	Recognizes colours	Knows full name		Copies with pencil
3 years	Dresses and undresses fully	Tells stories		Copies with pencil

1 immunization should be temporarily withheld if the child is suffering from any acute illness. Minor infections without fever or systemic upset are not reasons for withholding immunization;
2 a history of severe local or general reaction to a previous dose;
3 a family history of allergy is not a contraindication; and
4 a stable neurological condition, including a perinatal history or a family history of fits, is not a contraindication. Children with evolving neurological conditions may be immunized when the condition has become stable.

High-risk groups, such as Asian or Aboriginal neonates, are given 0.1 mL BCG (bacillus Calmette–Guérin) vaccine intradermally within the first week of life. Surveys in British children have shown that this vaccine is over 70% effective, with protection lasting at least 15 years.

Infants born to mothers who are hepatitis B surface antigen positive (and hepatitis B e-antigen positive) should receive passive immunization with hepatitis B immune gammaglobulin (200 iu) as well as active immunization with 10 µg of hepatitis B vaccine as soon after birth as possible, and again at 1 and 6 months.

Modification to immunization schedule for preterm infants

Generally, preterm infants are immunized according to their actual postnatal age and not their corrected age. Some extremely preterm infants are still too unstable to receive diphtheria–pertussis–tetanus (DPT), HIB and polio at 2 months, and immunization needs to be deferred for some weeks. Preterm infants should receive paracetamol (20 mg/kg) and may require separate monitoring for 24–48 h after injection because of the high risk of apnoea. Acellular pertussis vaccine has not been shown to reduce the incidence of apnoea in extremely preterm infants. As Sabin (polio) vaccine is a live attenuated virus, it is preferable for this to be given to preterm infants on the morning of discharge so that there is no risk

to other infants from the excretion of virus in stools.

Hepatitis B immunization for infants of < 2000 g birthweight should be delayed until 1 month or just prior to hospital discharge. Infants of birthweight < 1000 g should be immunized when they weigh a minimum of 2000 g or when they are 2 months old.

GROWTH

The maternal and child health clinic or the general practitioner should follow growth during the first year of life and plot length, weight and head circumference on appropriate percentile graphs.

The use of charts allows accurate assessment of these important parameters of physical growth. As a guide, term infants usually double their birthweight by 5 months and treble it by 1 year. The head circumference usually grows about 1 cm a month for the first 6 months, and then 0.5 cm a month for the next 6 months. Most babies increase their length by 20–30 cm (or 50%) in the first year of life.

POSTNATAL DEVELOPMENT

There is great variability in infant development. The rate of progress is influenced by many factors, including gestational age, nutrition, intercurrent illness, environmental stimulation and emotional support. Milestones in development can be considered in four groups: social, speech and language, gross motor and fine motor. The ages for the acquisition of these skills and milestones are approximate and there are wide variations between normal babies. Table 27.3 summarizes some of these important milestones. If there is evidence of significant developmental delay or cerebral palsy, the child should be referred to a child development centre for more comprehensive assessment by a multidisciplinary team. The totality of handicapping conditions in very low birthweight (VLBW) infants relates to corrected postnatal age and is illustrated in Fig. 27.1.

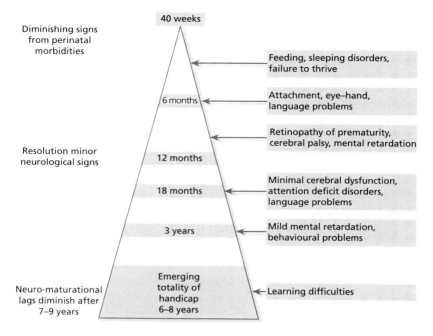

Fig. 27.1 Ages at which disabilities become evident in VLBW infants.

Definitions

Great care must be taken to use the terms 'handicap', 'impairment' and 'disability' correctly, so that comparisons can be made between different centres. The following are the internationally accepted World Health Organization (WHO) definitions.

IMPAIRMENT

Any loss or abnormality of psychological or anatomical structure or function.

DISABILITY

Any restriction or lack of ability (resulting from an impairment) in performing an activity in the manner or within the range considered to be normal.

HANDICAP

A disadvantage for an individual arising from a disability that limits or prevents the fulfil-

ment of a role that should be normal for that individual.

SPECIALIZED FOLLOW-UP CLINICS

Infants who are at risk for chronic handicapping conditions should be followed in special multidisciplinary clinics or by their paediatrician. Categories of infant that should be considered for specialized follow-up include:
1 those who were mechanically ventilated in the neonatal period;
2 VLBW infants (less than 1500 g birthweight);
3 those with severe perinatal asphyxia;
4 those with intracranial haemorrhage;
5 those with neonatal convulsions;
6 those with abnormal neurological examination at discharge;
7 infants who had major surgery.

The benefits of following up high-risk infants in specialized clinics include:
1 early diagnosis of problems enables early intervention and perhaps a better long-term prognosis;

Table 27.4 Complications in the first year of life in preterm infants

Medical	
Respiratory	Nasal congestion
	Exacerbation of bronchopulmonary dysplasia
	Recurrent wheezing
	SIDS
Cardiac	Patent ductus arteriosus
	Ventricular septal defect
Ophthalmic	Retinopathy of prematurity
	Strabismus
	Myopia
Auditory	Sensorineural hearing loss
	Conductive dysfunction
Surgical	Inguinal hernia, umbilical hernia, undescended testes, hydrocoele
Growth	Failure to achieve genetic growth potential
Gastrointestinal	Vomiting, gastro-oesophageal reflux, constipation, colic
Neurological	
Major	Spastic diplegia, hypotonia, hemiplegia, quadriplegia, hydrocephalus, microcephaly, mental retardation
Minor	Ataxia, incoordination and clumsiness, specific learning difficulties, attention deficit disorders, mild to moderate cognitive impairment
Miscellaneous	Child abuse, neglect, deprivation, behavioural disturbances, emotional disturbances, failure to thrive

2 evaluation of the perinatal factors that have an adverse effect on outcome, with subsequent modification of methods of perinatal intensive care;
3 evaluation of the long-term prognosis of high-risk populations of infants;
4 assessment of a cost–benefit analysis for perinatal intensive care.

Follow-up of preterm infants

The assessment of growth in preterm infants must always take into consideration the number of weeks of prematurity. Growth and development should be assessed according to the corrected age:

Corrected age = postnatal age – number of weeks infant is preterm

Data supporting this biological model suggest that, for infants less than or equal to 28 weeks' gestation, correction should be continued for 4 years; in those 29–31 weeks for 2 years; those 32–34 weeks for 1 year; and in those 35 weeks and beyond no correction is made for gestational age.

The healthy preterm baby who is appropriate for gestational age (AGA) should grow at the same rate as a term infant with the same growth patterns as low birthweight infants, i.e. regains birthweight at 2 weeks postnatal age and then accelerates, so that by the expected date of delivery the infant will be close to the expected weight of a term infant. At follow-up the height, weight and head circumference will be at or just below the 50th percentile for post-conceptual age.

Growth failure often occurs in small for gestational age (SGA) and sick preterm babies, who may receive inadequate nutrition for the first 4–6 weeks. In this latter group linear and head growth virtually cease, and even when adequate nutrition is established growth may remain suboptimal. The SGA infant usually loses little, if any, weight in the neonatal period and then rapidly gains weight to reach his potential growth percentile. This growth spurt may not be maintained, and a permanent deficit in somatic growth persists into childhood.

Growth of head circumference is often difficult to interpret in preterm babies. This is partly due to the scaphocephalic head shape. For 3–4 weeks after birth, growth in head circumference is suboptimal at about 0.2 cm/week; then follows a period of rapid head growth (catch-up brain growth spurt) at about 1 cm/week for 1–2 months; the head then grows at the normal rate of 1 cm/month for the first 6 months and then 0.5 cm/month for the rest of the first year of life.

Common problems identified in preterm infants at follow-up are shown in Table 27.4.

FURTHER READING

Ballard, R.A. (1988) *Pediatric Case of the ICN Graduate*. W.B. Saunders, Philadelphia.

Department of Health, Welsh Office, Scottish Home and Health Department (1996) *Immunization against Infectious Disease*. HMSO, London.

Harvey, D., Cooke, R.W.I. & Levitt, G.A. (eds) (1989) *The Baby Under 1000 g*. Wright, London.

Illingworth, R.S. (1983) *The Development of the Infant and Young Child. Abnormal and Normal*, 8th edn. Churchill Livingstone, Edinburgh.

28 Parent–infant attachment and support for parents experiencing perinatal loss

PARENT–INFANT ATTACHMENT

Following important observations in the 1970s by Klaus and Kennell (1982), it is now well accepted that a powerful parent–infant attachment ('bonding'), especially in mothers, has usually been established by the time of birth. Moreover, their research showed that little attention had been given to the possible effects on parents of the death of an infant who had had little or no opportunity for life. Since then there has been considerable literature on perinatal death, revealing that the care of recently bereaved parents leaves much to be desired. Thus, an understanding of the parent–infant process can help the doctor and other healthcare givers to minimize the devastating effect of perinatal loss, and also to understand the effects of prematurity and congenital abnormality on a family.

For mothers a bond is formed quite early in pregnancy, stimulated by hormonal changes, psychological preparation and fantasies about the unborn child. 'Nesting' behaviour is manifested by the preparation of a nursery and the purchase of baby clothes. For the father the attachment process is less recognizable during the pregnancy but heightens with the birth, enhanced by an involvement with the delivery and handling of the baby. A sense of pride and hope for the future ensues.

Steps in attachment

The actual process by which attachment bonds are formed is unknown, but the time periods listed below are believed to be essential to this process. The strength of the attachment during these stages may vary from one woman to the next.

1 Planning the pregnancy.
2 Confirming the pregnancy.
3 Accepting the pregnancy.
4 Onset of fetal movements (quickening).
5 Accepting the fetus as an individual.
6 The birth process.
7 Seeing the baby.
8 Touching the baby.
9 Caretaking.

Most research, however, has concentrated on early contact in the immediate postnatal period. Extrapolation from animal research has proposed that there is a 'maternal-sensitive' or 'maternal-critical period' which is the optimal time for a bond of affection to develop between a mother and her infant. There is little doubt that the importance of this immediate postnatal period has been overemphasized in humans.

Parents learn to love their infant at varying times during the pregnancy and after birth. Parents 'bond' to their adopted babies, yet there has been no 'maternal-critical period'. It is apparent that humans differ from animals in their patterns of bonding.

A mother initially demonstrates her attachment in several ways.

1 She is able to establish eye contact with the infant, who is in a state of arousal after birth.
2 If she is left alone with her naked infant, she may touch each part of the body with her fingertips.
3 A mother becomes overprotective of her infant in the first few days after delivery and becomes anxious about crying and minor difficulties. This anxiety may appear excessive to hospital staff and family around her.
4 Babies may mimic the facial expressions of their parents, e.g. protrude their tongues.
5 Breastfeeding may be used to comfort and pacify the infant.

Management factors that promote attachment

The parents together plan the pregnancy and attend antenatal educational and physiotherapy classes. The antenatal preparation of breasts and nipples will assist with subsequent breastfeeding. The father should support the mother during labour and witness the birth of the baby. Unless the baby is critically ill, the mother and baby should be permitted to respond to each other in their own time and manner. Unnecessary separation of infant and mother must be avoided. The infant should 'room in' with the mother for 24 h of the day and be taken out to the nursery at night only if the mother is ill, or if other mothers are being disturbed. Breastfeeding on demand, even at night, should be actively encouraged. However, if a mother fails in her attempts to breastfeed or does not wish to do so, she must not be made to feel inadequate or guilty or told she is an unnatural mother. Successful bottle feeding is much better than unsuccessful breastfeeding.

Risk factors for failure to produce attachment

Mothers who plan their pregnancies have good expectations of the outcome, breastfeed their babies and rarely subsequently maltreat them. Some of the risk factors that may have an adverse effect on bonding are listed below.

DURING PREGNANCY

1 Unsupported pregnancies.
2 Where the father was unfaithful or deserted the mother during pregnancy.
3 Frequent pregnancies with excessive workload.
4 Maternal depression during the pregnancy.
5 Loss of an emotionally significant person in relation to the pregnancy, e.g. the maternal grandmother, grandfather, a loved sibling, a child of the mother or even a close friend, especially when the mother was somewhat isolated.

6 Conception during a period of marital conflict.

DURING LABOUR AND DELIVERY

1 Being left alone and afraid in the labour ward, or when the mother perceived the staff as unconcerned.
2 When the birth itself was more painful or prolonged than was expected.
3 When breastfeeding was thrust upon the mother by the staff.
4 When the mother was unable to see the child after delivery, without explanation, or was told that the baby was damaged.
5 When the mother herself was damaged as a result of the birth.
6 When the father exhibited more interest in the infant than in his partner.

IN THE NEONATAL AND POSTNATAL PERIOD

1 Prematurity.
2 Congenital malformations.
3 Critically ill infants requiring neonatal intensive care.
4 Postnatal depression.
   Rejection is more likely to occur when the infant has problems in the perinatal period or requires neonatal intensive care. There is a discrepancy between the idealized, perfect baby and the real baby: under these circumstances the parents require careful counselling and support.

Failure of bonding or attachment

When bonding fails there is rejection or non-acceptance of the child. This may result in problems for both the child and the mother.

LONG-TERM PROBLEMS IN THE CHILD

1 *Child abuse.* Several studies have shown that preterm infants are over-represented among abused children. Approximately 30% of battered children are premature, yet the overall incidence of prematurity is 6%.

2 *Idiopathic failure to thrive.* Failure to thrive without organic cause is sometimes due to neglect or deprivation. Studies have revealed a fourfold increase among preterm infants and babies who require prolonged hospitalization in the newborn period.

3 *Temper tantrums, infant colic, feeding problems, sleeplessness and vomiting.* Behavioural and feeding disorders are more common when an affectional bond has not been formed.

4 *Inadequate personality and poor interpersonal skills.* Infants who have been deprived of love and affection may subsequently have emotional and personality disturbances. They may become abusing or neglecting parents as adults, and so the cycle may repeat itself.

PROBLEMS IN THE MOTHER

1 Hesitant, clumsy handling of the baby.
2 Anxiety states and depression.
3 Mother states that 'the baby belongs to the hospital or nursing staff'.
4 Feelings of inadequacy, disappointment, failure, deprivation and anger.
5 Mother may complain that the baby does not bond with her.

CARE OF PARENTS OF CRITICALLY ILL INFANTS

The modern intensive care nursery is a bewildering, frightening place to the parents of a recently delivered premature or sick infant. These parents often have feelings of extreme frustration, stress, guilt and helplessness and must be counselled sensitively. The total care of the high-risk neonate must include the parents. The approach to the parents is discussed in a chronological manner, from antenatal clinic through to discharge and follow-up.

Antenatal contact

Women with high-risk pregnancies should be introduced, prior to delivery, to a 'baby doctor', whom they will probably meet after the baby is born. It is also helpful to the parents if they have the opportunity to visit the neonatal intensive care unit prior to delivery, so that they are aware of the sights that will greet them when they first enter to see their own baby.

Labour ward

When condition permits, the baby should be given to the mother for suckling and skin-to-skin contact for as long as possible. The baby should be suctioned, dried and warmed prior to being handled by the mother. Even if the baby is critically ill, his condition should be explained and the mother should see him. The open visiting policy of the nursery should be explained to the parents.

Intensive care nursery

When the baby's condition is stable, the mother and father should come into the nursery to see and touch their baby. Careful explanations are given regarding abnormal signs (retractions, bruising, etc.) and equipment (monitors, incubators, respirator, umbilical arterial catheter, etc.).

Before entering the nursery the parents will take off their coats, watches, rings, etc. and roll up their sleeves to above the elbows. They will be instructed on hand-washing, and in some units will wear overgowns. Having adopted this careful technique, there is no evidence that parental visiting and handling of premature infants have influenced the incidence of bacterial infection or even colonization. The organisms that parents harbour are less virulent and exhibit less antibiotic resistance than the commensal organisms of hospital staff. There is every reason for the parents to be intimately involved with their critically ill infant from the outset. The premature infant has enough physiological problems already without adding attachment problems to the list. The parents are informed that they may visit or ring the nursery 24 h a day, and that both parents will be kept informed of the baby's progress. Consideration should be given to providing a pamphlet explaining the intensive care nursery and encouraging the parents to become actively involved in their child's care. A Polaroid photograph may help the mother to accept her baby for the day or two before she is able to visit the nursery. Occasionally, the baby may be placed in a portable incubator and taken to the mother.

Parents' first visit to the intensive care nursery

Parents should be greeted and welcomed to the nursery. Again, the equipment should be carefully explained. It is most important for the mother to be able to establish eye contact with her baby, and if appropriate the goggles used with phototherapy may be removed. Often the mother will have to look through the porthole to establish an *en face* position with her infant (i.e. align her head with her baby's). Some parents are very apprehensive of handling, and usually state that their baby is too fragile to touch.

The nursing staff must work through this anxiety with the parents and encourage them to touch, fondle and caress their baby. Once the parents realize that their baby can actually see them, respond to their voices and can be pacified by them, their attachment grows.

Parents' subsequent visits to the intensive care nursery

The parents should be encouraged to actively participate in their baby's care. They derive great satisfaction from holding the gavage syringe, changing napkins and sponging the baby. Even though in an incubator, the baby can usually come out briefly for a cuddle, provided care is taken to maintain body temperature and the patency of all attached tubes. This policy may also be adopted where mechanical ventilation is required.

Most mothers are only too happy to express their breast milk for their baby. The 28-week gestation infant needs the milk from his own mother's breasts. It is remarkably well tolerated, considering the immaturity of the gastrointestinal tract at that gestation, and may decrease the incidence of necrotizing enterocolitis (NEC) and infection. The mother will

need a great deal of empathy and support from staff members to continue breast expression for the 8–10 weeks before her infant will be able to suckle. The role of maternal milk in feeding the very low birthweight (VLBW) infant is discussed on p. 55. When the mother lives at a distance from the hospital the transport of breast milk may be difficult. Nevertheless, breastfeeding should be encouraged while she is in hospital, so that the benefits of colostrum may be obtained.

Babies as individuals

Notes attached to the baby's bed are encouraging to the parents, e.g. 'Mum is to feed me at 3 pm. I am looking forward to my first breastfeed. Love Billy.'

The parents are asked to provide the staff with the baby's name as soon as possible. An artist can then write the name in large print on the incubator. The baby should be referred to as 'Billy' or 'Susie' where possible, and *never* as 'it'.

Appropriate decorations and mobiles which may help parents adjust to a long hospital stay may be attached to incubators. Parents are encouraged to use the pastoral care personnel of the hospital, or else to bring their own minister of religion to baptize or administer rites to the baby.

How is my baby doing?

The staff should answer this question in a realistic but optimistic way. Never should an unduly pessimistic attitude be conveyed, as this will only encourage detachment from the child. It has been shown that even if the baby dies, the parents gain from having attached to their child. Their grief is physiological and appropriate. It is difficult to grieve appropriately for someone you have never known. When asked the above question, it is often useful to ask the parents how *they* think the baby is getting on. Caution should be exercised when making predictions about outcome, and a problem-orientated approach to the baby should be avoided. It is easy for the parents to become involved with the intricacies of oxygen therapy and oxygen tension, rather than the baby as a whole.

The social worker

The social worker plays an important role in the intensive care nursery. She should be introduced to the mother at the first visit and help to prepare her for the difficult period ahead. The social worker provides support, investigating the attitudes of parents towards the child, and at the same time may uncover social and economic problems. Consideration should be given towards keeping a parental contact chart recording telephone enquiries, visits and the specific involvement of parents during these visits. This helps with communication, especially between nursing shifts.

Babies transferred to hospital

Parents of babies transferred from other hospitals into the intensive care nursery have unique problems. Prolonged parent–infant separation is common. If possible, the mother should be transferred along with the baby; but this may separate mother from her husband and other children. If the mother cannot be transferred, a Polaroid photograph and daily progress reports should be provided. Whenever possible, the baby should be transferred back to the referring hospital for recovery care.

Preparation for discharge

Once the requirements for intensive care are over, the baby will still need monitoring, incubator care and gavage feeding. This can be a very frustrating time for the parents, who have already experienced so much. Early discharge for LBW babies can safely be practised and may promote attachment. Babies have been discharged to an optimal home situation with birthweights below 1600 g, provided they are feeding well, the mother is handling competently, that they are gaining weight steadily, and that adequate follow-up can be maintained (Derbyshire *et al.* 1982).

CARING FOR PARENTS OF AN INFANT WHO DIES

Birth and grief—a paradox

A birth is an event which is usually associated with joy and excitement. It is preceded by planning, expectations, dreams and hopes. For most people, having a baby brings with it changes in the family structure which affect each family member in a different way. The 9 months of the pregnancy are filled with adjustments in role for the mother, father and siblings, and with an awareness that a new life is growing within the mother. Grandparents and members of the extended family share in the preparations and hopes. In many families there may be ambivalent feelings. Perhaps the pregnancy was unplanned or unwanted, or the siblings may be reluctant to share their parents with a new baby.

Whatever the hopes and feelings, the news that the baby is dead comes as an unexpected catastrophe. For parents who have experienced miscarriage or a stillbirth, the fact that they have never known the baby can make their loss seem even more unreal and difficult to accept. When the baby survives for a short time, the parents have had an opportunity to experience their child as a living being.

Some of the common characteristics of normal grief are outlined below. The stages of grief are not necessarily in this order, and occupy a variable period of time. Culberg (1972) has suggested that a normal grief reaction lasts 6–9 months, although the most intensive phase lasts from 1 to 6 weeks.

1 'Shock'.
2 Emotional release.
3 Utter depression, loneliness and isolation.
4 Physical symptoms, e.g. choking, dyspnoea, empty feeling, weakness, fatigue, insomnia, loss of appetite.
5 Panic—about their own worth and the safety of other children.
6 Guilt.
7 Anger.
8 Inability to return to normal activities.
9 Overcoming grief.
10 Readjustment of life.

Management of parents of critically ill babies

Parents of critically ill children will all have their own special difficulties to overcome. However, guidelines of proven value in decreasing pathological grief and promoting normal reactions are given below.

1 The parents are encouraged to visit the nursery and handle the baby.

2 There should be frank discussions with the doctor regarding the chance and quality of survival of the infant.

3 Parents of critically ill babies should be visited by the hospital priest or chaplain and asked if they would like to have their child baptized.

4 Once death is imminent the parents are encouraged to cuddle the baby, who may die in their arms. Occasionally, this may even occur outside the nursery, and in some instances the infant may be taken home if this is the parents' wish.

5 The parents should, if possible, be permitted to express their emotions and feelings without the use of sedation.

6 If the mother is in the postnatal ward, she is offered the privacy of a single room and discharged early.

7 The staff should discuss death, autopsy and funeral arrangements with the parents at the earliest opportunity.

8 A health visitor or social worker may visit the parents at their home if this is thought to be desirable.

9 Preliminary autopsy results are discussed with parents as soon as they are available.

10 A follow-up appointment is made 8 weeks after the death to discuss the autopsy findings and causes of death, and for counselling for further pregnancies.

In spite of these attempts to support the parents, the death of a newborn infant, whether sudden or expected, imposes a severe stress on the family. A longitudinal prospective study of bereaved parents (Vance *et al.* 1991) has shown that parental distress, as manifested by anxiety and depression, is greatest at 6–8 weeks. Although the timing of the follow-up appointment should not be changed, those who carry out the interview should be aware of this.

Bereavement counsellors and perinatal support groups

Beneficial support, additional to that provided by doctors, nurses and social workers, can be provided by trained bereavement counsellors or from other parents who have experienced and recovered from perinatal loss, e.g. Stillbirth and Neonatal Death Support Group (SANDS). Invaluable support may also be provided by books (e.g. Kubler-Ross 1975, 1977) and resource packages (e.g. Murray 1993) that help parents to understand the grieving process.

REFERENCES

Culberg, J. (1972) Mental reactions of women to perinatal death. In: *Psychosomatic Medicine in Obstetrics and Gynecology* (ed. D. Morris), pp. 326–329. S. Karger, New York.

Derbyshire, F., Davies, D.P. & Bacco, A. (1982) Discharge of preterm babies from neonatal units. *British Medical Journal*, **284**, 233–234.

Klaus, M.H. & Kennell, J.H. (1982) *Parental–Infant Bonding*, 2nd edn. C.V. Mosby, St Louis.

Kubler-Ross, E. (ed.) (1975) *Death. The Final Stage of Growth*. Prentice-Hall, New Jersey.

Kubler-Ross, E. (ed.) (1977) *On Death and Dying*. Tavistock Publications, London.

Murray, J. (1993) *An Ache in Their Heart* [kit]. University of Queensland, Department of Child Health, Brisbane.

Vance, J.C., Foster, W.J., Najman, J.M., Embelton, G., Thearle, M.J. & Hodgen, F.M. (1991) Early parental responses to sudden infant death, stillbirth or neonatal death. *Medical Journal of Australia* **155**, 292–297.

FURTHER READING

Boyle, F.M. (1997) *Mothers Bereaved by Stillbirth, Neonatal Death or Sudden Infant Death Syndrome*. Ashgate, Aldershot.

29 Ethical issues in the treatment of critically ill newborn infants

Ethical problems arise in the interaction of persons and these involve the welfare or freedom of humans. They occur when one person or group of persons acts in ways that impair the welfare of another person or group of persons.

The traditional medical ethic is to act in ways that benefit the patient and which do no harm to the welfare or freedom of the patient.

The four major principles of ethical reasoning particularly relevant to newborn infants are:
1 beneficence;
2 non-maleficence ('first do no harm—*primum non nocere*');
3 autonomy;
4 equity or distributive justice.

Good ethics can only be exercised if the medicine practised is correct. Good ethics requires accurate medical facts, and even sound ethical reasoning will not rescue a decision based on false assumptions. The medical profession must act in favour of preserving human life. With the advances in medical technology has come a greater public awareness of neonatal intensive care.

An individualized approach to management is advocated, but institutional guidelines are also necessary. Institutional guidelines are preferable to governmental and legal guidelines.

Most neonatal ethical dilemmas fall within the following four areas.

1 *When not to resuscitate at birth*. Unfortunately, junior physicians are often in the acute situation and may not have the relevant knowledge to make such a decision. Institutional guidelines are necessary to cover all situations. Mistakes can undoubtedly be made in those first few vital seconds, and if there is any doubt one must err on the conservative side of resuscitation. A decision can be reversed later on. Currently recommended indications for failure to resuscitate at birth would include very few conditions:

(a) anencephaly;
(b) other severe central nervous system malformations;
(c) multiple absence of sense organs;
(d) absence of fetal/neonatal heartbeat > 10 min.

Infants with conditions such as suspected chromosomal anomalies (triploidy, trisomy D, E), perinatal lethal renal disease and lethal skeletal disorders should probably be resuscitated and then fully assessed and investigated so that a rational decision can be made with all relevant information available.

2 *'How small is too small?'—or when not to resuscitate on gestational age or birthweight criteria*. Human nature being what it is, we are straining to push back the frontiers of viability, to improve our statistics, and tend to accept death as failure.

Hospitals should develop guidelines based on their own survival and outcome data. An approach would be to attempt resuscitation on all infants over 600 g (22–23 weeks' gestation) and/or ≥ 24 weeks' gestation, and for selected infants between 500 and 600 g, depending on past obstetric history, the likelihood of infection, birth trauma and severity, initial asphyxia and parental wishes. Present indications suggest that infants less than 600 g and of an appropriate weight for gestational age and those less than 24 weeks' gestation and with fully fused eyelids are unlikely to survive even with intensive care in centres of neonatal excellence (Fig. 29.1).

Survival rates for extremely low birthweight infants admitted to intensive care nurseries in 1997 in Australia and New Zealand are shown in Table 29.1 (Donoghue *et al.* 1999).

Saying that the neonatologist will attempt full resuscitation and subsequent intensive care for all infants ≥ 24 weeks' gestation and/or ≥ 600 g does not mean that the obstetrician

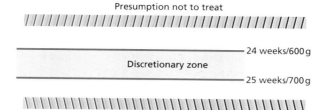

Presumption not to treat

24 weeks/600 g

Discretionary zone

25 weeks/700 g

Presumption to treat

Fig. 29.1 How small is too small? Or when not to resuscitate on birthweight or gestational age criteria.

Table 29.1 Survival to discharge by gestational age and birthweight for live born infants. The data for Australia and New Zealand refers to 1997 and only includes babies admitted to NICUs.

| Gestational age (weeks) | % Survival at discharge | | Birthweight group (g) | % Survival to discharge (Australia and New Zealand) |
	Australia and New Zealand data	UK data*		
23	43	11	500–599	50
24	59	26	600–699	63
25	74	44	700–799	81
26	82	—	800–899	86
27	92	—	900–999	93

* UK national figures for survival to estimated date of delivery after extremely premature birth. (From the Epicure Study, 1995. Unpublished data, with permission of N. Marlow, 1999.)

must necessarily do *everything possible* for all these pregnancies, as he or she has two people to consider, not just the neonate. At times there will be a dichotomy in the aggressiveness of care between obstetrician and neonatologist.

3 *Major congenital malformations.*

(a) *Severe but not life-threatening abnormalities.* These babies will be given all appropriate medical and nursing care to promote survival and minimize later disability.

(b) *Lethal abnormalities*: e.g. anencephaly, trisomy D, E, encephalocoele. Babies receive good nursing care to keep them comfortable, warm, free of hunger and relieved of pain. No active means are taken to shorten life. At times these babies are discharged home under the parents' care. Parents and family receive ongoing counselling and support.

(c) *Potentially lethal conditions which may be associated with severe handicap*, e.g.:

(i) neural tube defects (myelomeningocoele, hydrocephalus, encephalocoele); and

(ii) birth asphyxia with evidence of severe hypoxic–ischaemic encephalopathy.

Life support measures may be instituted while the infant is fully assessed and all necessary information obtained. Parents are progressively counselled so that they are fully aware of the clinical condition, such as sequelae and the management options available.

4 *Withdrawal of life supports.* The situation regarding possible withdrawal of life supports arises under different circumstances:

(a) clear-cut cases, e.g. confirmation of bilateral renal agenesis, trisomy 13 or 18, triploidy, irreversible cervical cord injury. To continue ventilation for these lethal conditions would be futile and under the circumstances would constitute 'extraordinary care';

(b) irreversible brain death following hypoxic–ischaemic injury;

(c) preterm infant with progressive bronchopulmonary dysplasia, grade IV cerebroventricular haemorrhage or post-haemorrhagic hydrocephalus.

These cases may be clear cut when the infant can be recognized as dying despite maximal assistance, and death seems inevitable.

The question of whether life support systems should be withdrawn for very low birthweight (VLBW) infants demonstrating a large cerebroventricular haemorrhage with intra-parenchymal extension is a frequent dilemma.

SELECTIVE WITHDRAWAL OF NEONATAL INTENSIVE CARE

Reasons for considering withdrawal include:
1 prognosis too bad:
  (a) short-term survival;
  (b) long-term outcome;
2 therapy too burdensome.
The decision-making process involves:
1 accurate and complete medical facts:
  (a) subspecialist consultation;
  (b) scientific documentation;
2 consultation with hospital ethicist (if available) or independent consultant;
3 in-depth case conference:
  (a) medical–moral–ethical discussion.

PARENTS IN THE DECISION-MAKING PROCESS

Although parents are usually the best-qualified advocates for their infant, they should not shoulder the burden entirely but rather a shared decision should be made.

All 'proxy decision' makers, whether they be parents, physicians or Courts of Law, must be fully informed and cognizant of the relevant facts.

The hospital and the State recognize their responsibility to provide appropriate care for all newborn infants and, in the unusual situation of conflict when parents prefer no active treatment, the wishes of the parents may be overridden to sustain life. The reverse situation (i.e. parents wishing the continuation of life supports and medical staff wishing to withdraw) occasionally arises and must be handled compassionately.

CIRCUMSTANCES UNDER WHICH THE PARENTS' WISHES MIGHT BE OVERRULED, OR WHEN PARENTS ARE INCAPABLE OF DECISION MAKING

1 Exchange transfusion or urgent blood transfusion for Jehovah's Witness infants.
2 Operation for duodenal atresia/oesophageal atresia in Down syndrome infants.
3 Institution of life support systems in 'good-prognosis' preterm infants with severe respiratory distress syndrome (RDS).

ROLE OF CASE CONFERENCE

A suggested approach to deal with issues regarding the withdrawal of life support is the case conference. This involves all relevant staff (medical, nursing, allied health, pastoral care) and parents to work through the complex series of medical, social and ethical issues.
Purpose of conference:
1 ensures staff comfort with the decision;
2 enhances communication between staff;
3 to develop a future care plan:
  (a) further information (investigation);
  (b) time frameworks;
4 guidance for counselling parents;
5 process for withdrawal of life supports;
6 staff understand decision-making process;
7 opportunity for all opinions to be expressed.

COMMUNICATION OF WITHDRAWAL OF LIFE SUPPORT

1 The attending physician clearly annotates the medical facts in the chart.
2 At times a second neonatologist is consulted and their opinion is documented in the chart.
3 Rarely the Hospital Ethics Committee is convened if there is ethical uncertainty.
4 The decision-making process is annotated in the chart.
5 Communication of the decision to relevant

persons, e.g. Charge Nurse, Director of Nursing, Medical Superintendent.

6 Cases with unique aspects are documented in detail and archived by the Ethics Committee.

CARE OF PARENTS

1 The parents, preferably together, receive progressive counselling from the neonatologist.

2 Ongoing support is provided by nursing staff, social workers and pastoral care staff.

3 Parents are informed of the case conference and are counselled afterwards.

4 Life and death decisions are made jointly by the neonatologist and the parents—the final decision is parental.

THE ROLE OF INSTITUTIONAL ETHICS COMMITTEE

1 Develop and ratify institutional guidelines.

2 Advisory and consultant body.

3 Educative role for staff.

4 Disseminate information.

5 Absolve attending physician from decision-making process when necessary.

6 Resolve differences of opinion.

There are no algorithms readily available that one can follow simply each time an ethical dilemma arises: rather, one must work through a complex series of moral, religious, cultural and legal issues to reach an acceptable conclusion (Freed & Hageman 1996).

REFERENCES

Donoghue, D. (1999) *Australian and New Zealand Neonatal Network 1997*. AIHW National Perinatal Statistics Unit, Sydney.

Freed, G.E. & Hageman, J.R. (eds) (1996) Ethical dilemmas in the prenatal, perinatal and neonatal periods *Clinics in Perinatology*, 23.

FURTHER READING

Goldsworth, A., Silverman, W., Stevenson, D.K., Young, E.W.D. & Rivers, R. (eds) (1995) *Ethics and Perinatology*. Oxford University Press, New York.

30 Procedures

Where possible a procedure should be witnessed at least twice and then performed under supervision before it is attempted without supervision. In ill infants some of these procedures may be potentially harmful, even when performed by experienced staff. Ensure that all equipment is prepared and that assistants are familiar with the procedure. Maintain adequate thermal care. Do not persist beyond three failed attempts—seek a colleague's help or take a break and try again.

BAG-AND-MASK VENTILATION

It is important for any nurse, midwife or doctor who is involved in the delivery or care of newborn infants to learn how to use a bag and mask for emergency assisted ventilation. Two types of bags are commonly used in labour wards and neonatal units: the Laerdal or Ambu type (Fig. 30.1) and anaesthetic bags. The Penlon (Cardiff) bag was previously extensively used but has now been superseded.

The Laerdal bag is self-inflating with a blow-off valve set at 40 cmH$_2$O. It is easy to deliver high-pressure inflation to the baby's lungs with this bag, with inspired O$_2$ close to 100%. Oxygen flow only occurs when the bag is compressed or the baby inspires with the face mask applied. For free O$_2$ flow to the baby's nostrils disconnect the bag from the delivery valve.

There are several different types of face mask in different sizes to suit premature and full-term infants. The two most commonly used are:
the Bennett mask. This is round and clear and fits snugly over the nose and mouth; and
the Laerdal mask. This is also round, with a single silicone plastic flange to create a good seal with the infant's face.

It has been shown that the Laerdal mask gives the best seal and leaks less air than any other type (Palme *et al.* 1985).

Technique (Fig. 30.2)

1 Place infant supine with neck extended (sniffing position), on a firm surface, and aspirate the airway.
2 Place face mask firmly over the nose and mouth with an O$_2$ flow rate of 4 L/min.
3 Hold face mask on firmly (but do not occlude nares) and hold the jaw forwards.
4 Inflate at a rate of about 30–40 breaths/min.

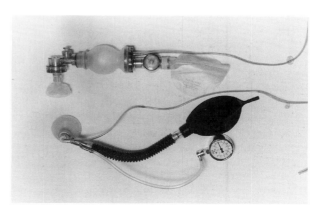

Fig. 30.1 Laerdal (upper) and anaesthetic bagging systems with Laerdal face masks.

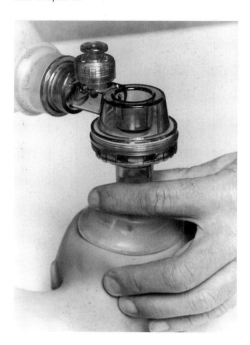

Fig. 30.2 Bag-and-mask ventilation. Note fingers extending neck and holding mask securely.

Make sure there is good chest wall movement, good air entry on auscultation of the lungs, and improvement in the infant's colour. If chest wall movement is poor, check position of the neck and that the airway is clear. Frequently, the insertion of an appropriate infant pharyngeal airway (Guedel) will improve air entry. The bag should be inflated only sufficiently to produce good chest wall movement. Damage can be done to the infant's lungs by overvigorous bagging. If there is no improvement in condition after bagging for 1–2 min, the infant will need intubation.

The anaesthetic bagging system uses a 500-mL bag and T piece attached to a manometer measuring pressure in cmH_2O. Inspiratory and expiratory pressures can be accurately controlled by regulating gas flow and by thumb occlusion of the bag (or by gate clamp). Operators using this system must give their total concentration, as it is easy to inadvertently give very high inspiratory and/or expiratory pressures.

INTUBATION OF THE TRACHEA

There are two basic types of endotracheal tube.

'Shouldered' or tapered (Cole's or Warne's). These tubes are designed so that the shoulder will not pass through the glottic region and thus the tip will lie above the carina. Too much force may push the shoulder through the cords, leading to glottic or subglottic injury. Use tube sizes 10, 12 and 14 for a 1.5, 2.5 and 3.5 kg infant, respectively.

Uniform-diameter tube (Portex, Shiley). These tubes are designed for prolonged intubation and intubation of infants less than 1.5 kg birthweight. Use sizes 2.5, 3.0 and 3.5 mm for infants weighing 1.0, 2.0 and 3.0 kg, respectively.

Orotracheal intubation

1 Select tube size and insert the introducer almost to the end of the tube and bend it slightly. Check laryngoscope, suction apparatus, bag, mask and adaptor.
2 Place baby on a firm surface, suck pharynx and nares and ventilate by bag and mask for 30 s.
3 Place baby's head in 'sniffing' position by extending the neck by traction under the infant's jaw. Ensure the face is in the midline. An assistant may press directly on the cricoid cartilage to push the glottis up into view.
4 Pass laryngoscope blade gently along right side of mouth and pull tongue and epiglottis forward by exerting traction parallel to the handle of the laryngoscope (*not* by tilting the blade upward) (Fig. 30.3).
5 Aspirate the airway again and pull the laryngoscope blade back until the epiglottis and vocal cords come into view (Fig. 30.4).
6 Pass endotracheal tube about 2 cm beyond the vocal cords, remove the introducer and apply gentle insufflation of the lungs. Table 30.1 gives the approximate distance for tube insertion, but the position of the tip of the tube should always be checked radiologically after each

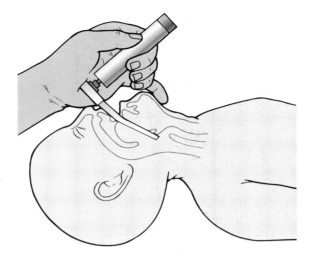

Fig. 30.3 Laryngoscopy. The laryngoscope blade displaces the tongue and lifts the epiglottis anteriorly to expose the cords. (Reproduced with permission of Baillière Tindall.)

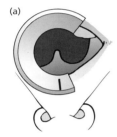
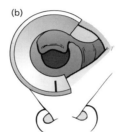
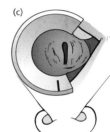

Fig. 30.4 The stages of intubation. Visualization of the uvula and oropharynx (a). The epiglottis is seen with the oesophagus beyond it (b). The cords are seen (c).

Table 30.1 Recommendations for neonatal intubation

Infant's weight (g)	Tube diameter	Distance (cm)	
		Nasal tube (anterior nares to mid-trachea)	Oral tube (lip to tip)
500–750	2.5	7.5	6.5–6.8
750–1250	2.5	8.5	6.8–7.3
1250–2000	3.0	9.5	7.3–8.0
2000–3000	3.5	10.5	8.0–9.0
3000–4000	3.5	11.0–12.0	9.0–10.0

intubation. It should be situated 0.5 cm above the carina or mid-trachea.

Nasotracheal intubation

This is often used for long-term intubation as fixation is more satisfactory.

1 Select tube and check Magill's forceps. An introducer is not used. Visualize the back of the mouth with a laryngoscope.

2 Endotracheal tube is gently passed down the right nostril until it just appears behind the soft palate.

3 The tip of the endotracheal tube is picked up

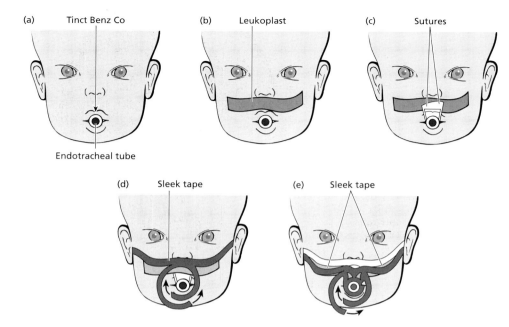

Fig. 30.5 A method of fixing the endotracheal tube for long-term ventilation. This can be used for oral or nasal tubes.

by the Magill's forceps and placed gently between the vocal cords. The assistant pushes the tube down the trachea as the operator guides it with Magill's forceps.

Fixation of the endotracheal tube

Each unit has its own methods for securing an endotracheal tube. It is most important that the tube is fixed securely on to the face to avoid accidental extubation, and also to ensure that the infant's sensitive skin is not traumatized by the procedure.

TAPING THE TUBE

Tincture of benzoin compound is first applied to the infant's upper lip and, when this has dried, plaster tape is laid on the lip. Thin strips of tape are then wound around the tube and then on to the plaster (Fig. 30.5). The use of a soft adherent pad protects the skin.

Some units apply a plastic guard ring around the outside of the endotracheal tube and then suture this to the tube by silk thread penetrating both the ring and the tube. Care must be taken not to narrow the lumen of the tube by the suture, so that suction cannot be easily performed. The plastic guard ring may then be plastered to the upper lip or attached at either end to a bonnet over the infant's head (Fig. 30.6).

Routine endotracheal tube care

Individual units must develop their own protocols to prevent pooling of secretions and promote overall lung expansion. Active chest physiotherapy techniques (vibration, cupping or contact-heel percussion) are indicated only when positioning and suction methods fail to maintain a clear chest.

Extubation procedure

This should be done with the resuscitation trolley at hand and after correcting anaemia and treating apnoea as necessary. Prophylactic treatment with aminophylline or caffeine may aid successful extubation. Extubation should be planned, preferably in the morning, to pro-

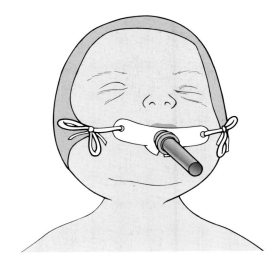

Fig. 30.6 Alternative method for fixing the endotracheal tube using a plastic flange tied to the infant's bonnet. A suture is inserted through the cuff of the flange and the tube to secure it.

vide the best chance of success. Individual units must develop their own protocols.

1 Careful positioning, and suctioning for 6 h prior to extubation.

2 Cease feeds 6 h before extubation and insert an intravenous (i.v.) drip.

3 Extubate while inflating lungs with an anaesthetic bag.

4 Gently suction the pharynx and nares.

5 Lay baby semiprone with the right lung uppermost.

6 Place in headbox with humidified O_2 at 5% greater concentration than before extubation, or insert nasopharyngeal continuous positive airway pressure (CPAP) tube in infants < 1250 g birthweight.

7 Perform chest X-ray 6 h after extubation, or earlier if symptoms are severe.

8 Active chest physiotherapy with cupping is indicated in the presence of a moist chest or evidence of any collapse on X-ray.

9 Withhold feeds for at least 12 h after extubation.

NASOPHARYNGEAL INTUBATION FOR CONTINUOUS POSITIVE AIRWAY PRESSURE

Nasopharyngeal intubation for CPAP is a form of management used for ventilatory support following endotracheal extubation or to support infants with recurrent apnoea of prematurity. One technique for the placement of a nasopharyngeal CPAP tube is described. A widely used alternative is the infant neural CPAP driver (p. 120), which uses short nasal prongs.

Technique

1 Select a soft Portex tube of appropriate size to pass snugly through the anterior nares.

2 Measure distance from the tragus of the ear to the nostril and cut the tube to that length.

3 Attach circuit adaptor.

4 Lubricate the tube with a small amount of xylocaine ointment, then pass it through the nostril and backwards along the floor of the nose until only 1.5 cm remains out of the nose.

5 Check the position of the tip of the tube in the nasopharynx by visualizing the oropharynx with a laryngoscope. Advance the tip of the tube until it can just be seen in the pharynx, and then withdraw it slightly so that it disappears from view—this is the correct position—and tape the tube in place.

6 Set the appropriate oxygen concentration and flow rate (this must not exceed 5 L/min).

7 The nasopharyngeal tube will require changing every 24 h to prevent obstruction. Occasionally, more frequent changes may be

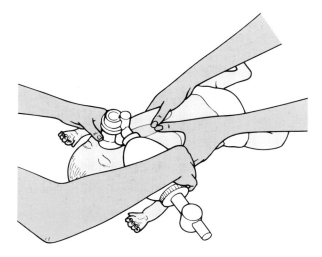

Fig. 30.7 External cardiac massage over the lower third of the sternum. Simultaneous ventilation is also necessary as shown.

necessary, but this should only be done on the orders of a consultant neonatologist or senior physiotherapist. The tube should be passed into alternate nostrils with each change to minimize trauma.

EXTERNAL CARDIAC MASSAGE

This is necessary for cardiac arrest or severe bradycardia not responding to suction, oxygenation and ventilation.

1 The hands are placed around the chest with the fingertips around the back and the thumbs over the middle to lower third of the sternum (Fig. 30.7). The sternum should be depressed about 1.5–2.0 cm 100 times/min. Every third depression should be followed by a lung inflation.

2 Constantly check the effectiveness of massage by observing colour, perfusion and pulses, and briefly stop massage every so often to auscultate the heart.

DRAINAGE OF A PNEUMOTHORAX

If there is a sudden deterioration in an infant with respiratory distress, whether receiving mech-anical ventilation or not, a pneumothorax should be considered and the following carried out.

1 Auscultate. Is air entry different between the two sides?

2 Transilluminate the chest using a cold fibre-optic light source. A pneumothorax will cause the affected hemithorax to glow. In very tiny babies the whole chest may transilluminate normally because of the thin chest wall.

3 If the baby is not *in extremis*, perform an urgent chest X-ray.

4 If the condition is critical and a pneumothorax is strongly suspected, a therapeutic thoracocentesis is performed by placing a 19G butterfly needle into the second intercostal space in the midclavicular line. It is essential that the other end of the butterfly tube is attached to a three-way stopcock (turned off) and to a 20-mL syringe. Remember that blindly needling the chest may itself produce a pneumothorax.

5 Once the infant's condition is stable, an intercostal catheter is inserted with aseptic precautions (see below).

6 After securing the catheter do a check X-ray to ensure adequate evacuation of air.

Placement of a pneumothorax drain

There are two positions for drainage insertion:
1 anteriorly in the second intercostal space in the midclavicular line (Fig. 30.8a);
2 laterally in the fifth or sixth intercostal space in the anterior axillary line (Fig. 30.8b).

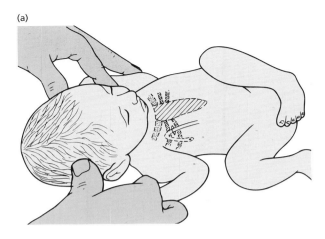

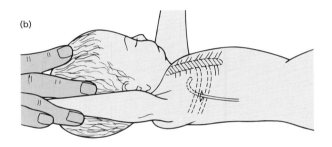

Fig. 30.8 Pneumothorax drainage. (a) Insertion of a pleural drain anteriorly through the second intercostal space in the midclavicular line. (b) Insertion of a pleural drain through the fifth intercostal space in the anterior axillary line.

The anterior position appears to be the most successful in draining pneumothoraces, but it is important to avoid trauma to the infant's nipples and unsightly scarring. The procedure is described below.

1 The skin is cleansed with alcohol, prepared with povidone-iodine and infiltrated with local anaesthetic (1% xylocaine).

2 A deep incision is made in the second intercostal space in the midclavicular line on the affected side. The intercostal muscle should be breached by the scalpel blade.

3 An Argyle size 10 pleural catheter with trocar is introduced through the chest wall and pleura. The catheter and trocar should be cross-clamped with a pair of forceps 2 cm from the tip to prevent overinsertion. The catheter is introduced in the direction of the lung apex for a distance of 3–5 cm. Once the tip is in the pleural cavity about 2 cm, the trocar is withdrawn and quickly attached to the Heimlich valve. The catheter is then advanced a further 1–2 cm.

4 The catheter is secured with a pursestring suture and strapped to the chest wall with a bridge of Micropore tape or plastic adhesive dressing such as Tegaderm (Heimlich).

A flutter valve is very useful instead of an underwater seal if the pneumothorax occurs before transportation of the infant. However, if the flutter valve becomes wet with blood or moisture, the surface tension between the two rubber leaves will significantly increase the pressure required to open the valve. For this reason, we prefer underwater drainage. If blood is present in the chest, a pump is used to apply low negative pressure to the other side of the underwater seal. For a more laterally sited catheter it is important that the catheter be angled anteriorly, as posteriorly positioned catheters are more likely to obstruct.

Removal of intercostal catheter

The chest tube is clamped when there has been no bubbling for 24 h, and it is removed after a further 12–24 h if there is no deterioration clinically or reaccumulation of the pneumothorax on chest X-ray. Take care that air is not sucked into the chest after catheter removal. The intercostal catheter is removed slowly and pressure applied to the site. The skin edges can be closed with Steristrips and an adhesive dressing applied to the site. Pursestring sutures can leave unsightly scars.

ABDOMINAL PARACENTESIS

Approaches may be midline or lateral. The bladder should be empty for this procedure.
1 Midline: a 21G needle is inserted vertically throughout the abdominal wall 1–2 cm below the umbilicus.
2 Lateral: the needle is inserted into right or left iliac fossa lateral to the rectus abdominis, taking care to avoid a grossly enlarged liver and spleen and inferior epigastric artery.

Large collections will drain freely but may be enhanced by dependent positions.

PERICARDIAL ASPIRATION

This procedure is indicated for cardiac tamponade due to pneumopericardium or a large pericardial effusion or haemorrhage.
1 Use a 23G needle connected to a three-way stopcock and a 10-mL syringe.
2 Enter under the thorax to the left of the xiphisternum and advance upwards and to the left at 45° to vertical and 45° to the midline while applying gentle suction.
3 The pericardium is entered to a depth of 1 cm and air or fluid withdrawn.

UMBILICAL VESSEL CATHETERIZATION

Umbilical arterial catheterization is performed for intermittent sampling of arterial blood and continuous monitoring of arterial Po_2 and blood pressure. Catheter size:
1 3.5FG for infants less than 1500 g;
2 5FG if greater than 1500 g.

There are two common positions for placement of the tip of the umbilical artery catheter:
1 high: in the aorta at the level of the diaphragm (T10);
2 low: below the level of the renal arteries (L4–L5). This position has a greater risk of thrombosis (Wesstrom *et al.* 1979).

An estimate can be made on how far to pass the catheters on the basis of the distance in centimetres between the umbilicus and the shoulder tip. The length to be inserted can then be read directly from Fig. 30.9.

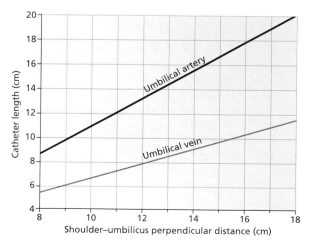

Fig. 30.9 Chart showing the distance to insert umbilical artery catheter (high position in aorta at or above diaphragm) and umbilical vein catheter based on the infant's shoulder-to-umbilical distance. (Adapted from Dunn 1966.)

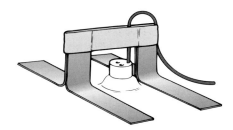

Fig. 30.10 Securing the umbilical catheter using Micropore tape.

Technique

1 Measure the shoulder-to-umbilicus distance and estimate the distance to pass the catheter from Fig. 30.9. The calculated distance is for placement in the aorta at T10.

2 Use full surgical scrub technique with gloves, gown and mask. Cleanse cord and abdominal wall with alcohol and povidone-iodine.

3 Apply a piece of ribbon gauze around the cord before cutting the cord with a scalpel. Cut cord horizontally about 1 cm above the abdominal wall. Identify the three cord vessels and dilate the mouth of one of the arteries with a pair of fine iris forceps or dilator.

4 Attach a three-way stopcock and a syringe of normal saline to the catheter and flush it with heparinized saline solution. Cannulate the artery and introduce the catheter the calculated distance. Check position of catheter radiologically.

5 The catheter is secured *in situ* using a purse-string suture (3–4 bites) and taped to the abdominal wall using a 'bridge' or 'goalposts' (Fig. 30.10).

6 The catheter is connected to an infusion pump and to a pressure transducer for blood pressure monitoring. Circulation to the lower limbs is closely observed.

7 An A-P abdominal X-ray is taken to locate the catheter tip. If the catheter is sited too low for high position it must not be advanced but may be withdrawn to the low position.

Umbilical venous catheterization is enjoying a resurgence in very low birthweight (VLBW) infants:

1 urgent resuscitation in the labour ward;

2 venous access for fluid administration in VLBW infants;

3 exchange transfusion. A 5FG catheter is used and should be placed in the inferior vena cava (IVC) if possible (although only 70% will pass through the ductus venosus). The location of the catheter tip should always be checked radiographically;

4 lack of venous access, e.g. hydrops fetalis;

5 central venous pressure (CVP) monitoring;

6 performance of balloon septostomy for transposition of the great arteries (TGA).

Technique

EMERGENCY RESUSCITATION

1 Secure a cord tie snugly at the base of the umbilical cord (do not pull tight).

2 Make an incision halfway through the superior aspect of the cord 0.5 cm from its base to expose the umbilical vein but avoiding the arteries.

3 Insert a 5FG umbilical arterial catheter into the vein. Distance to be passed for position in IVC is calculated from Fig. 30.9 after measuring acromioclavicular–umbilical distance. If it is not possible to withdraw blood, then the site of the catheter should be checked by injecting 2 mL of normal saline.

4 Tighten cord tie and tape catheter to the baby's abdomen.

ELECTIVE INSERTION

1 Preparation as for umbilical artery.

2 Distance inserted is calculated from graph.

3 Umbilical vein must be clearly distinguished from two umbilical arteries. Rarely is it necessary to spend much time on dilatation, but clot may need to be removed.

4 Check position before suturing pursestring as catheter can easily slip out.

EXCHANGE TRANSFUSION

The indications for exchange transfusion are:

1 hyperbilirubinaemia—unconjugated variety;
2 septicaemia—this may be useful in the early overwhelming variety, e.g. group B β-haemolytic streptococcus;
3 disseminated intravascular coagulation;
4 inborn errors of metabolism;
5 intoxications;
6 to correct anaemia (especially hydrops fetalis).

The blood should be less than 48 h old, ABO compatible with mother and infant and rhesus negative. If the baby is critically ill, blood may be buffered with trishydroxyaminomethane (THAM) 3.5% to correct the pH. The volume to be exchanged is usually 180 mL/kg for a double-volume exchange.

Techniques

1 *Isovolaemic*. Blood is removed from the umbilical artery and given via the umbilical vein.
2 *Single catheter*. Preferably umbilical vein, but the artery may be used.
3 *Peripheral vessels*. A peripheral artery catheter and venous cannula are used.

Donor blood is warmed via a heating coil in a water bath. Generally, 10 mL aliquots are used. Calcium gluconate 10%, 1 mL diluted in 10 mL of blood, is given after every 100 mL of transfusion. The first 10 mL aliquot is sent for SBR, haematocrit (Hct), FBC, electrolytes, proteins, glucose-6-phosphate dehydrogenase (G6PD), liver enzymes, serology, etc. The heart rate, blood pressure, temperature and respirations should be monitored continuously throughout the exchange transfusion. A careful record is kept of all blood sampled and transfused. At the end of the exchange transfusion, blood is sent to the laboratory for haemoglobin, total and direct bilirubin, electrolytes, calcium, sugar and blood culture.

Do not feed the infant for at least 2 h before and at least 4 h after exchange transfusion. Instead give maintenance i.v. fluids.

Complications of exchange transfusion

Vascular: air/clot embolization, thrombosis
Cardiac: dysrhythmia, volume overload, arrest
Electrolyte: hyperkalaemia, hypernatraemia, hypocalcaemia, acidosis
Infective: bacteraemia, hepatitis B, cytomegalovirus (CMV)
Other: hypoglycaemia, necrotizing enterocolitis (NEC).

Dilutional exchange transfusion for polycythaemia (p. 210)

The indications for an isovolaemic dilutional exchange transfusion are:
1 a venous Hct greater than 70% in an asymptomatic baby; and
2 a venous Hct greater than 65% in a symptomatic baby.

Use fresh frozen plasma or salt-rich 4–5% albumin:

Volume to be exchanged = infant's
Hct – desired Hct × kg × 90

The exchange transfusion should take about 30 min and must be performed via a blood vessel with a good blood flow (usually an umbilical vein).

PERIPHERAL ARTERIAL CATHETERIZATION

Cannulation of either the radial or the posterior tibial artery is probably less hazardous than cannulation of the umbilical artery, but for some operators is more technically difficult.

Technique

1 Palpate the vessel and visualize it with a fibreoptic cold transillumination light.
2 Collateral circulation is assessed by the Allen test. The wrist is held firmly on the radial side and the blood squeezed out of the hand. If the colour returns rapidly to the hand while pressure is maintained on the radial artery, it is safe to cannulate the radial artery.
3 The wrist is cleansed with alcohol and povidone-iodine. The transillumination light can be held under the wrist while a 22G cath-

eter is advanced slowly in the direction of the radial artery at an angle of about 20° to the skin. Once blood is seen in the clear plastic chamber the catheter is advanced a further 0.5 mm, and then, while advancing the catheter slightly, the stylet is withdrawn. The index finger is placed over the radial artery to prevent blood loss.

4 The catheter is attached to an extension tubing, three-way stopcock with Luer lock adaptors, and connected to an infusion pump with heparinized saline set at 1–2 mL/h (1 U heparin per mL of solution). The catheter should be attached to a pressure transducer. Under no circumstances should drugs, blood or any other solutions except normal saline be infused through this line. The catheter must be firmly strapped and taped to an armboard, which is immobilized. Sometimes N/2 (0.5 N) saline is acceptable.

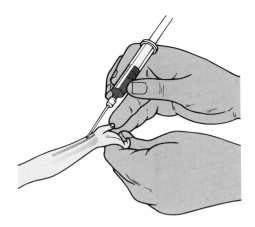

Fig. 30.11 Technique for radial artery sampling. The needle transects the artery and is then withdrawn whilst aspirating the syringe.

draw the needle. Apply pressure over the artery for at least 3–4 min.

INTERMITTENT ARTERIAL SAMPLING

This may be performed most safely from the radial, posterior tibial or superficial temporal arteries. The brachial and femoral arteries are less acceptable as limb ischaemia may occur. Femoral artery puncture is particularly hazardous because of the risk of haemorrhage and infection.

Technique

1 Palpate the vessel.
2 Prepare either a 25G needle with a clear barrel or a 25G short butterfly and attach to a mL syringe which has been lightly coated with heparin (1000 U/mL).
3 Cleanse skin with an alcohol/chlorhexidine swab and insert the needle at an angle of 30° to the skin surface (Fig. 30.11). The landmark at the wrist is just proximal to the proximal crease and lateral to the flexor carpi radialis tendon. Transfix the artery and then withdraw the needle slowly until blood spurts into the syringe.
4 Remove 0.3 mL of blood and then with-

BLOOD SAMPLING

Venepuncture

The antecubital fossa vein is the first choice, followed by peripheral veins, scalp veins and external jugular veins.
1 Visualize and palpate the vessel. Apply a tourniquet proximal to the vessel (an appropriately fitting rubber band is adequate for the scalp). Cleanse the skin with alcohol/chlorhexidine swab.
2 Use a 21 or 23G needle with a 2-mL syringe but avoid using excessive suction. Blood will usually drip fully from the needle into a specimen container.

SCALP VEIN

1 It will generally be necessary to shave the scalp, so avoid using a scalp vein if possible.
2 Use a 23G butterfly needle.

EXTERNAL JUGULAR

This is inappropriate for very small infants and infants with respiratory distress syndrome (RDS).

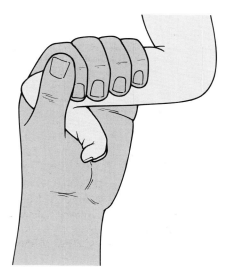

Fig. 30.12 Method for holding the heel prior to blood sampling.

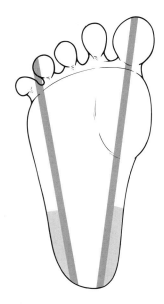

Fig. 30.13 Heel-prick specimens should only be taken from the shaded areas of the foot.

1 Hyperextend the head and lower it below the shoulder level. Make the infant cry to extend the vein. It may be useful to use a needle bent slightly at the hilt.

2 Insert a 23G needle into the vein and aspirate blood. At the completion of the procedure, sit the baby up and exert pressure over the puncture site for at least 3 min.

Heel-prick capillary blood sampling

Most laboratory tests can be carried out readily on small quantities of blood. In newborn infants capillary blood obtained from a heel prick is usually the method of choice. Up to 1 mL of blood can be sampled by this method.

1 Wash hands carefully and clean the heel with a 70% alcohol Mediswab.

2 Hold the leg around the ankle with thumb and fingers (do not hold the leg around the calf or shin as this may cause extensive bruising) (Fig. 30.12).

3 Prick the heel with a disposable lancet or autolet, on the most medial or lateral portion of the plantar surface (see hatched areas on Fig. 30.13).

Heel punctures should be performed on the plantar surface of the heel, beyond the lateral and medial limits of the calcaneus, marked by these lines. The heel prick should not be deeper than 2 mm, and should not be on the posterior curvature of the heel, nor through previous sites that may be infected.

4 Collect the blood into a plastic microcontainer capillary blood tube held horizontally.

It may be necessary to squeeze the foot beforehand to get a good flow of blood. Warming the foot with a warm wrap may improve the blood supply.

Blood culture

It is always necessary to have a nurse in attendance for this procedure. Use a full aseptic technique. Avoid drawing blood from indwelling catheters: it is preferable to take blood from a peripheral vein.

TECHNIQUE

1 Wash hands before undertaking any invasive procedure such as blood collection.

Table 30.2 Tubes and blood volumes required for culture

Patient category	Adult aerobic (grey top)	Paediatric aerobic (pink top)	Anaerobic (orange top)	Isolator (yellow top)
Neonates (icn/scn)	x	0.5–3 mL	x	0.5–1.5 mL
Babies (nurseries)	x	1–3 mL	1–3 mL	x
mothers	10 mL	x	10 mL	x

2 When a blood culture is drawn by venepuncture, a peripheral arterial stab etc., strict aseptic technique must be adhered to.

3 Swab skin with 70% alcohol and allow to dry, or else wait 1 min. This is to remove surface grease and dead skin cells. Repeat procedure with another 70% alcohol swab. This is to disinfect the skin. It is essential to use two separate swabs and allow the skin to dry (or wait 1 min) after each.

4 After removing the covering cap on the blood culture bottle, the rubber bung should be swabbed with 70% alcohol and then allowed to dry, as the rubber bung is not sterile. The same procedure should be used if a yellow-top isolator blood tube is being used in ICN.

5 After skin preparation with 70% alcohol, every effort must be undertaken to prevent contamination by examining fingers. Use a sterile glove or else swab the fingertip with 70% alcohol.

6 After obtaining the sample of blood, the needle must be removed and a new needle used to inoculate the blood equally into each blood culture bottle (or yellow-topped isolator tube if in ICN).

7 Volumes of blood to collect are indicated in Table 30.2.

8 Record the site where the blood was collected from (i.e. venous, arterial, central line, arterial catheter, etc.).

9 Blood culture bottle inoculation must occur *before* blood is placed into any other tubes or into a blood-gas analyser to avoid contamination.

Note. Under no circumstances must blood inoculation follow the performance of an arterial blood gas, or even blood being placed into clotted or unclotted collecting tubes. This is to prevent contamination of blood cultures.

Insertion of a silastic long line

This is a useful technique and is not difficult to perform. The following equipment is required:
1 a 19G butterfly with the plastic tubing cut off close to the needle;
2 a 30-cm length of fine 2FG silastic catheter; and
3 a 25G butterfly needle with its plastic tube intact.

This procedure must be carried out using strict aseptic precautions and the operator should be fully masked and gowned. The veins in the antecubital fossa, long saphenous or superficial temporal veins are the most suitable for cannulation. The area is exposed and thoroughly cleansed with alcohol and povidone-iodine. Before inserting the 19G butterfly, the length of silastic tubing necessary to place the tip in the right atrium is estimated and a mark made on the tube at the required length. The 19G butterfly is inserted into the vein as for venepuncture. When blood is seen to drip out of the needle, the silastic catheter is threaded through the inside of the 19G butterfly until the mark is reached. The 19G butterfly is then removed from the catheter and a 25G needle carefully inserted into the lumen of the catheter. The whole line should then be gently flushed with heparinized saline. Occasionally, the connector needle perforates the fine catheter tubing at the join and the dressing becomes moist. To avoid this complication great care must be taken to prevent movement at this connection site by using a wooden spatula and carefully taping the connector and three-way stopcock. The entry site is then scrubbed with povidone-iodine, secured firmly with sterile adhesive strips, and covered with a sterile transparent dressing (e.g. Opsite). The

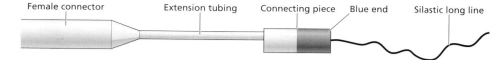

Fig. 30.14 Silastic catheter for long peripheral intravenous line insertion.

site of the catheter tip in the peripheral vein is marked on the skin for monitoring purposes. If a limb vein is used, the limb is immobilized by splinting. Before commencing the infusion the position of the catheter tip should be checked to ensure it is in a central vein by priming the silastic line with radio-opaque dye. If it is in too far it may be pulled back to a more suitable position.

INSERTION PROCEDURE

The following refers to the insertion of the Vygon silastic long line (Fig. 30.14).

The Vygon silastic long line contains the following:
1 19G butterfly needle;
2 30-cm length of fine silastic catheter, marked at 5-cm intervals;
3 a connecting piece with extension tubing.

Suitable veins are those in the antecubital fossa, the long saphenous at the ankle or knee, and superficial temporal veins. The axillary vein is often visible in extremely preterm infants and may be used, although care should be taken as it lies perilously close to the axillary artery.

Prior to scrubbing up, a tape measure should be used to estimate the length of silastic tubing necessary. For veins in the upper limb and scalp, the tip should lie in the right atrium. For veins in the lower limb, the tip should lie in anywhere in the IVC to the right atrium.

The operator scrubs up and gowns. The long line is connected by inserting the metal end of the silastic line into the blue end of the connector piece and then tightly screwing the connector piece together. The three-way tap is attached to the female connector and the whole system primed with heparinized saline. The tap is turned off to the long line with the syringe still attached.

The area over the chosen vein is exposed, cleansed using medicated (Persist Plus) swabs, and draped.

The butterfly needle is inserted into the vein as for venepuncture. It is crucial to the success of the procedure that the needle is inserted cleanly. The best way of achieving venous occlusion is for the assistant to squeeze the limb proximally with his or her hands under the drapes. This also helps in holding the limb still. When blood is seen to drip out of the needle, the assistant should be asked to relax the grip as a fast flow of blood from the needle makes insertion of the silastic catheter difficult. The silastic catheter is threaded through the inside of the butterfly needle using fine forceps. The needle itself is almost 5 cm long, and so the catheter tip reaches the needle tip when the first mark on the catheter is visible at the end of the needle. This is where resistance may be encountered, and patience and perseverance may be required before the catheter is felt to enter the vein and advance up it. The catheter is then advanced using the forceps until the desired length has been inserted, bearing in mind that the length at the skin is 5 cm less than the length at the end of the needle. The line is flushed and then the butterfly needle removed. This is achieved by unscrewing the connector piece and removing the metal end of the silastic catheter, and then pulling the needle out of the skin and threading it back over the silastic catheter to discard it. As the needle is removed, pressure should be applied to the puncture site to prevent the catheter being pulled out of the vein, and also to effect haemostasis. The silastic catheter is then re-inserted into the connector piece, which is tightened. The metal part should be inserted into the blue end as fully as possible, as this is the weak link in the long line. The line is flushed and the tap to the line turned off.

Haemostasis is effected using gauze and applying pressure. This may take 5–10 min owing to the size of the puncture wound. If haemostasis cannot be achieved, a tiny square of Algoderm may be used.

The area around the puncture site is cleansed of blood using medicated (Persist Plus) swabs. The silastic catheter outside the vein is coiled around on the skin and the whole area covered with a sterile transparent dressing (e.g. Opsite 3000 or Tegaderm Plus). Do not include the connector piece under the sterile dressing as it is bulky and sterility under the dressing will not be maintained.

Taping is important. The blue part of the connector must be taped to the baby using brown tape. If the blue connector is allowed to move with respect to the catheter, the metal end can puncture the silastic tubing. This is the weakest point of the whole long line. Ensuring that the metal end is fully inserted into the blue end of the connector also helps to prevent catheter puncture.

Immobilization of the limb is not absolutely necessary, although an armboard may be useful if the long line has been inserted in the antecubital fossa to prevent kinking of the catheter and infusion problems when the infant bends his arm.

SPECIAL INSTRUCTIONS

1 Maintain patency by flushing the line with heparinized saline until an X-ray can be taken.
2 Do not attach to infusate until position is confirmed by X-ray and medical review.
3 Record the date and time of insertion on a sticker and place on the armboard or around extension tubing.

OBSERVE FOR COMPLICATIONS

1 Site—blood loss/leakage.
2 Redness.
3 Exudate.
4 Temperature instability.
5 Oedema.
6 Induration.
7 Reduced perfusion of limb.

The above should be reported to the medical officer.

LUMBAR PUNCTURE

The indications for lumbar puncture (LP) may be diagnostic (suspected meningitis and intracranial haemorrhage, convulsions, unexplained apnoea, metabolic screen and syphilis) or therapeutic (progressive ventricular dilatation).
1 A full surgical scrub technique is necessary with gloves, gown and mask.
2 An experienced nurse needs to hold the baby in the left lateral position with the head, hips and knees well flexed. The back needs to be completely parallel to the edge of the table. Make sure the airway is not obstructed.
3 The skin is cleansed with povidone-iodine and alcohol. Generally a 22G LP needle with stylet is used. Some operators prefer a 23G butterfly needle, but this does not possess a stylet and there is a greater risk of a dermoid cyst developing at the site in later years.
4 Use lumbar spaces L3–L4 or L4–L5. The needle is directed towards the umbilicus. Once the subarachnoid space is penetrated, the stylet is removed and cerebrospinal fluid (CSF) is allowed to drip into each of three bottles (Fig. 30.15). Sometimes the needle needs to be gently rotated to check for CSF flow. It is easy to push the needle too far into the anterior vertebral venous plexus.
5 Measurement of lumbar CSF pressure may be necessary in infants with posthaemorrhagic ventricular dilatation (see p. 224). This can be done by attaching a Luer locking pressure transducer directly to the hub of the needle or by a manometer tube. Pressure measurements are only valid if the infant is breathing quietly and not crying. The head and trunk must be flat and in the same plane, and the infant not too tightly curled up.

Occasionally, sampling may more easily be obtained with the baby sitting up.
6 CSF should always be sent for cell count, Gram stain and culture and glucose and protein estimations. Other tests may include viral

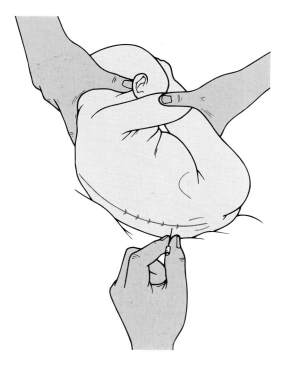

Fig. 30.15 Technique for lumbar puncture in the newborn.

studies, syphilis serology, fluorescein staining and counterimmune electrophoresis.

VENTRICULAR TAP

Rarely, a ventricular tap will be needed to diagnose ventriculitis or intraventricular haemorrhage, or to perform a ventriculogram or instil antibiotics. Generally, the procedure will be performed by a neurosurgeon or other experienced staff.

1 The baby is placed in a supine position with the nose upwards and the neck and face parallel to the mattress.

2 After the scalp has been shaved a full aseptic technique should be used. A long 20G or 22G LP needle with stylet is gently inserted at the lateral angle of the anterior fontanelle and angled towards the medial canthus of the eye on the same side (Fig. 30.16).

3 Once the skin and dura have been pierced, the stylet may be removed and the needle gently advanced until CSF wells up from the needle.

4 CSF from the ventricles should be collected by allowing it to drip into sterile bottles.

SUBDURAL TAP

In the past this was a common diagnostic procedure, but with the advent of better computed tomography (CT) and ultrasound scanning it should generally be reserved for therapy and not diagnosis.

1 Full aseptic technique should be used after scalp shaving. The baby lies on his back and the operator stands at the baby's head.

2 A 20G or 22G subdural needle with stylet is inserted at the lateral angle of the anterior fontanelle and pushed in a distance of 5–7 mm at right angles to the skin.

3 After the needle has passed through the dura (a slight change in resistance is felt), remove the stylet and wait for fluid to emerge. Normally only a few drops will be obtained. If serous fluid is present, probably not more than 10 mL should be withdrawn at one time. If pure

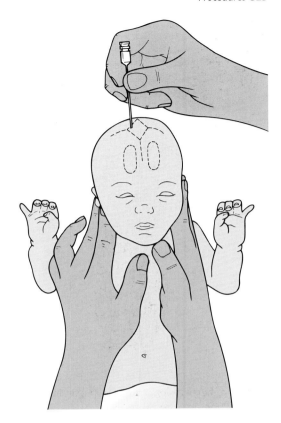

Fig. 30.16 Ventricular tap through the anterior fontanelle using a styletted needle.

blood is obtained from a subdural haematoma, leave the needle *in situ* until the blood stops dripping.

4 Do not attach a syringe and aspirate subdural fluid.

5 When collection is complete withdraw the needle and apply pressure over the puncture site.

Frequently the procedure will need to be repeated on the other side with a new needle.

URINE COLLECTION

This may be performed by a 'clean-catch' bag method, suprapubic aspiration or urethral catheter.

Bag collection

A clean-catch bag sample of urine may provide useful information. However, an inexpertly collected sample provides confusing or misleading information.

1 Cleanse a wide area of the perineum and penis with sterile saline-soaked swabs using a no-touch technique. In females the vulva will need to be separated, but the foreskin must not be retracted in males although it needs to be cleaned.

2 Wait for the perineum to dry before attaching a sterile urine collecting bag. Sometimes the application of tincture of benzoin enhances the adhesion of bag to skin.

3 Inspect the bag periodically, and as soon as the baby has voided remove the bag and immediately pour the urine into a universal sterile container.

4 Send the sample to the laboratory immediately. If there is any delay in transporting the sample, refrigerate it.

5 If no urine has been obtained after 1 h, the

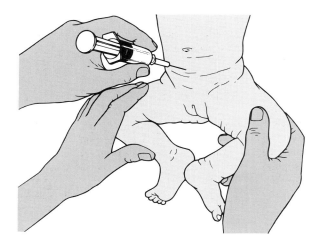

Fig. 30.17 Suprapubic aspiration of urine from the bladder. The needle should be aimed slightly superiorly in the midline and 0.5 cm above the pubis.

skin should be cleansed again and a fresh collecting bag applied.

Suprapubic aspiration

The indications for this procedure are an inconclusive culture from a bag specimen, a critically ill child or the presence of vulvovaginitis or balanitis when urinary tract infection is suspected.

1 The bladder must be full prior to commencing the procedure.
2 A wide area of skin over the lower abdomen is prepared with povidone-iodine solution and alcohol.
3 A 21G needle attached to a 10-mL syringe is used to puncture the skin 1 cm above the pubic symphysis in the midline.
4 The needle is advanced into the bladder, angled slightly upwards to the perpendicular. As the needle is slowly advanced gentle suction is applied. The needle usually only needs to be advanced 1.5–2.0 cm below the skin surface (Fig. 30.17).

EXAMINATION OF STOOLS FOR REDUCING SUBSTANCES

When testing stools for evidence of sugar intolerance, a strict technique must be carried out. Only fluid stools should be tested. Try to obtain 10 drops of liquid stool and add 20 drops of water. If a smaller volume of stool is obtained, make sure that exactly double the volume of water is added. This is a semiquantitative test and there must always be two parts water to one part liquid stool. Add 15 drops of the water/liquid stool mixture to a Clinitest tablet, then wait 15 s for a colour change and match the colour with the colour chart on the bottle.

Table 30.3 Interpretation of clinitest tablet

Trace = 0.25%
+ = 0.5%
++ = 0.75%
+++ = 1%
++++ = 2%

Generally ++ or greater represents sugar intolerance and stool should also be tested for pH and sent for identification of the reducing substance by chromatography.

PERITONEAL DIALYSIS (PD)

The indications for PD in the newborn include:
1 uraemia (plasma urea > 40 mmol/L);
2 hyperkalaemia (serum potassium > 7.5 mmol/L);
3 severe metabolic acidosis due to renal failure;

4 inborn errors of metabolism (see p. 179);

5 inadvertent drug overdose;

6 water overload.

PD can be attempted in infants without major abdominal pathology such as NEC or recent laparotomy. A urinary catheter should be inserted to empty the bladder. A 19G intravenous cannula is inserted through the right iliac fossa into the peritoneal cavity, and warmed dialysis fluid is instilled to fill the cavity. This allows the PD catheter to be more safely introduced, with a lower risk of damaging the bowel.

The PD cannula is then inserted at a point midway between the umbilicus and the left anterior superior iliac crest, and secured with a pursestring suture. An isotonic dialysis solution (1.36% glucose) is used for biochemical and metabolic indications. A hypertonic solution (3.86% glucose) is used for fluid overload, but hyperglycaemia is a risk when this solution is used.

Dialysis is undertaken in the following sequence:

1 allow the fluid to drain from the peritoneal cavity;

2 for each cycle, run in 20–30 mL/kg of pre-warmed dialysis fluid over 10 min;

3 allow this to remain in the cavity for 20–30 min so that dialysis occurs;

4 let fluid drain out under gravity for 20 min. Each cycle therefore lasts about 1 h;

5 accurately record the volumes in and out; and

6 perform microscopy of the dialysate every 24 h to detect infection.

REFERENCES

Palme, C., Nystrom, B. & Tunnell, R. (1985) An evaluation of face masks in the resuscitation of newborn infants. *Lancet* **1**, 207–210.

Wesstrom, G., Finnstrom, O. & Stenport, G. (1979) Umbilical artery catheterization in newborns. 1. Thromboses in relation to catheter type and position. *Acta Paediatrica Scandinavica* **68**, 575–581.

FURTHER READING

Barr, P. (1992) *Newborn Intensive Care*. Royal Alexandra Hospital for Children, Sydney.

Dunn, P.M. (1966) Localisation of the umbilical catheter by post mortem measurement. *Archives of Disease in Childhood* **41**, 69–74.

Fleming, P.J., Speidel, B.D., Marlow, N. & Dunn, P.M. (eds) (1991) *A Neonatal Vade-Mecum*, 2nd edn. Edward Arnold, London.

Halliday, H.L., McClure, G. & Reid, M. (eds) (1989) *Neonatal Intensive Care*, 3rd edn. Baillière Tindall, London.

Robertson, N.R.C. (1993) *A Manual of Neonatal Intensive Care*, 3rd edn. Edward Arnold, London.

31 Pharmacopoeia

The neonatal pharmacopoeia is presented in three sections: general, antimicrobials and standard infusions. It is suggested that this pharmacopoeia be used in conjunction with the more detailed neonatal drug information obtained from references listed in Further Reading.

GENERAL

Drug	Dose	Interval	Route
Acetazolamide (Diamox)	25–100 mg/kg	6–8 h	Oral, i.v.
Adenosine	50 µg/kg Double dose every 2 min 0.25 mg/kg		Bolus every 2–3 min i.v.
Adrenaline 1/10 000	0.1–0.3 mL/kg/dose	Once	e.t.t., i.v., i.c. Cardiac arrest
Adrenaline (neb.)	0.2 mL diluted 2 mL saline	2–6 h	Inhalation
Albumin 4–5% 25%	10–20 mL/kg 1–1.5 g/kg	12–24 h 12 h	i.v. i.v.
Alcuronium	Loading 200–300 µg/kg Maintenance 100–200 µg/kg	p.r.n.	i.v.
Aminophylline	Loading 6 mg/kg Maintenance 4.5 mg/kg	Infusion over 20 min 8 h	i.v. i.v.
Amiodarone	5 mg/kg/dose	Infusion over 1 h	i.v., oral
Atropine	20–30 µg/kg/dose	Once	s.c., i.v.
Beclomethasone nasal drops (Aldecin, Beconase)	1 drop	6–8 h	Intranasal
Bicarbonate (8.4% solution)	2 mmol/kg once Give diluted	2 min for arrest or 1 h infusion	i.v.
Budesonide (Pulmicort)	200 µg Aerochamber spacer	8–12 h	Ventilator Face mask
Caffeine citrate	Loading 20 mg/kg Maintenance 2.5–5.0 mg/kg/day	24 h	i.v. i.v., oral
Calcitriol	0.05 µg/kg	24 h	i.v., oral
Calcium gluconate	Maintenance 300 mg/kg/day Replacement 100 mg/kg/day	24 h p.r.n.	Oral, i.v. Slow i.v.
Caloreen	2–6 g/kg/day	Feeds	Oral

Drug	Dose	Interval	Route
Captopril	0.1–1.6 mg/kg/day	6 h	Oral
Carbamazepine (Tegretol)	10 mg/kg	24 h	Oral
Carbimazole	2.5 mg/kg/day	8 h	Oral
Chloral hydrate	15–25 mg/kg/day	p.r.n.	Oral, i.m.
Chlorthiazide	20–40 mg/kg/day	12 h	Oral
Chlorpromazine	2–3 mg/kg/day	6 h	Oral
Cisapride	0.75 mg/kg/day	6–8 h	Oral
Clonazepam	Loading dose (full term) 0.25 mg/kg	Once	Oral, i.v., i.m.
	Maintenance 0.1 mg/kg/day	12 h	Oral, i.v., i.m.
Cholecalciferol	600 iu/day	Once	Oral
Cimetidine	10 mg/kg/day	Once	Oral
Cortisone	0.25–2.5 mg/kg/day (depends on indication)	8 h	Oral
Cromolyn (Intal)	80 mg/kg	6 h	Inhalation
Cyclopentolate (Cylogyl)	1 drop 0.5% before exam	24 h	Ocular
Dexamethasone	Loading 0.5–1 mg/kg	Once	i.v., oral
	Maintenance 0.1–0.5 mg/kg	8 h	i.v., oral/day
Diazepam	Loading 0.5 mg/kg/dose	Once	i.v., oral
Diazoxide	5 mg/kg/dose	12–24 h	i.v., oral
Digoxin	See p. 197		
DOCA	1 mg	24 h	i.m.
Edrophonium	1 mg/kg/dose	Once	i.m., i.v.
Ethacrynic acid	1 mg/kg/dose	Once	i.m., i.v.
Exosurf	5 mL/kg (65 mg/kg DPPC)	Once (repeat once in 12 h)	e.t.t.
Fentanyl	2 µg/kg/dose	4–6 h	i.v.
Ferrous gluconate	30 mg/day	24 h	Oral
Ferrous sulphate	50 mg/day	24 h	Oral
Fibrinogen	500 mg/kg	Once	i.v.
Flecainide acetate	3–6 mg/kg/day	12 h	i.v., oral
Fludrocortisone	0.05–1 mg/day	24 h	Oral
Fluoride	4 drops/day	24 h	Oral
Folic acid	0.25 mg/kg	24 h	Oral
Frusemide	1–2 mg/kg/day	12 h	i.v., oral
Gaviscon	1–2 g/100 mL/feed	2–4 h	Oral

Cont'd on p. 328

Drug	Dose	Interval	Route
Glucagon	Bolus 100 µg/kg	Once	i.v., s.c., i.m.
	Infusion 5–10 µg/kg/h		i.v.
Granulocyte colony stimulating factor (G-CSF)	5 µg/kg/day	24 h	i.v., s.c.
Heparin	600 U/kg/day	4 h	i.v.
Hydralazine	0.5 mg/kg/dose (start)	Once	i.v., oral, i.m.
	2–3 mg/kg/day (max.)	8 h	
Hydrocortisone	10–25 mg/kg/dose	4–6 h	i.m., i.v.
Ibuprofen	10 mg/kg/dose	24 h	i.v.
Indomethacin	0.2 mg/kg/dose (3 doses only)	12 h over 30 min	i.v., rectal
		24 h	
	or 0.1 mg/kg/day	daily—6 doses	i.v., rectal
Insulin	0.25 U/kg	p.r.n.	i.v., i.m.
Kayexalate	1 g/dose	Once	Rectal repeat 6 h
Ketamine	2–5 mg/kg/dose	Once	i.v.
Konakion MM Paediatric drops	2 mg/dose repeat 1 month if breastfed	Birth, 4–7 days	Orally
Lignocaine	1 mg/kg	Once over 10 min	i.v.
	then 1 mg/kg/h	Infusion	
Lorazepam	0.05–0.1 mg/kg/dose	6 h	i.m., i.v.
Magnesium sulphate 50%	250 mg/kg/dose	Once or twice	i.v., i.m.
Mannitol 20%	0.5–1 g/kg over 20 min	p.r.n.	i.v.
MCT oil	0.9–1.8 mg/kg/day	8 h	Oral
Methadone HCl	0.3–0.4 mg/kg/day	24 h	Oral
Methyldopa	25 mg/kg/day	8 h	Oral
Methylene blue	1–2 mg/kg/dose	Once	Oral
Metoclopramide	0.1–0.2 mg/kg/dose	Once	i.v.
	0.1–1.0 mg/kg/day	8 h	Oral
Midazolam	0.1 mg/kg	Once	i.v., oral, nasal
Morphine	0.1 mg/kg/dose	8 h p.r.n.	i.m.
Mylanta	6 mL/dose	6–8 h	Oral
Naloxone	0.1 mg/kg (0.4 mg/mL)	Once (= 0.25 mL/kg)	i.v., i.m.
Neostigmine	3 mg/kg/day	8 h	i.m., i.v.
Pancuronium	0.1 mg/kg/dose	4 h p.r.n.	i.v.
Paraldehyde	0.15 mg/kg/dose	4 h p.r.n.	Deep i.m.
	0.3 mg/kg/dose	4 h p.r.n.	Rectal
Pethidine	1 mg/kg/dose	4 h p.r.n.	i.m., i.v.
Phenobarbitone	Loading 20 mg/kg/dose	Once	i.v.
	Maintenance 6 mg/kg/day	12 h	i.m., oral

Drug	Dose	Interval	Route
Phenytoin	Loading 20 mg/kg/dose Maintenance 5 mg/kg/day	Once 12 h	i.v. Oral
Phosphate (Sandoz)	2–4 mmol/kg/dose	6 h	Oral
Phytomenadione	1 mg/dose	Once	i.m.
Potassium chloride	2–3 mmol/kg/day	p.r.n.	i.v., oral
Procainamide	5–15 mg/kg/day	Once	Only i.v.
Promethazine	0.25–1.0 mg/kg/dose	6 h p.r.n.	i.m., i.v., oral
Propylthiouracil	5–10 mg/kg/day	8 h	Oral
Propranolol	0.1 mg loading slowly 0.75–2.0 mg/kg/day	Once 8 h	i.v. Oral
Prostigmine/atropine (mix 0.5 mg prostigmine with intervals 0.2 mg atropine)	0.2 mL/dose	Repeat twice at 5 min	i.v.
Protamine sulphate	1 mg/100 U heparin/dose	Once	i.v.
Purified protein fraction	10 mL/kg	Infusion	i.v.
Pyridoxine	Diagnostic 50 mg/kg Maintenance 5 mg/kg/day	Once 24 h	i.v. Oral
Ranitidine	1–2 mg/kg/day 3–4 mg/kg/day	8 h 8–12 h	i.v. Oral
Silver nitrate 1%	2 drops each eye	Once	Ocular
Sodium chloride	2–5 mmol/kg/day	24 h	Oral, i.v.
Somatostatin	3–10 µg/kg/day	6–8 h	s.c.
Spironolactone	2–3 mg/kg/day	8–12 h	Oral
Survanta	100 mg/kg (4 mL/kg)	Once (repeat once)	Intratracheal
THAM (3.5%)	2–3 mL/kg/dose	p.r.n.	i.v.
Theophylline	Loading 5–7 mg/kg Maintenance 3 mg/kg/day	Once 8–12 h	Oral Oral
Thiopentone	1 mg/kg/h	Infusion	i.v.
Thyroxine	0.025–0.05 mg/day	24 h	Oral
Verapamil	0.1–0.3 mg/kg	Daily	Oral
Vitamin A	600–1500 U/dose	24 h	Oral, i.v.
Vitamin B_{12}	50–100 µg/dose	Monthly	i.m.
Vitamin C	25–50 mg/kg	Daily	Oral
Vitamin E	25 iu/day	Daily	Oral
Vitamin K_1	0.5–1.0 mg/dose	At birth	i.m., repeat p.r.n.
Zinc sulphate	300 µg/kg	Continuous infusion	i.v.

ANTIMICROBIALS

Antibiotic agents

Drug	Total daily dose	Interval	Route
Amikacin	7.5 mg/kg preterm 22.5 mg/kg term	24 h preterm 8 h term	i.v. over 30 min
Amoxycillin	50–100 mg/kg	12 h	i.v., i.m., oral
Ampicillin	50–200 mg/kg	12 h	i.v., i.m., oral
Cefotaxime	50–100 mg/kg	6–12 h	i.v., i.m.
Ceftazidime	60–100 mg/kg	12 h	i.v., i.m.
Ceftriaxone	50 mg/kg	24 h	i.v., i.m.
Cefuroxime	50–100 mg/kg	12 h	i.v.
Chloramphenicol	25 mg/kg	12 h	i.v., i.m.
Co-trimoxazole (Bactrim, Septrin)	0.6 mL/kg	12 h	Oral, i.v.
Erythromycin	30–50 mg/kg	8–12 h	i.v., oral
Flucloxacillin	25–50 mg/kg	6–12 h	i.v., oral
Fusidic acid	20 mg/kg 50 mg/kg	12 h	i.v. Oral
Gentamicin	2.5 mg/kg/dose	> 1.5 kg 12 h 1.0–1.5 kg 18 h < 1.0 kg 24–36 h	i.v., i.m.
Imipenem	45 mg/kg	8 h	i.v.
Isoniazid	10 mg/kg	12 h	Oral
Kanamycin	< 2 kg 15 mg/kg > 2 kg 20 mg/kg	12 h	i.v., i.m.
Meropenem	20–30 mg/kg	12 h	i.v.
Methicillin	15 mg/kg load 50 mg/kg	12 h	i.v.
Metronidazole	15 mg/kg	12 h	i.v., oral
Moxalactam	100 mg/kg	12 h	i.v., i.m.
Netilmicin	6 mg/kg	12 h	i.v., i.m.
Penicillin G	50 000–100 000 U/kg (1 000 000 U = 600 mg)	12 h	i.v., i.m.
Pipracillin	100 mg/kg	12 h	i.v.
Rifampicin	10 mg/kg	12 h	i.v., p.o.
Spiramycin	100 mg/kg	12 h	p.o.
Ticarcillin	Loading 100 mg/kg Maintenance < 2 kg 225 mg/kg > 2 kg 300–400 mg/kg	12 h	i.v.

Drug	Total daily dose	Interval	Route
Tobramycin	5 mg/kg	12 h	i.v., i.m.
Vancomycin	30 mg/kg	12 h	i.v.

Antiviral agents

Aciclovir	15–30 mg/kg	6–8 h	i.v., p.o., topical
Ribovarin	6 g in 300 mL water (nebulized over 12–18 h)	24 h	Aerosol
Vidarabine	15–30 mg/kg (over 12–24 h)	24 h	i.v.
Zidovudine	8 mg/kg	6 h	p.o.
	6 mg/kg	6 h	i.v.

Antifungal agents

Amphotericin	0.25–1 mg/kg (max. accumulation 35 mg/kg)	24 h (over 6 h)	i.v.
Liposomal amphotericin	0.5–5 mg/kg	24 h (over 1 h)	i.v.
Ketoconazole	5–10 mg/kg	12–24 h	p.o.
Flucytosine	100–150 mg/kg	6–12 h	p.o.
Fluconazole	3–6 mg/kg	24 h	i.v., p.o.
Miconazole	30 mg/kg	8 h	i.v.
Nystatin	400 000 U	6 h	p.o.

STANDARD INFUSIONS

Drug	Concentration	Amount to be added (total volume 30 mL)	Required dose	Infusion rate
Dobutamine	250 mg/20 mL	2.88 mL/kg	10–20 µg/kg/min	0.5 mL/h
Dopamine	200 mg/5 mL	0.9 mL/kg	10–20 µg/kg/min	0.5 mL/h
Doxapram	20 mg/mL	3 mL/kg	1 mg/kg/h	0.5 mL/h
Insulin	0.1 U/mL	0.03 mL/kg	0.05–0.2 U/kg/h	1 mL/h
Isoprenaline	3 µg/mL	90 µg/kg	0.05–1.0 µg/kg/min	1 mL/h
Magnesium sulphate	80 mg/mL	3 mL/kg	20–50 mg/kg/h	1 mL/h
Midazolam	5 mg/mL	0.12 mL/kg	10 µg/kg/h	0.5 mL/h
Morphine	5 mg/mL	0.12 mL/kg	10 µg/kg/h	0.5 mL/h

Cont'd on p. 332

Drug	Concentration	Amount to be added (total volume 30 mL)	Required dose	Infusion rate
Nitroprusside	0.3 mg/mL	0.9 mg/kg	0.5–4.0 µg/kg/min	1 mL/h
Prostin VR (PGE$_1$)	500 µg/mL	0.04 mL/kg	0.01 µg/kg/min	1 mL/h
Tolazoline	1 mg/mL	30 mg/kg	1 mg/kg/h	1 mL/h

Abbreviations: dose, per dose; e.t.t., endotracheal; /h, per hour; i.c., intracardiac; i.m., intramuscular; i.v., intravenous; /kg, per kilogram weight; /min, per minute; p.o., per os (by mouth); s.c., subcutaneous.

FURTHER READING

Bhatt, D.R., Reber, D.J., Wirtshafter, D.D., Parikh, A.N. & Thomas, J.C. (1997) *Neonatal Drug Formulary*, 4th edn. NDF, Los Angeles.

MIMS Annual (1998) 22nd Australian edn. MIMS Australia, Sydney.

Neonatal Formulary. The Northern Neonatal Network Pharmacopoeia (1998) 10th edn. BMJ Books, London.

Index